Health, Medicine & Politics

in Ireland 1900-1970

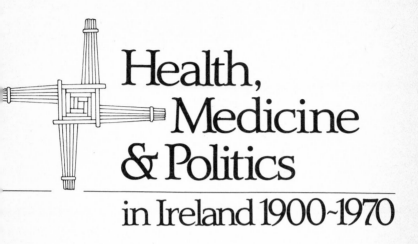

Health, Medicine & Politics

in Ireland 1900–1970

Ruth Barrington

Institute of Public Administration

First published 1987

by the Institute of Public Administration
57-61 Lansdowne Road, Dublin 4,
Ireland.

Barrington, Ruth
    Health, medicine and politics in Ireland, 1900-1970.
    1. Health planning — Government policy — Ireland
    i. Title
    362.1'09417   RA395.I7
    ISBN 0-906980-70-4
          0-906980-72-0 pbk

Design by Della Varilly
Index by Sarah O'Hara
Typeset in 12/13 Bembo by
Printset & Design Ltd, Dublin
Printed by Criterion Press Ltd, Dublin.

Contents

To my father, Tom Barrington, who gave me the idea for this book and my husband, John Delap, who gave me the opportunity to write it.

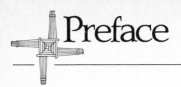# Preface

HOW DID WE come to have one of the best health services in the world? No one has answered this question. Some aspects of the development of health and medicine in Ireland have received a great deal of attention, most notably in John Whyte's *Church and State in Modern Ireland* and Ronan Fanning's *Independent Ireland*. But the significance of the Mother and Child scheme and other controversies for the evolution of health services was not their primary concern. Brendan Hensey's *The Health Services of Ireland* is essential reading for any student of health policy but it does not pretend to be an historical work. The neglect of the topic is strange given the attention it has received in other countries but it is not the only strand of Irish social history that has been under-explored. This book tries to answer the questions: what are the origins of our current arrangements for preventing and treating illness and what forces shaped the Irish health services?

I had two worries when setting out to answer these questions. The first was that the sources would be inadequate to unravel the mystery. This fear was groundless as the problem was not so much a shortage as a surfeit of material. The problem was to concentrate on the main stream and resist the temptation to explore tributaries.

A second worry was that the story would be too dull to be of interest to the general reader. It was a surprise, therefore, to discover a story so full of human interest. The great achievement of building a healthy society and a comprehensive system of medical care was the result of the vision, commitment and energy of determined men and women who saw a need and set out to respond to it. In the period covered by this work, the major infectious diseases — tuberculosis, typhoid, typhus, diphtheria, polio, syphilis, gastroenteritis — were either eradicated or controlled with incalculable effects for human wellbeing. Infant mortality was reduced from a rate of over 100 deaths per 1,000 births to 18 per 1,000 births. Medical services of a high quality were made available throughout the country and charges for treatment either removed or heavily subsidised. The entanglement of health issues with the political, economic and social life of the nation gives the story a wider interest than might appear at first sight.

What purpose, apart from satisfying personal curiosity and the recounting of an interesting story, does a narrative of this kind serve? In a recent article, Richard Kearney threw some light on the importance of history to our present pre-occupations. Narrative, he argues:

> by creatively interpreting the past ... serves to release new and hitherto concealed possibilities in understanding one's history; and by critically scrutinising the past it can wrest tradition away from the conformism that is always threatening to overpower it. (The Irish Times, 4 November 1986)

Understanding the change that has taken place in our society's approach to the prevention and treatment of illness between 1900 and 1970 opens up the concealed possibilities of the past. Events did not have to happen in the way they did. Other solutions could have been found; critical situations might have been handled differently with different long term effects. That things turned out the way they did says a lot about Ireland in those seventy years: about the passionate desire to create a better, more healthy society; the fierce determination to protect traditional values; the capacity for leadership and great political skill; and conversely, about intransigence and political ineptness.

Understanding how present arrangements developed should also protect against conformism. Conformity, by claiming the imprimatur of the past, raises what may have been the result of expediency to absolute principle. It discourages innovative thinking or adaptation to new challenges. An uncritical understanding of the ideas which shaped present practice breeds the kind of practical men that J.M. Keynes referred to, who believe themselves to be quite exempt from any intellectual influences but who are usually slaves of some defunct economist. It may come as a surprise to some readers to see just how long some 'new' ideas about health and medicine have been around. This book will serve a useful purpose if it helps to widen our understanding of current health services by 'creatively interpreting' the intellectual foundations on which they are built.

Every author relies on the support, encouragement and advice of many people. Without such support, encouragement and advice, this book would not have been written. To my father, Tom Barrington and husband, John Delap, I owe the greatest debt. The dedication on the frontispiece is in recognition of their contribution by way of ideas and encouragement. I am particularly grateful to Professor Brian Abel-Smith, of the London School of Economics, who, as supervisor for the thesis which formed this book, was always encouraging and perceptive in his advice. The Departments of Health and the Public Service facilitated my research by granting me two years special leave of absence from the civil service and by contributing towards my university fees. I hope they consider the finished product worth the investment. Colleagues in the Department of Health, especially Jerry O'Dwyer, Joe Robins and Oliver Hogan, were always supportive, in the best traditions of the Department. Professors David Donnison and Basil Chubb helped direct my studies and provided valuable introductions. Professor Chubb also read and commented on an early draft. Professor John Whyte made my research much easier by giving me notes of interviews he had made with prominent people when researching his *Church and State in Modern Ireland*, for which I am extremely grateful. Dr James Deeny gave me access to his private papers and stimulated my research in many ways. Dr Helen Burke's suggestions at various stages were particularly helpful and Professor Kathleen Jones, John Collier and Margaret Hayes gave me many comments which greatly improved the text.

One of the most satisfying aspects of writing the book was the opportunity it gave me to meet people who have played a prominent part in shaping our present health services. The energy and enthusiasm which they had brought to the task in their youth and middle age was still evident in their later years. To those who granted me the privilege of an interview or helped me in other ways, I am very grateful.

The research for the book was carried out in many different libraries. The assistance I received from the State Paper Office in Dublin Castle and Trinity College was outstanding. I am also grateful to the Bodleian Library, Oxford, the British Library of Economics and Political Science, the Public Record Office and the Library of the British Medical Association in London, the Brotherton Library, Leeds, Bradford University Library, and the National Library and the Library of the Royal College of Surgeons in Dublin. I was continually impressed by the courtesy extended by librarians and archivists to demanding students of esoteric subjects.

Others helped me indirectly. Professor Dale Tussing widened my perspective by opening up new ways of looking at health services. Conversations with Dermot McCarthy, Michael Kelly and James Raftery deepened my understanding of the relationship of health, medicine and government. I am grateful for the hospitality and encouragement of friends who made my research less lonely, especially Nuala O'Hare, Don Grant, Derek Nash, and Miriam and Neil Collins. The Hugh Parry Hall, London provided me with accommodation whenever I needed it.

It might be thought that as an official of the Department of Health since 1975, I had access to material not generally available to the public. To avoid accusations of privileged access, I decided from the beginning of my research to consult only documents and sources that were available to the general public. The one advantage my official experience gave me was, perhaps, to make the interpretation of some documents a little easier. The reason for stopping the story in 1970 is in deference to the convention that serving civil servants should not comment critically on events with which they may have been connected. Needless to say, all opinions expressed in the book are my own.

The manuscript was typed by Anne Coogan. Her accuracy, speed and good humour made it a pleasure to work with her. I am grateful to the Institute of Public Administration, and Jim O'Donnell in particular, for agreeing to publish the typescript. The comments of the two readers for the IPA were particularly helpful. Sarah O'Hara helped transform a thesis into a book by her commitment and attention to detail. My thanks are also due to Iain MacAulay and Kathleen Harte for their contribution to the book's production.

Although this is an Irish story, it is part of a wider saga of how the health and medical services of the Western world were transformed in this century. For those readers unfamiliar with Irish history, geography and terminology, I have included in the Appendix a map of the country, a chronology of the main political and economic events referred to in the text and a glossary of Irish political terms.

R.B.
April 1987.

1
Health, Medicine and Irish Society in 1900

THE SUCCESS OF MEDICINE in overcoming many of the illnesses which blighted or cut short the lives of previous generations is one of the remarkable developments of this century. Equally remarkable is the way in which access to medical care, with little or no regard to a person's ability to pay, has become in most Western societies one of what Hugh Heclo calls the 'social rights of citizenship'.[1] This study examines how government in Ireland expanded its responsibility for the treatment of the physically ill between 1900 and 1970, to the extent that access to medical care had by 1970 become a social right of citizenship. This expansion was the result of forces common to many countries – the effects of medical advances, the growth of democracy and the increased willingness of government to promote the welfare of its citizens – mediated by conditions peculiar to Ireland.

In 1900, the important influences on health and medicine in Ireland included social and economic conditions, the limitations of government responsibility for protecting health and treating illness, the organisation of medical services for the poor and the distribution of power. Amongst the most powerful actors were the Irish administration, the arm of contested British rule in Ireland; the Irish Party, representing the nationalist majority and pledged to the achievement of Home Rule; the medical profession, on the brink of great therapeutic advances but weak and divided as a

1

profession; and brooding behind every aspect of Irish life, the immense influence of the Catholic Church.

Social and Economic Conditions

By comparison with other European countries, Ireland at the turn of the century was a 'demographic freak'.[2] The population of 4.46 million in 1901 showed a decline of 45 per cent on the figure recorded in the census of 1841. The decline would continue at a slower rate until the late 1960s. The birth rate, which remained steady and high at 23 births per 1,000 people in the last decades of the nineteenth century and the death rate, which declined to about 17 per thousand people in 1901, should have resulted in a natural increase in population. However, emigration turned the natural increase into an overall decline. Between 1848 and 1914 5.5 million people left the country.[3] The annual loss through emigration at the turn of the century was between 30,000 and 40,000 people.

Emigration had become an 'economic and social necessity' because neither Ireland's dominant agricultural base nor its underdeveloped industry could support the natural increase in population.[4] Those who stayed behind married seldom and late. In the early years of this century, the average age at which men married was 33 and women, 28. In 1911, an extraordinary 26 per cent of women aged 45-54 had never married.[5] The high birth rate is all the more remarkable given the relatively small numbers of married women.

Economic growth in Ireland in the late nineteenth century was amongst the slowest in Western Europe.[6] Belfast and the Lagan valley was the only region where industry had developed to a scale comparable to the main industrial regions of Europe. The other Irish cities relied largely on trade for their prosperity. Trade with Britain dominated the Irish economy. In the early years of this century four-fifths of exports went to Britain and about two-thirds of imports came from Britain.[7]

The disparity in comparable income between Britain and Ireland was great. Income per head in Ireland was £34 in 1911 and in

Britain, £60.[8] However, looked at in a wider context, Ireland's position was more favourable. An estimate of GNP per capita for 28 countries in 1913 puts Ireland in the tenth highest place, with Britain in fourth place.[9] If Ireland was a more prosperous place in 1900 than in 1840 it was not because national income increased significantly, but largely because emigration had reduced the number of people to be supported by an inadequate economy. Although the wages of skilled and unskilled workers improved somewhat towards the end of the century, the wages were considerably below those paid in Britain and, in the words of F.S.L. Lyons, 'were insufficient to conceal the existence of deep abysses of poverty'.[10]

Medicine and Illness in 1900

In 1900 few worried about the extent to which government should ensure access for all to a high standard of medical care. This was partly because the scientific discoveries of the nineteenth century, in anaesthesia, bacteriology, pathology, radiology were only beginning to make an impact on medical practice. The major infections and surgical conditions remained unconquered. The limitations of medicine were reflected in attitudes to doctors and to medical intervention. Hospitals, for example, were less places of cure than refuges of last resort for those with untreatable illness. They were places for the poor whose inadequate housing or family circumstances did not permit a minimum standard of nursing care. Most people were born and died at home.

Those who could afford medical fees preferred to be treated at home by physicians and even surgeons, although by the beginning of this century, private nursing homes attached to voluntary hospitals were becoming increasingly popular with the middle classes. In an age before antibiotics, those who could keep their distance from the poor and their infections, did so. The well-known Dublin maternity hospitals, institutions associated with a higher success rate than other hospitals, were used almost exclusively by the poor.[11] Women of more substantial means were delivered at home.

People did not expect the state to provide for more than a

3

minimum level of medical care for the population. Government in these islands had not yet accepted a general responsibility for the health of the population, nor a duty to make medical facilities available to all at little or no cost to the patient. Those who could afford to, paid their doctors' fees directly. The fees charged by Irish general practitioners varied but 5s or 6s was not uncommon, with a reduction to 2s 6d for working class patients.[12] At a time when building labourers in Irish cities earned about 20s a week, medical fees could be a major financial headache for working class families.[13] Those on modest incomes might contribute to a benevolent or friendly society which employed doctors to look after their members and such societies were popular with working men and women in the main cities. The out-patient departments of the voluntary hospitals in Dublin, Belfast, Cork, Waterford and Limerick gave medical attention at little or no cost to working people and their families, but under physical conditions which left much to be desired. Only the medical care of the very poor and the control of infections associated with poverty were considered to warrant public intervention. These responsibilities were known to contemporaries as 'medical relief' and 'public health' respectively.

Medical relief

The responsibility of public authorities for the medical relief of the poor had its origins in the eighteenth century when the Irish parliament passed legislation encouraging the provision of an infirmary for the relief of the infirm and diseased poor in each county and borough, to be financed by public and philanthropic effort.[14] By 1841, there were 39 infirmaries funded by county grants and public subscriptions, each one staffed by a qualified surgeon and governed by a committee, the members of which had the right to nominate poor persons for admission.[15] The surgeon of the infirmary enjoyed considerable prestige locally and usually had a large private practice in addition to his responsibilities to the poor in the infirmary. After 1898, the infirmaries came under the control of the newly created county councils. Some were well-equipped surgical hospitals by the standards of the day but others could hardly be distinguished from the workhouse infirmaries.[16]

Government assumed more extensive responsibility for the medical relief of the poor in the nineteenth century in the elaborate mechanism of the poor law and the dispensary medical service. Modelled on its English predecessor, the Irish poor law was introduced in 1838 against the advice of the Whately Commission which had made a study of Irish poverty at the government's request.[17] In the next thirteen years, 163 workhouses were built despite enormous administrative difficulties.[18] The workhouse was intended as a last refuge for all forms of destitution. Each workhouse served a poor law union whose affairs were controlled by a board of guardians, consisting of elected local representatives and ex-officio members. Most significant of all, an unpopular system of local taxation, the poor law rate, was introduced by which the charge of relieving poverty in a union fell on the property owners of the area. For the first time, an organised system of relief from destitution, paid for by local taxation, was made available to the poor in Ireland. As local government activity in the nineteenth century increased, the poor law rate was extended to finance a wide range of local activities, including public health measures.

The Irish poor law differed from its English antecedent. In particular, the Irish poor law placed a much greater emphasis on medical relief. This was done partly as a concession to the Whately Commission which, in its recommendations on relieving poverty, had stressed the importance of organised medical relief for the poor.[19] Irish poor law guardians were charged by law to give priority of admission to 'destitute poor persons as by reason of old age, infirmity or defect may be unable to support themselves'.[20] Legislation also obliged the Poor Law Commissioners to report on the number of dispensaries and hospitals, in addition to workhouses, which were required for the relief of the sick poor.[21] Unlike workhouses in England and Wales, Irish institutions were built with an infirmary for male and female patients and a medical officer was appointed to supervise its operation.

In 1862, the workhouses were formally opened to sick persons who were not destitute.[22] Boards of guardians were also empowered to provide for any poor person requiring medical or surgical aid in a county infirmary or voluntary hospital and to pay the cost of sending such persons for treatment.[23] In 1867, an annual parliamentary grant was introduced which met half the salary of the workhouse medical officer and of medicines dispensed by him. The effect of these measures, combined with demographic and economic changes in the late nineteenth century, was to increase greatly the proportion of sick persons relative to other inmates in Irish workhouses, rising from about a sixth in 1852 to a third in 1905.[24]

Each workhouse was under the control of a 'master', with a 'matron' responsible for the female inmates and nursing of sick inmates. 'Nursing' for the most part consisted of the attention of female inmates who were fit enough to work. In the 1860s, nursing orders of religious sisters began to attach themselves to workhouses and where they did so, helped improve the care of the sick poor.

Little was done apart from these moves, to ensure that the conditions of workhouse infirmaries improved apace with rising standards of living in the late nineteenth century or with more progressive attitudes to hospital treatment. Most workhouse infirmaries were primitive. If inmates of the infirmaries were not necessarily classified as paupers, they had to endure the same conditions as paupers: workhouse diet, clothes and rules, the unceilinged roofs, unplastered walls, straw mattresses and the absence of running water and sanitation. 'Respectable' people shunned the workhouse infirmaries because of the association with the poor law. In 1906 the Viceregal Commission on Poor Law Reform (discussed in Chapter 2) found that 'the wards and arrangements existing in most Workhouses in Ireland are quite unfit for the treatment of surgical or even medical cases according to any modern standard'.[25]

The poor law was not designed for the comfort of the destitute, and despite creating some vested interests around it as time passed, remained intensely unpopular with the common people. The institutionalisation of poverty in the workhouse was equally disliked in Britain but in Ireland there was the added dimension that the system was 'alien' — designed to meet British conditions and imposed against expert advice on an unwilling populace. The virtual collapse of the system during the famine years of 1845-9 under the pressure of unprecedented levels of disease and destitution on the one hand, and the undermining of the rating system by the bankruptcy of many landowners on the other, did nothing to endear the new system to popular consciousness.

In 1900 the Irish poor law was 62 years old, an unpleasant, expensive but apparently indispensable fact of life. The workhouse provided a last resort for the infirm elderly and poor of all ages with chronic or terminal illness whose families or employers would no longer support them. Despised as it may have been by the respectable poor, the workhouse at least provided a minimum safety net for the destitute. Discontent with the system was mainly expressed by the ratepaying electorate who objected to supporting provisions originally designed for a population of eight million but which by 1901 had shrunk to less than half that number. To ratepayers and their representatives this was clear evidence of waste and extravagance.

The dispensary service

The creation of the Irish dispensary service in 1851 was one of the most innovative responses to meeting the medical needs of the poor in any country in the last century. Its introduction owes much to the ideas and persistence of Denis Phelan, a surgeon and assistant Poor Law Commissioner, who campaigned tirelessly for a medical poor law oriented towards the out-door relief of the sick poor. He was impressed by the network of medical dispensaries subsidised by landlords which developed with little official support in the 1820s and 1830s. Phelan persuaded the Poor Law Commissioners of the merits of a scheme to divide the country into dispensary districts each with a salaried medical officer whose first priority was to treat the poor, and who was responsible to the board of guardians of the poor law union.[26] The cost of medical relief would be met from the rates and overall control would rest with the Poor Law Commissioners. But the system of medical relief he proposed would not, unlike admission to workhouses, be confined to the destitute poor but be accessible to anyone who could not afford to pay for medical aid for themselves and their families.[27]

Attempts were made in the 1840s to introduce a scheme of dispensary medical relief but the experience of the Great Famine, while emphasising the need for such relief, made anything but emergency provisions impossible. The Famine may, however, have contributed to the speed with which the dispensary system was subsequently introduced because it impressed those in authority with the need for such a service and because the destruction of the rural economy in many areas made medical practitioners receptive to the idea of an organised and salaried service. In 1851 the necessary legislation was passed and by May 1852 the island had been divided into 723 dispensary districts, each with one or more medical officers under the general control of the poor law guardians.[28] Midwives to attend poor women at confinement were also appointed in many dispensary districts at the ratepayers' expense.

The timing of the dispensary service was fortuitous as it took advantage of the trends in medical education and registration which led to the appearance of the 'general' practitioner, a doctor trained in medicine, surgery and midwifery. While the Poor Law Commission had little choice but to recruit existing doctors to staff the new service initially, many of whom would not have had such broad training, it insisted that all new recruits have recognised certificates in medicine, surgery and midwifery, many years before these were made legal requirements for medical registration.[29]

Each dispensary doctor was appointed to office following election by the board of guardians. Under the terms of the appointment, the doctor had to attend every sick person in the district possessing a dispensary ticket. Tickets were provided for each episode of illness by a poor law guardian and were of two kinds; a black ticket entitling the holder or his dependants to attend the doctor at the dispensary and a red ticket, known to doctors as a 'scarlet runner', entitling the holder to attendance in the patient's home. The doctor was usually obliged to dispense medicines, although in the main urban areas apothecaries were recruited to provide this service. In return, the medical officer received a salary, which by 1907 averaged £116 a year, ranging from less than £90 to £150 per annum.[30] The doctor was free to devote the remainder of his time to private practice, the amount of which varied enormously from place to place. Many were also the medical officers to the workhouses.

The dispensary doctors quickly accumulated other duties. In 1864, they were made responsible for vaccinating children against smallpox and for registering births and deaths in their districts. In 1874 they became medical officers for health (MOH) for their districts, for which they received a further salary, which by the early 1900s averaged £19 a year.[31] The arrangement did little to improve environmental conditions for public health, since the obligations of the MOH often conflicted with the interests of private practice and it was noted that they were paid 'to hold their tongues and take no notice of dirt and disease within their districts'.[32]

The advantages of the dispensary service were many. It provided medical relief to the poor in their homes and at dispensaries throughout the country and in places which normally could not have supported a doctor. It benefited the better off in remote areas as the doctor's salary was in effect a subsidy to their care. It was relatively cheap; the entire cost was met from the rates until 1867 when a parliamentary grant paid half the salary of the medical officer, a midwife (if appointed) and medicines dispensed. The over-production of Irish medical graduates ensured that candidates for the hundred or so vacancies which arose each year in the service were as 'plentiful as blackberries in September'.[33] Towards the end of the century, the dispensary service provided a structure around which a home nursing service for the sick poor grew, through the work of the Lady Dudley and Jubilee Institute nursing organisations.

The disadvantages of the system were mainly and increasingly felt by the medical profession. By the turn of the century, the grievances of the eight hundred dispensary doctors — about one-third of the registered medical practitioners in Ireland — had become one of the celebrated causes in medical circles in these islands. Salaries and conditions were the main grounds for complaint. The absence of an incremental salary scale in every district, of a right to a pension depending only on satisfactory service and the lack of promotion opportunities within the service were further sources of frustration. Much of the dispensary doctors' anger was directed at the boards of guardians which controlled many aspects of their professional lives. The decision to pay a doctor a pension, for example, was at the discretion of the guardians. The doctors claimed that guardians were too generous with dispensary tickets, giving them to people who would afford to pay fees but who had to be cultivated before the next election. The scope for friction increased after 1898 when the franchise for elections to the board of guardians was greatly extended. The appointment of the medical officer, one of the main prerogatives of the guardians, was also the occasion for the exercise of patronage, sectarianism and favouritism by guardians who numbered up to a hundred in some unions. One official commentator on the service did not mince words:

> The existing method of selecting candidates, under which the professional qualifications are ignored, and political opinions, religious belief, and local influence are the only questions considered, is quite sufficient to ruin any service.[34]

At a time when entry to the army and navy medical corps was by written competitive examination, the selection methods of the Irish dispensary service seemed anomalous.

The extent to which medical officers engaged in other activities to the detriment of their medical duties was also a cause for concern:

> Whether from the inadequacy of their salaries, or an insufficient sense of their responsibilities, Medical Officers in some districts engage in farming, horse dealing, and other pursuits ... in many instances the standard of sobriety is below what it ought to be.[35]

Others noted the prevalence of 'the dispensary manner' which

10

'chills off the peasantry' and allowed the doctor time to attend the races and the local hunt.[36]

The dispensaries where the poor queued to see the doctor also left much to be desired. Few were purpose built, the normal practice being to rent a room in a small house in a town or village at which the poor would attend for treatment at the fixed dispensary hours. One visiting medical commentator was taken aback by the conditions he found:

> Anything more cheerless than the average Irish dispensary fabric it is difficult to imagine even in the towns, but the outlying depots in dispensary districts in the remote parts of the unions are, as a rule, wretched, comfortless, and unfit for the examination of patients ... it is pitiful to see their air of discomfort.[37]

Private patients were normally seen at the doctor's house. It was taken for granted that private and public patients should be seen in separate premises since 'respectable' people feared catching infections from the poor.

None of the faults in the workhouse infirmaries or in the dispensary service were beyond the remedy of practical people with the necessary commitment and money. Yet, while there was a willingness to maintain the system, the commitment to developing it to the standard required by a new generation seems to have been lacking. Reluctance to increase the rates was an obstacle as was the low priority afforded in Irish public life to medical relief of the poor.

One exception to this pattern of neglect was the initiative to provide a nursing service for the sick poor in their homes. Money raised in Ireland to celebrate Queen Victoria's jubilee was used to establish an institute of nursing which trained women to nurse the sick poor at home. The nurses, known as 'Jubilee nurses', were employed by local committees who raised the money for their salaries. The initiative worked well in more prosperous areas with active local committees but the poorest areas seldom had the benefit of a Jubilee nurse. In 1903, the Countess of Dudley gave her name to a nursing service for the poorest or 'congested' districts of the western seaboard. The Lady Dudley nurses were trained and supervised by the Jubilee Institute and worked under the direction of the dispensary doctor. The Jubilee and Lady Dudley nurses, without any support from public funds, provided a valuable and unique nursing service to the sick poor. But the service was uneven and depended entirely on local initiative. The number of district nurses employed in 1917 was 174, of which only 21 were employed as Lady Dudley nurses in the congested districts.[38]

Public health

The public health movement, a product of Victorian sanitary engineering and administrative zeal, aimed to prevent and contain outbreaks of infectious disease which were endemic in these islands and which posed a particular threat to the increasingly urbanised population of Great Britain. The first significant steps to control infectious diseases in Ireland were taken in the late 1840s during the Famine when the Poor Law Commissioners were given powers to contain outbreaks of infectious diseases, particularly typhus and cholera.[39] Subsequent legislation extended the powers of local sanitary authorities to build sewers and protect water supplies and to appoint sanitary inspectors to supervise the implementation of public health legislation.[40] The Public Health Act, 1878, which provided the country with a framework to control infectious disease comparable to that of England's, gave local authorities the power to destroy unsound food, supervise slaughter houses and isolate persons suffering from certain notifiable infectious diseases.

The problem in Ireland was that few local authorities approached the problem of eradicating infectious disease with determination. The gap between reality and the statute book was great. Although the death rate from the principal epidemic diseases – smallpox, typhus fever, typhoid, measles, diphtheria, whooping cough, scarlet fever, diarrhoea – declined from 2.8 to 1.5 per thousand between 1882 and 1906, it was still well above the rate of .9 per thousand for England.[41]

Much more serious was the scale of death from tuberculosis, which was not then classified as an infectious disease under public health legislation. Until Koch's work on the *tubercle bacillus* became widely known at the end of the century, the disease was thought to be hereditary. With a death rate of 2.68 per thousand in the early 1900s and claiming more than 11,500 lives a year, the disease was by far the most common cause of death among Irish people, accounting for nearly twice as many deaths as all other infectious diseases combined.[42] It was particularly disturbing that mortality from the disease in Ireland showed no signs of the long term decline apparent in England and Scotland.[43] The disease was associated with poverty, poor diet and bad housing, but the relationship was not causal. The absence of accommodation to isolate those in the advanced stages of the disease, concealment of what was considered to be a family 'weakness' and the widespread habit of spitting greatly increased the opportunities for spreading infection. The disease was particularly feared since most of its victims succumbed between 15 and 25 years of age. The Women's National Health Association, founded in 1907 by the energetic Lady Aberdeen, the wife of the formal head of British rule in Ireland, did much to educate people about preventing the disease and to provide sanatorium beds but they met much apathy and resistance. An attempt, largely inspired by the Association, to have the disease made notifiable in the Tuberculosis (Ireland) Bill, 1908 foundered on popular opposition to compulsory notification, expressed through a veto by the Irish Party at Westminster.

The material poverty in which so many Irish people lived was a major reason for low standards of health. But so too was the apathy with which public health issues were treated in Ireland. A commitment to improving the situation could have overcome many shortcomings in the law and administration but elected representatives in Ireland did not seem to set much store by the utilitarian notion that the whole community benefited from fresh water, clean streets and good housing. Few things struck the visitor to the country more than the dirt and squalor of many Irish cities, towns and villages. In the early years of the century a number of inquiries and commissions looked into the sanitary affairs of Dublin, Belfast and Waterford.[44] Their conclusions reflected badly on the commitment of the authorities of the cities to carry out their responsibilities. Apart from Belfast, there was little immediate improvement as a result of these reports. Dublin was notorious for its poverty, appalling tenements, filthy streets, high death rate and the lack of interest of its citizens in preventive health. A similar lack of interest could be found all over the country as the Reports of the Local Government Board for these years testify.[45] If the Local Government Board tried to use its authority to force action, it was accused of being anti-democratic and unrepresentative. While public health officials were well aware of the problems and of the responsibility on public authorities to improve the situation, one is left with the impression that the poverty and squalor of much of Irish life, combined with the relaxed tempo of Irish administration and the reluctance of local bodies to undertake improvements which would increase local taxation, were a match for their best efforts.

Dramatis Personae

The voluntary hospitals and the medical profession

Although in the business of giving medical relief to the poor, the voluntary hospitals in Dublin, Belfast, Cork, Waterford and Limerick ran their affairs independently of any public relief schemes. The only link between the state and these hospitals was through an annual grant voted by parliament towards their upkeep, a legacy from the days of the Irish parliament in the eighteenth century. This grant was not used to influence the activities of the hospitals in any way.

The first voluntary hospitals, or medical charities as they were then called, were established by philanthropic individuals or groups of doctors in the eighteenth century in response to a genuine concern for the condition of the sick poor and to the growth of a more clinical, hospital-based approach to the teaching of medicine. The movement began in Dublin with the establishment of the Charitable Infirmary, Cork Street in 1718, followed by Dr Steevens' Hospital in 1720, Mercer's Hospital in 1745, the Rotunda Lying-in Hospital in 1745 and the Meath Hospital in 1753. In addition to these facilities for the poor, the hospitals were associated with medical schools, providing clinical material to train young doctors and develop expertise which might be put to more profitable use among the wealthy later on. Doctors on the staff of the hospitals were not remunerated for their services, but appointments were eagerly sought because of the entry such appointments gave to private practice, the income from medical tuition and the potential for referral of private patients by former students. In 1902 a well-informed commentator blamed the 'over hospitalising' of Dublin on the tendency of doctors to establish hospitals 'not because they were needed by the poor or diseased but for professional interests, as a connection with a hospital of repute is of vital importance to professional men' and because 'denominations wished for management by governors of their own communion'.[46] More recently Eckstein has remarked of the voluntary hospital system, it was 'a most subtle combination of direct charitable service for indirect financial reward and no doubt it was a happy arrangement for the voluntary hospitals and their poorer patients'.[47] Apart from the poor under their care in the hospitals, these specialist doctors treated, almost exclusively, the wealthiest section of Irish society, their fees being beyond the means of most people.

Initially Protestant or non-sectarian in character, the consequences of a rising Catholic bourgeoisie, of increasing numbers of Catholic doctors and the growth of the nursing orders of religious sisters following Catholic Emancipation in 1829, encouraged the establishment of Catholic hospitals such as St Vincent's in 1835, the Mercy in Cork in 1857 and the Mater Misericordiae hospitals in Dublin and Belfast. In an increasingly denominational age, these hospitals self-consciously set out to provide for the spiritual as well as the medical needs of their Catholic patients.

By 1900, it was apparent that the role of the voluntary hospitals, and of county infirmaries to a lesser extent, was changing. There was an increasing willingness of those who could afford to pay the cost of medical treatment to be admitted to 'pay beds' or private accommodation closely associated with the hospitals.[48] As demand for hospital accommodation grew and financial pressure on the hospitals increased, a conflict arose between the hospitals' traditional commitment to the poor and the need to remain financially solvent.

The voluntary hospitals, both Catholic and Protestant, enjoyed great prestige, through their boards of management, subscribers and medical staffs. Their physicians and surgeons were the leaders of the medical profession in Ireland, dominating medical organisation, medical teaching and the affairs of the professional colleges such as the Royal Colleges of Physicians and Surgeons. These hospitals, with relatively high standards of medical, surgical and nursing care, set the standard by which the county and workhouse infirmaries were judged by contemporaries.

Medical organisation

The Medical Registration Act, 1858 established a common medical register for Great Britain and Ireland of persons qualified to practise as doctors and a general medical council to supervise medical education and professional practice. The Act strengthened links between Irish and British doctors through a common register and representation on the Medical Council. Despite this framework, the organisation of the profession in Ireland differed significantly from that in Britain. The biggest difference was that about half of the 2,200 registered medical practitioners in Ireland were employed as dispensary or workhouse medical officers. If the surgeons to the county infirmaries and the medical officers of the lunatic asylums are included, the number of doctors paid by the public purse was extremely high. One medical commentator noted that 'in Ireland, to a greater extent than in any other civilized country, the care of the sick population devolves upon state supported functionaries'.[49] The low level of industrial development in most of the country and the existence of the dispensary system, meant that, unlike Britain, contract work by doctors with friendly societies of working men was of much less importance to Irish doctors.

The Irish Medical Association and the British Medical Association, both founded in the 1830s, represented the interests of the profession in Ireland. The Irish Medical Association was almost exclusively concerned with improving the terms and conditions of dispensary and poor law doctors but even among such doctors its membership was not large. It made efforts in the early years of the century to improve salaries and conditions of dispensary doctors by calling on medical solidarity to 'black' posts which did not carry the minimum terms of employment approved by the Association. This policy seems to have met with only limited success, as the medical journals of these years continually complain of the extent to which doctors ignored the Association's policy and competed for posts with salaries well below those recommended by the IMA, even to the extent of some doctors buying the votes of the guardians.[50] Attempts to reorganise the Association after 1905 led to organisational stalemate and a marked drop in membership.[51]

The members of the British Medical Association, on the other hand, tended to be the leading specialists and private general practitioners, concerned more with scientific matters than the terms and conditions of employment of poor law doctors. Criticism of the lack of interest in the struggle of Irish dispensary doctors led the BMA to undertake its own examination of conditions in Ireland in 1904 and to proposals for the reorganisation of the poor law medical service into a state medical service for the poor.[52] In 1905 the BMA set up a permanent Irish committee and established formal links with the IMA with the aim of achieving a state medical service in Ireland. A suggestion that the two associations should combine was, however, resisted by the IMA which argued that a separate organisation was needed to deal with the very different problems of doctors in Ireland.[53]

The profession was far from being a seamless robe and doctors were as much divided by the different conditions in which they worked as united by the ties of professional solidarity. The salaried dispensary doctor and the specialist attached to a voluntary hospital with a large private practice inhabited different worlds. Nor did the profession as a whole enjoy the kind of public recognition to which it aspired. It was a source of disappointment to medical practitioners that their profession ranked below the church, the law, the naval, military and civil services, and trade in terms of income and social status.[54]

Medical science had not yet made the advances which would bring greater public recognition in its train. While individual doctors by virtue of their expertise, family or political connections may have exercised considerable influence, the power of the profession as a whole was weak compared to that of the main interests in Irish society at the time, the Irish administration, the Irish Party and the Catholic Church.

The Irish administration

Since the Act of Union of 1800, Ireland had been governed as a part of the United Kingdom of Great Britain and Ireland. Administratively, the union was never complete and much of the country's affairs continued to be run from Dublin, rather than London. The most powerful figure in the Irish administration was the Chief Secretary, who was usually a member of the British Cabinet. The Chief Secretary had the unenviable task of reconciling British and Irish interests in Ireland, maintaining the balance between the interests of the unionist minority and nationalist majority, the Catholics and Protestants and landlord and peasant. The Chief Secretary presided over a formidable bureaucracy, which in 1906-7 numbered 67 boards, offices and departments employing 100,000 persons.[55] Mistrusted by the majority of the population, considered by nationalists to be unrepresentative and extravagant, its importance sprang from its responsibility for law and order and control of patronage, public relief and grants.

One of the important responsibilities of the Chief Secretary was his office of President of the Local Government Board for Ireland. The Local Government Board stood at the apex of the poor law, dispensary and public health structures. Since 1898, the Board had been placed at the head of the new democratic system of local government, giving it an interest in all the activities carried out by the newly formed county councils and borough councils. Between 1898 and 1908, 22 new Acts affecting the Board were passed, doubling the estimated 70,000 papers handled annually by officials of the Board.[56] By 1914 the staff of the Board numbered about 230, three times as many as in the mid-1890s.[57]

While the Chief Secretary was the titular head of the Board, real power lay with the Vice-President, a permanent official and to a lesser extent with the four other commissioners of the Board, one of whom was a medical commissioner. The Vice President from the beginning of the period under discussion until 1921 was Sir Henry Robinson. Sir Henry was a seasoned public servant with an intimate knowledge of the Irish poor law and dispensary system and an adroit 'courtier' to the many Chief Secretaries he served in his long career.[58] Beatrice Webb described him as 'the most agreeable of companions' but with characteristic perspicacity identified his lack of a 'philosophy of life or government' and over-riding concern to keep his Chief Secretaries out of trouble as his main shortcomings.[59]

If Sir Henry had few ideas of his own for reforming the system, he had clear views about the nature of the Board's purpose and functions. The Board had on its side considerable legislative and administrative controls over the affairs of local authorities, particularly poor law authorities, and substantial Exchequer grants towards the cost of local services. For Sir Henry, local government was largely a tussle between the central authority of the Board and the local authority. According to one source he described the relationship as 'a sort of war that went on between them all the time' and that while the Board could not get local government to march, it could 'compel it to shamble'.[60]

The Irish Party

Dominating the Irish political landscape was the Irish Parliamentary Party, led by John Redmond, dedicated to the overriding goal of Home Rule. In the 1880s under the leadership of Charles Stewart Parnell it was a radical party, but by the early 1900s it had developed a more respectable and conservative air. The strategy of the Party was opportunist: to bring about a situation in Westminster where it held the balance of power between the Liberals and Conservatives and to use Home Rule as the price of its support for the Liberals. During the barren years when this strategy was unworkable, the Party campaigned for legislation to improve the economic and social

19

conditions of the country, principally in the fields of land reform, housing and university education. Not all members of the party by any means were interested in these issues. It was a small number who voiced the issues at Westminster and lobbied the Irish administration. Among the more prominent were John Dillon, Joseph Devlin, John Clancy and James Lardner, either because they were liberal by nature or because they represented working class constituencies.

The Irish Party was in the difficult position of being the elected representatives of the majority of the people without the power to govern, while the Irish administration had the prerogatives of government but lacked legitimacy in the eyes of the majority. The situation called for compromise on both sides if the country was to be governed. The Party's relationship with the Irish administration was, as a result, ambiguous. On the one hand, the administration represented everything which the nationalists hoped Home Rule would replace – an inefficient, expensive and unrepresentative officialdom.[61] On the other hand, in the short term, the administration was the main source of power, patronage, grants and favours. With the Liberal victory in 1906, and particularly after the Liberals were dependent on the Irish vote to stay in power between 1910 and 1914, the Party exercised considerable influence over the conduct of government in Ireland.

The Church

Without a formal place in Irish political and administrative life, the Catholic Church nonetheless exercised enormous influence. The importance which Irish Catholics of all social classes attached to their faith was remarkable by any standards. Part of the reason for the Church's hold over the people was its support for the aspiration for political independence provided this was achieved by peaceful means.[62] The Church had helped maintain a sense of national identity and solidarity at a time when the political aspirations of the majority seemed thwarted. It had come to terms with successive generations of the nation's leaders and in return it expected those leaders to promote and protect its vital interests, particularly in matters of public morality and education. How defensive the Church could be on such matters is illustrated by the ease with which Cardinal Logue, the head of the Hierarchy, could openly advocate civil disobedience in 1911 if the government went ahead with proposals to secularise the marriage ceremony in Ireland.[63] The relationship between the Hierarchy and the Irish Party was not, however, a straightforward one as individual bishops exercised considerable autonomy and differed in the extent to which they supported the Party. Both the Hierarchy and the Party were usually careful not to tread openly on each other's vital interests.

The Irish Church was extremely conservative on social and economic issues, even by the standards of Catholics in other countries. The attitude of the Church in the early part of this century has been described by Emmet Larkin as 'reflexive rather than reflective, insular rather than cosmopolitan', leaving it 'ill equipped, institutionally and intellectually, to meet the growing complexities of a rapidly changing society to which it was being introduced'.[64] Because they reflected the predominantly rural and farming ethos of Irish life, priests and bishops could immediately identify with the struggle of the Irish farmer to gain possession of his land. They viewed the struggle of organised workers, on the other hand, to improve their pay and conditions of work as socialism to be opposed by every means possible.[65]

Because of the close association of Unionism and Protestantism in Ireland, the Church leaders were particularly sensitive on denominational issues and felt the need to protect their flock from opportunities for proselytising by providing medical care in Catholic- run institutions. Cardinal Cullen, a dominant influence on the Irish Church in the second half of the nineteenth century, hated the workhouses and did his best to promote Catholic institutions for the Catholic poor.[66] The influence of the Irish Hierarchy over government policy prior to independence was limited by the fact that it had to operate within the wider context of the United Kingdom, with differing traditions of Catholicism. One attraction of Home Rule for the Irish Church was that as the church of the vast majority of the people, it would greatly increase its scope for creating a truly Catholic climate in which the faithful would be protected from anti-Catholic influences.

Conclusion

At the beginning of this century, Ireland had, by the standards of the day, an extensive system of medical relief for the poor, particularly in the dispensary service, and an impressive legal and administrative structure to protect the population against infection. However, practice often fell short of aspiration and a combination of poverty and inertia combined to make the risks to the health of the Irish greater than elsewhere in the United Kingdom. More fundamentally, government responsibility for health and medical care was limited to providing a safety net for the poor and controlling the outbreak of certain infectious diseases. In the main cities, public measures of medical relief for the poor were supplemented by the independent activities of voluntary hospitals. Public measures for medical relief were sorely in need of overhaul but neither public health nor medical relief was a priority of government or society in 1900. Dissatisfaction with existing arrangements was motivated less by philanthropy than by the perceived extravagance of the system, the grievances of the dispensary doctors and a struggle for power between elected local authorities and the 'unrepresentative' Local Government Board for Ireland. The medical profession was poorly organised and was hardly a force by comparison with the power and influence exercised by the chief interests of the day — the Irish administration, the Irish Party and the Catholic Church. For different reasons, none of these interests was particularly concerned with raising the standard of the nation's health.

Major scientific, political and social forces were stirring at this time, however, which would profoundly alter the relationship between government, the medical profession, other interest groups and the people, in Ireland as in other Western countries. Firstly, the capacity of medicine and the medical profession to combat human illness was about to increase dramatically. Secondly, access to medical care based on need rather than ability to pay was soon to be considered as a right of all citizens, one of the social implications of the political equality promised by democracy. Thirdly, government, in response to the aspirations of the newly enfranchised classes, was prepared to accept a much greater responsibility for the welfare of its citizens than heretofore. It is no coincidence that the convergence of these trends made the extension of government responsibility a controversial issue in many countries, with government wishing to extend access to medical treatment to all or most of the population and the medical profession and other interests resisting state encroachment on their autonomy and privileges. The precise nature of the conflict and the subsequent outcome would vary with the history and particular conditions of each country. In Ireland, the mediating factors included the earlier arrangements for medical care, the preoccupation of Irish society, up to 1921, with the achievement of independence, the constraints of an underdeveloped economy, the close association of the country with the wealthier and more cosmopolitan British society and the relative power of organised interests in Irish society, in particular, the Catholic Church. The growth of public responsibility for the medical treatment of the physically ill between 1900 and 1970 in Ireland created tensions which led to conflict, on occasions dramatic conflict, between government and the interests affected.

2
Proposals for Reform
1903~1911

THE RECOGNITION THAT the poor law was an inadequate and expensive way of tackling poverty and medical relief led to an intense preoccupation with reform in Ireland and Britain. Between 1903 and 1909, two major reviews were undertaken of the poor law and medical relief system in Ireland, by the Viceregal Commission on Poor Law Reform and by the Royal Commission on the Poor Laws and Relief of Distress.[1] The two Commissions reached the same conclusions on many issues but disagreed fundamentally on others. The Royal Commission was itself deeply divided, a minority producing a report which made a greater impact than that of the majority.[2]

The recommendations of the Commissions were, however, overshadowed in the short term by initiatives for reform based on more radical assumptions than even those entertained by the minority of the Royal Commission. While poor law reformers attempted to make the provisions for the poor more humane and to reduce administrative complexity, the radicals of the 'new liberalism' wanted to prevent as many people as possible falling into the net of poverty in the first place. The provision of pensions for the elderly and insurance against ill health and unemployment epitomised the approach of the new school of thought under the powerful leadership of David Lloyd George at the Treasury and Winston Churchill at the Board of Trade.

The Viceregal Commission

The Viceregal Commission was established in May 1903 to find ways of reducing the cost to ratepayers of supporting the sick and destitute poor. The Commission was asked to recommend 'a more economical system for the relief of the sick, the insane and all classes of destitute poor in Ireland' with the object of 'reducing or adjusting local taxation without impairing efficiency in administration'.[3] Within the constraints of efficiency and economy, the Commission was also asked to consider better arrangements for the inmates of workhouses and the need for additional accommodation for the sick poor.[4]

The influence of the Local Government Board can be seen in the appointment of two of the three members; the chairman, William Lawson Micks was a Commissioner and Dr Edward Coey Bigger a medical inspector with the Board. The third member was politician George Murnaghan, member for mid-Tyrone. Despite the bureaucratic bias, the Commissioners refused to interpret the terms of reference narrowly, and in their Report cautiously recommended radical changes in the organisation and administration of the poor law; their recommendations for the treatment of the sick were particularly significant.

The Commission was critical of the way in which the poor law system was introduced into Ireland and of its English origins. The mixed workhouse was singled out as the most objectionable feature of the system. Most reformers in Britain also found the workhouse an unnatural solution to relieving poverty but it was easier for the Irish Commissioners to justify the closure of the mixed workhouse because of its 'foreign' origins. This view was not shared by the many guardians who gave evidence before the Viceregal Commission, presumably because the workhouse was a symbol of their authority and generated business for the farmers and shopkeepers in the surrounding area.

The importance of the county as a unit of local administration was clear from the Commission's report. The Commissioners always invited evidence from the representatives of the county or borough councils before those of the guardians. They compared

25

the management of lunatic asylums by the county councils very favourably with the guardians' management of the workhouses. A good number of witnesses suggested the county councils take over the functions of public health from the smaller rural and urban districts, on the English model. The prominence given to the county, at the expense of the union and board of guardians, shows how quickly the scheme of local government initiated in 1898 had taken root and what opportunities it offered for improving medical and other services.

The growing importance of hospital treatment was obvious from the evidence. Describing hospitals as 'the repairing shops of the community', one doctor commented on the growing number of people availing of hospital accommodation.[5] When Mr Murnaghan asked a Naas Guardian, 'Might you not carry this question of hospitals too far; is not the natural place, if one can afford it when he gets sick, his own home?', the reply was:

> The doctors are inclined to think that with trained nurses and scientific appliances and daily and nightly attendances ... the best place is the hospital ... if it is a surgical case it is often better treated in rooms attached to a hospital as is universally done in Dublin.[6]

A major theme of the Viceregal Commission's report was specifying the benefits of modern hospital development by improving medical, nursing and physical facilities in the provinces. There was general agreement that the same hospitals should be open to all who needed treatment and that those who could afford to pay should do so, and in return receive some extra comforts. This view represented a radical and novel approach to hospital development.

The Commissioners were very critical of the conditions they found in most workhouses and many county infirmaries. The poor condition of the buildings, the scarcity of trained nurses and the employment of pauper inmates to attend the sick (a practice disapproved of by the Local Government Board) were major causes for concern. Even the better county infirmaries did not have a resident house surgeon; giving an indication of the scope for improvement.

The Commission also wished to see the workhouse and county infirmaries concentrate on the treatment of the acutely ill. Of the 13,750 patients in the workhouse infirmaries on 11 March 1905, the Commission estimated that less than half were proper cases for sick wards. The others were aged and infirm rather than acutely ill. They recommended that in future 'only the sick in need of medical care or skilled nursing should be admitted into hospital'.[7]

Developments in transport during this period lengthened the distance which sick people could be expected to travel to hospital. By 1914, Ireland had one of the densest rail networks in the world, with 3,500 miles of track.[8] A train permitted a sick person to travel in relative comfort to a distant hospital for an operation, a journey which would have been unthinkable on foot or in a trap. It allowed doctors and nurses to move quickly to control outbreaks of fever or to treat emergencies. By the time of the Viceregal Commission, the motor car was becoming a familiar sight on Irish roads. One far-sighted witness foresaw the day when motor ambulances would bring patients from the district hospitals to the county hospital for surgery,[9] while another called for an ambulance service to cover each county.[10] The development of transport made it possible to raise the question of whether it was possible to 'centralise the sick', a question which would grow in importance in later years.[11]

The seriousness of the problem of tuberculosis was clear from the evidence presented. Many young people were dying because of the lack of suitable accommodation and the reluctance of people to take precautions against spreading infection.[12] One medical witness emphasised the need to fight the disease on a broad front, arguing that the decline in mortality from tuberculosis in England was due to better feeding, rising wages, better housing and factory conditions, improved drainage, ample hospital accommodation and a more efficient public health service. He warned against over-estimating the effects of sanatorium treatment alone in combating the disease. The eradication of the disease in Ireland, he argued, called for direct measures such as the provision of sanatoria, notification of the disease, suppression of spitting, improved public health and also for indirect action to improve the social condition of the people.[13]

27

The cornerstone of the Commission's recommendations was the closure of the mixed workhouses. Destitution could no longer justify the herding together of the sick, the aged, the harmless lunatic, the single mother and destitute child into one building. The Commission recommended that the needs of each group be met in separate accommodation: county and district hospitals for the sick, sanatoria for the consumptive, asylums for the lunatics and epileptics, almshouses for the elderly and infirm, nurseries for single mothers and labour houses (under the Prisons' Board) for 'vagrants, ins and outs, ne'er-do-wells'.[14]

In the case of the sick, the Commission recommended that hospital services be removed from the scope of the poor law altogether; that they be organised as a county hospital service, catering for all people requiring hospital accommodation. It envisaged a network of district hospitals equivalent in number to those already existing in the workhouses but based on separate accommodation. A dispensary medical officer would be responsible for the medical care of the patients, referring serious cases to the county hospital, in the proposed county ambulance. The county infirmary would become the county hospital and 'the chief hospital in the County and just as accessible to the poor as the Union Infirmary is at present'.[15] Nurses would be trained in the hospital for the whole county and medical staff of the county hospital would visit the district hospitals for consultations.

Mr Micks and Dr Coey Bigger recommended that the cost of running this new hospital service be met from a rate charged on the county or county borough. They saw this as a step towards the adoption of a national rate, with central control by an elected body over local expenditure, to promote greater efficiency and uniformity of standards.[16] Mr Murnaghan disagreed with a county rate 'which all experience shows has a tendency to high expenditure beyond the means of a country so poor and of such scanty resources as ours'.[17]

The formation of a state medical service was perhaps the most radical recommendation of the Commission: a new medical structure to reform the dispensary service and staff the new county hospital system. The proposed scheme would incorporate all medical posts at county and district hospitals and dispensaries and posts of medical officer of health, with entry by competitive examination. All posts would be salaried and the service would be controlled by a medical council with power to assign and promote medical officers and determine superannuation. Private practice would be permitted, except in populous areas where appointments would be on a full-time basis. It was a bold recommendation designed to reconcile the needs for an improved medical service for the poor with the demands of the medical profession for improved conditions of service.

The Viceregal Commissioners stopped short of recommending the abolition of the boards of guardians, an administrative change which would have complemented their proposals for a county hospital and state medical service. The abolition of the workhouses, the union poor rate and the transfer of responsibility for dispensary medical officers would remove their chief administrative functions. Perhaps because of the political repercussions of recommending their abolition, the Viceregal Commission refrained from drawing the logical conclusion about their future.

The Commission commented that 'there is no health question of greater importance to Ireland at the present time than the prevention and cure of tuberculosis'.[18] It advocated that the disease be fought on a broad front, on the lines of the evidence presented to it.[19] It recommended the provision of sanatoria as a 'public duty', to be maintained by county councils.

The Royal Commission

The Viceregal Commission's report, while well received in Ireland, was overshadowed by the announcement at the end of 1905 of the appointment of a Royal Commission to investigate the workings of the poor law and the relief of distress throughout the United Kingdom. The Commission was set up as one of the last acts of Balfour's Conservative government in response to widespread dissatisfaction in Britain with the poor law. The majority of members were naturally more concerned with conditions in Britain, particularly in England and Wales, and no detailed investigation of Irish conditions was undertaken. Because of the existence of the Viceregal Commission, the Royal Commission decided not to collect any fresh evidence but to accept the recommendations of its predecessor unless these conflicted with the scheme of reform it might propose.[20]

There were two Irish members of the Royal Commission, Sir Henry Robinson and Dr Denis Kelly, Bishop of Ross. They found themselves in the formidable company of Beatrice Webb, Dr Arthur Downes, Charles Booth and eleven other members under the chairmanship of Lord George Hamilton. By his own account, Sir Henry and the Bishop contributed little to the Commission's thinking: their purpose was to make sure that reforms agreed by their colleagues were adapted to Irish conditions.[21] Following a visit to the country by the Commissioners, Sir Henry and the Bishop of Ross drafted the Report on Ireland which was agreed by the members (at least the majority) with very little amendment.[22]

The members of the Royal Commission, who completed their work in 1909, could not agree to a unanimous report. Both Sir Henry Robinson and Bishop Kelly agreed with the more conservative majority and the *Report on Ireland* is an adaptation of the principles agreed by the majority, with some modification, to Irish conditions. The minority believed that the principles of their report applied equally well to Ireland, and used developments in Ireland to demonstrate their case against the majority.

The majority report of the Royal Commission accepted many of the recommendations of the Viceregal Commission but incorporated them in a different framework for reform. There was agreement that the mixed workhouse was 'foreign to the sentiment of the country' and should be abolished.[23] But the Royal Commission drew different conclusions from the break-up of the workhouse system. As the area of the union was considered too small to support a number of specialised institutions, it recommended the establishment of a new local authority, the Public Assistance Authority, to be co-terminous with the county and borough councils. It recommended that the boards of guardians be abolished and their functions transferred to the new authorities.

The public assistance authority would finance its services by levying a rate over the area of the county or borough.

In one respect, this recommendation was more radical than those of the Viceregal Commission as it did away with the boards of guardians and transferred poor and medical relief to an administration based on the county. In other ways, some of the Royal Commission's recommendations were regressive by the standards of the Viceregal Commission and were criticised as such in the Minority Report. The Viceregal Commission wanted to dissociate health services from the workhouse and poor law regulation, to develop a modern hospital service open to everyone who was sick and to integrate the dispensary, hospital and public health services into a state medical service. The Majority Report of the Royal Commission, on the other hand, did not accept the need to separate health services from 'public assistance', which to many was a new name for the old poor law. They recommended that the dispensary and public health service should be brought directly under the new public assistance authority. This made for administrative convenience, but it meant that 'public assistance' rather than medical need would be the criterion for the new authority's intervention.

The Majority Report of the Royal Commission on Ireland shows much less understanding of health and medical problems than the earlier Commission, possibly because there was no direct medical contribution to its Report.[24] It endorsed the recommendations for a county hospital system, but without much enthusiasm, and its comments on tuberculosis hardly reflected the seriousness of the problem. It rejected the evidence that many doctors in the dispensary service had low incomes. It pointed out that public expenditure on medical salaries and drugs in Ireland was just over half of the equivalent expenditure in England, despite the fact that Ireland had only one-eighth of England's population and wealth, and that the average salaries from public funds paid to poor law medical officers in England and Scotland were substantially less than those received by their Irish colleagues.[25] The Royal Commission dismissed the grievances of the dispensary medical officers but its case is not convincing. It confused income from public funds with total income and made no allowance for the different organisation of general practice in the two countries or the ability of people to pay their doctor.

The Irish medical profession made clear its support for a state medical service, as recommended by the Viceregal Commission, in a letter of 13 August 1907 from the Irish Committee of the British Medical Association to the Royal Commission.[26] However, the Royal Commission dismissed the views of the Viceregal Commission, the medical profession and the Medical Commissioner of the Local Government Board, Dr Stafford, on a state medical service. The reasons given were the cost to the Exchequer and the Commission's reluctance to deprive local authorities of their rights to select and control medical officers.[27] It substituted the notion of a 'county medical service' whereby the public assistance authority would employ all the medical officers in the county and suggested that this change would correct many of the defects in the dispensary and poor law services. It did not, however, accept the idea of entry by competitive examination or any increase in the Exchequer's contribution to medical salaries. Other defects in the system could be remedied by 'raising the standard of general education of candidates who enter on medical studies, and in improving the tone and spirit of the medical schools'.[28]

This peremptory refusal by the Royal Commission to endorse a state medical service raises one of the tantalising, unanswerable 'ifs' about the development of Irish medical services. Up to this time, doctors had had more to fear from the tyranny of local representatives than from the state. The opportunity of reorganising public medical services presented itself before the state had accepted a greater responsibility for the medical care of the population and before it threatened the interests of the profession in a fundamental way. As that threat increased in the coming decades, a state-organised medical service would soon be viewed by the profession as a new form of slavery to be fought at all costs. An opportunity to avert or deflect that conflict in Ireland was missed in 1909.

The Royal Commission preserved the unique character of the dispensary service, despite the fact that it differed from its recommendations for medical relief in Britain. Early in the *Report on Ireland*, the majority conceded that the dispensary system 'is a more comprehensive system of Medical Relief for the Poor than has existed hitherto in Great Britain'.[29] They accepted that medical clubs, provident dispensaries, trade and benefit societies hardly existed in Ireland and that in rural society it would be impossible to organise such organisations to pay for medical care. For these reasons they did not recommend the reorganisation of medical relief in Ireland on the basis that people would contribute in advance to dispensaries or provident societies on a regular basis to cover the cost of their medical care. Not for the last time would the dispensary system seem preferable to any other method of organising general practitioner services for the poor and the working classes.

Minority Report

The Minority Report of the Royal Commission disagreed with the majority in their view that services for the poor, sick, aged, unemployed and children should continue to be managed by a single authority, the new public assistance authority. The minority described this arrangement as 'a swollen Poor Law' under a different name.[30] They argued that 'the function of preventing and treating disease among destitute persons cannot in practice, be distinguished from the prevention and treatment of disease in other persons' and that what was demanded was 'not a division according to the presence or absence of destitution, but a division according to the services to be provided'.[31]

On the basis of these principles, the minority recommended the abolition of the centralised poor law authority and the transfer of its functions to specialised bodies; the abolition of the boards of guardians and the transfer of their functions to county and borough councils which would be, as far as illness and disease were concerned, public health authorities. They recommended that treatment should be given on the basis of medical necessity, irrespective of a patient's economic condition. Fees would be recovered subsequently by a registrar of the health authority when appropriate.

The minority expressed caution in advocating their scheme for Ireland but justified themselves by pointing out that Ireland had already gone far down the road towards separating medical treatment from poor relief and pointed to the recommendations of the Viceregal Commission to justify their case.[32] It would seem in retrospect that the recommendations of the Viceregal Commission on the organisation of health services were closer to those of the minority. Without any explicit ideological commitment, the Viceregal Commissioners had arrived at a similar view of the specialised function of health to that of the articulate and socially committed minority. If in the short term the recommendations of the Majority Report were more influential, those of the minority and the Viceregal Commission had more impact in the long term.

Many of the ideas which were to influence the development of the Irish health services were formulated by the reports of these Commissions. Although little was done immediately to implement the Commissions' recommendations, the ideas were 'in the air' to be used by a future generation of policy makers as solutions to problems as they saw them.

Health Insurance

It would be surprising if politicians were not confused by the conflicting recommendations presented to them for the overhaul of the poor law. But even as the Viceregal and Royal Commissions were sitting, a different approach to the problems of poverty was gathering momentum, one which ignored the poor law and concentrated attention on helping the working class maintain its independence during sickness, unemployment and old age. The reforms proposed by the dynamic Liberal government which came to power in 1906 were novel in the British context where some attention had been given to protecting the working classes against poverty. In Ireland, where the issue was hardly discussed, the liberal reforms came as a surprise. The centrepiece of these reforms was the Health Insurance Act, 1911.

The British scheme of health insurance was the brainchild of

David Lloyd George, Chancellor of the Exchequer. He wanted a system of insurance to give people reasonable protection against medical costs and loss of income due to sickness and unemployment. He wanted also to help working people with the additional costs associated with childbirth and to offer protection against the ravages of tuberculosis. All this had to be paid for by a reasonable level of contribution and underpinned by a solvent insurance fund. The scheme was to have an element of compulsion, workers were to contribute directly, the state would make a contribution and the friendly societies were to be involved in the administration of the scheme. Significantly, none of the Treasury officials who formulated the Bill seems to have had any knowledge of Irish affairs or problems.

In the absence of a state scheme, the friendly societies in Britain gave workers a measure of protection against medical expenses and loss of earnings during illness. The six million members of the 2,500 or so societies received these benefits in return for a small weekly contribution. Each society contracted one or more doctors to provide attendance and medicines for its members at an inclusive capitation fee. This 'contract work' was eagerly sought by doctors early in their careers as a stable source of income and as a means of making their names known but the low fees offered — about 3s to 4s per member a year — and the interference of the societies was bitterly resented. The power exercised by the friendly societies over their professional lives was considered by general practitioners to be, in the words of Richard Titmuss, 'an intolerable infringement on their liberty to practise medicine'.[33]

Friendly societies existed only on a limited scale in Ireland. The most active were the Hearts of Oak, the Irish National Foresters and the benefit section of the Ancient Order of Hibernians but their members were largely confined to the 'respectable' working classes in and around Belfast and Dublin. The small size of the industrial workforce and the existence of the dispensary service limited their growth. The exact number of members was unknown but was probably of the order of 40,000.[34]

The National Health Insurance Bill, as introduced by the Chancellor on 4 May 1911, provided for two main categories of contributor — compulsory and voluntary.[35] Compulsory contributors included most wage earners between 16 and 65 years of age whose contributions would be deducted from their wages each week by employers. The contribution payable by male workers was 4d a week or 'the price of two pints of the cheapest beer per week or the price of an ounce of tobacco'.[36] In addition, the employer would pay 3d and the state 2d a week. Self-employed persons who wished to join the scheme could do so as voluntary contributors, paying both the worker's and employer's share of the contribution. No upper income limits were set for manual workers who would be compulsorily insured nor for voluntary contributors. Non-manual workers earning more than £160 a year were not obliged to insure although they could do so on a voluntary basis. Those workers obliged to contribute who could not or would not join a society were to be known as 'the deposit contributors'. They would pay their contributions through the post office and their benefits would be administered by local health commitees. The Chancellor explained that this group of contributors would include the 'bad risk', the cantankerous worker and the casually employed. The Chancellor estimated that 11.7 million workers throughout the United Kingdom would be covered by the provisions for health insurance.

The first benefit to which contributors would be entitled was 'medical benefit', entitling the worker to free medical attendance by a general practitioner and free medicines. The Chancellor admitted that the current arrangements for medical treatment through the friendly societies were unsatisfactory and that the doctors had a case for an increased capitation rate.[37] Secondly, contributors would be entitled to 'maternity benefit' to cover the cost of medical and nursing attendance at childbirth. Insured workers would be entitled to 'sickness benefit' if unable to work due to illness, on production of a medical certificate. If still unavailable for work at the end of six months, a worker would be entitled to a permanent 'disability benefit'. Finally insured persons would be entitled to a 'sanatorium benefit', which would provide workers with free maintenance in a sanatorium or hospital while undergoing treatment for tuberculosis. These benefits were described as the minimum to which a contributor was entitled and which the agencies working the Bill were obliged to provide.

The local health committees proposed under the Bill would have other functions in addition to administering benefits to the deposit contributors. They could, if an approved society requested, take over the administration of medical benefits on behalf of its members. They were also charged with the administration of the sanatorium benefit for the county. A committee, with the approval of the county council and the Treasury, could sanction expenditure on sanatoria, half the money coming from the Treasury and the other half from the rates.

That, in summary, was the insurance scheme against illness proposed by the Chancellor. With the provisions in the second part of the Bill giving some protection against unemployment, it was a major step towards freeing the working class from the destitution brought by events over which they had little or no control. The attraction of insurance lay in the way it averaged the risks of illness, unemployment and childbirth throughout a working person's life and throughout the community. The worker would be afforded protection and society would benefit from a decline in poverty and dependence on the poor law. The insurance scheme was based on the well established principles of self-help and provision for the future and was given a sound financial basis. It would be difficult to oppose the Bill in principle.

In his introductory speech, the Chancellor made no reference to how the Bill would be applied to the different circumstances of Ireland. In particular, he did not say how a health insurance system based on friendly societies would work where such societies covered only a small proportion of the labour force.

Conclusion

The 1903 – 11 period was one of intense scrutiny of the poor law and medical relief for the poor and witnessed, at least in Britain, a surge of interest in the wider questions of poverty and its prevention. There was no shortage of ideas about what ought to be done or commitment to carry out reform. If the poor law had been reformed in Britain at this juncture, Ireland would have followed suit, perhaps with some adaptation to local conditions. But the radical Liberal government was not interested in reforming the poor law, preferring to tackle social problems from a different perspective. Since the Irish administration, and particularly the Local Government Board, was not noted for its reforming zeal, major reform of the poor law had to await a more dynamic native government. In the meantime, the country was confronted with Lloyd George's Health Insurance Bill, a humane and reforming measure but one which was not designed for Irish conditions and which raised, in a fundamental way, the issue of the state's responsibility for the medical treatment of the working classes.

3
Medical Benefit
1911~1913

THE REFORM PROGRAMME of the Liberal government posed a dilemma for the Irish Party. The majority of its members had little sympathy with the economic and social measures designed to alleviate the hardships of the British working classes and were hostile to the steep rise in taxation required to fund the programme. Yet the same tax proposals led to a showdown in 1910 between the government and the House of Lords and to the removal in 1911 of the Lords' absolute right of veto. The last constitutional obstacle to Home Rule was removed. The Liberal government, dependent on the support of the Irish Party, began drafting a scheme of Home Rule. Although John Redmond considered aspects of the Liberal social legislation to be extravagant and unsuited to Irish conditions, he could not withdraw his support from the government and had to rely on his party's considerable influence to adapt the measures to Irish circumstances.

This strategy was brought to a fine art with the Health Insurance Bill, 1911. It was, Redmond conceded, 'a noble and magnificent effort ... to deal with the very worst of our social grievances', but he entered the standard Irish Party caveat about its suitability to Ireland.[1] The Irish Party approved the Bill in principle, against the advice of some members who felt that it would be wiser to wait for a lead from Irish public opinion, and established a committee to prepare amendments to modify the Bill's application to Ireland.[2] The most active members of the committee were Joseph Devlin and John Clancy, representing large industrial constituencies, and James Lardner, who was appointed secretary. Devlin and Lardner were also closely associated with the two largest friendly societies in Ireland, the Ancient Order of Hibernians and the Irish National Foresters. Redmond appointed Lardner and Clancy as the Party's negotiators with the Treasury. The committee got to work in Dublin at the end of May.

The Irish Clauses

The health insurance provisions of the National Health Insurance Bill were prepared in great haste and the Irish clauses were agreed very late in the day. No consideration seems to have been given to Irish conditions until the end of March 1911 when Lloyd George instructed his officials to get the assistance of the Irish Office to adapt the provisions of the scheme to the different organisation of local government in Ireland.[3] The person deputed by the Irish Office to assist the Treasury was Sir Henry Robinson, a man who did not accept the need for reform of medical relief in Ireland (see Chapter 2).

The Irish situation proved extremely complicated, with the question of medical benefit giving most difficulty. How would insurance work where there were few friendly societies and where a dispensary service already provided free medical care for many of those who would be insured under the new Act? The Irish provisions, as drafted by Robinson and agreed with the Chancellor, were finalised just two days before the Bill was introduced.[4]

Section 59 of the published Bill contained the Irish clauses.[5] It was clear from the section that the government was not going to carry out a radical reorganisation of Irish general practice as a result of the introduction of medical benefit. The dispensary system would be left intact with the new insurance scheme grafted on to it.

Some of the blame for the subsequent course of events must rest with Sir Henry and the Treasury. They took the option of least possible change, despite the Irish doctors' commitment to overhauling the dispensary service. To be fair to Sir Henry, he was hardly given the time in which to prepare a new scheme even if he had the inclination. But his views as expressed in the Majority Report of the Royal Commission on Ireland and later on in this controversy suggest that he saw no need to reorganise medical relief in Ireland.

The minority of Irish workers who were members of friendly societies would receive their medical benefit in the same way as in Britain. A different system, however, would operate for deposit contributors. They would be treated by dispensary doctors paid a yearly sum 'as may be prescribed' by the health committees. It is hard to escape the conclusion that the rate for treating deposit contributors would be lower than the rate to be agreed between the government and medical profession for treating members of approved societies.[6] Since a large number of Irish workers would be deposit contributors, medical benefit for the Irish would be provided on the cheap. The bargaining power of dispensary doctors was weakened by the provision that remuneration would be 'fixed by the rules' or 'prescribed', not 'arranged' as in the main text of the Bill. A further consequence of Section 59 was that private practitioners were excluded from treating deposit contributors, which could mean a significant drop in private practice. If medical benefit held attractions for the medical profession in Ireland, it was not apparent from Section 59. Finally, the clear distinction between poor law medical relief and insurance medical benefit, so essential to the thinking of Lloyd George, would be blurred in Ireland by restricting deposit contributors to attendance by dispensary medical officers and to a supply of drugs from the poor law guardians.

Section 59 also contained what in retrospect was a most significant clause allowing approved societies to opt out of providing medical benefit, if they found that they could not make arrangements on reasonable terms for the administration of the benefit to their members. The explanatory memorandum accompanying the Bill asserted that this clause aimed to 'protect the societies against unreasonable demands from the salaried dispensary doctors'.[7] So far as Ireland was concerned, medical benefit was not intended to be a minimum and compulsory benefit which approved societies were obliged to provide.

No figures were provided publicly by the government for the number of persons who would be insured in Ireland. Unofficial estimates ranged from 800,000 to 1.3 million.[8] The schedules to the Bill excluded persons employed in the army and navy, teachers, civil and public servants, and persons employed without payment by small farmers. Those employed in non-manual jobs earning more than £160 a year and the casually employed were exempted from the compulsory provisions of the Bill, although they could become voluntary contributors. The self-employed, a relatively large group in Ireland, were also exempted from compulsory contributions, although they too could become voluntary contributors. The biggest groups in Ireland likely to be affected by the compulsory provisions of the Bill were about 150,000 general and agricultural labourers, 170,000 domestic servants, 613,000 industrial workers, and 30,000 shop assistants and commercial clerks in private business.[9]

The initial reaction to the Bill in Ireland was hostile. The humanitarian purpose of its provisions was overshadowed by accusations that it represented a further incidence of penal taxation by a callous British government without real benefit to the people of Ireland. The *Irish Independent* led the campaign of opposition to the Bill, resting its case on the burden of contributions on Irish industry, the potential insolvency of a Home Rule government, and the inappropriateness of its provisions to Irish conditions. There were calls for Ireland's exclusion from the Bill.

The Second Reading

The Bill was read for the second time on 24 May 1911. By this time MPs had had an opportunity to study the Bill and to take preliminary soundings from their constituencies and the interests they represented. John Clancy, speaking for the Irish Party, welcomed the Bill as 'the latest of a series of efforts made in the last generation to cope with the evils and miseries which have been produced by generations of class legislation in the interests of the rich'.[10] He was quick to defend the Bill from its critics in Ireland. He described the living conditions of the poor in Irish cities as 'simply shocking' and disagreed with those who argued that the expense of the scheme would be ruinous for industry.[11] The problem, as he saw it, was how far this measure suited the particular needs of Ireland. The scheme was designed for industrial conditions, not for the predominantly rural and agricultural Irish conditions. He asked for time to consider the Bill and to decide how far separate treatment was necessary. Provided the government accepted the modifications which the Party would suggest, the Party would support the application of the Bill not only to Britain but also to Ireland.

The initial warm reception of the Bill in Parliament soon gave way before the pressure of what Lloyd George called the 'vested interests in disease and death'.[12] The Conservative Party had discovered that many workers did not share Lloyd George's view of insurance as the panacea for their problems and objected strongly to paying the contributions. The political atmosphere was poisoned by the passage of the Parliament Bill, which went before the House of Lords in the early summer, and by the talk of Home Rule which would follow its enactment into law. Between May and December 1911, Lloyd George negotiated his Bill through the House, buying off, conciliating and occasionally overruling the demands of the interests affected. The Irish Party was one of the major interests to be appeased. According to a close associate, Lloyd George played the game brilliantly, he 'made promise after promise, did one dodge after another'.[13]

Apart from the Irish Party, the other interests to be appeased were the friendly societies, the industrial insurance companies, the medical profession and the labour movement. British doctors, after a late start, had woken up to the far-reaching effects the insurance proposals would have on general practice and were determined to secure the best possible conditions for themselves. The seriousness with which Lloyd George viewed their objections is reflected by the fact that most of his speech in the second reading is devoted to soothing ruffled feathers. In that speech he made it clear that his opening offer was a capitation fee of 6s for each patient on a doctor's panel, a figure that was neither 'fixed or final'.[14] The fee was a matter for negotiation and was not written into the Bill.

On 31 May, the British Medical Association (BMA) held a special representative meeting in London to discuss the Bill as a result of which the Association committed itself to 'six points': an income limit of £2 a week for those entitled to medical benefit, choice of doctor, the exclusion of the friendly societies from the administration of medical and maternity benefit, local flexibility in the method of remunerating doctors, adequate remuneration and strong medical representation at all levels of the new administration.[15] The only resolution passed by the meeting that affected Ireland was one demanding equal representation for the medical profession with the county councils on the local health committees. Every registered medical practitioner in the United Kingdom was invited to sign an undertaking that he would not enter into any agreement for giving medical attendance and treatment to any person insured under the Act unless the conditions of service were in accordance with BMA policy.

The Chancellor addressed the doctors on the second day of their special meeting. He was asked if it was the government's intention to retain Ireland under the Bill and if so, whether the funds for the administration of medical benefit would be applied equally and in the same way in Ireland and Great Britain. He avoided answering the first question directly by referring to the dispensary service and to the Irish phenomenon (which he claimed he had only discovered while preparing the Bill), that 'well-to-do' people in rural areas had no objection to applying for a dispensary ticket. 'In Ireland the problem is not to set up a separate independent medical attendance, but to pay the parish doctor more than he is getting now'.[16] The question should be settled by Irishmen themselves, he declared, and the problems of Irish doctors by Irish doctors as he did not understand the problems. However, on the application of medical funds, he said the same amount would be available to pay Irish as British doctors, but as to its distribution, they would have 'to fight that out themselves'.[17]

The first problem for the Irish medical profession was to

understand how the Bill affected them. Their representative associations did not advise them well in this respect. The supplement to the *Journal of the British Medical Association* which reprinted the text of the Bill omitted the Irish Section 59. On 30 May, the Irish Committee of the BMA sent a misleading letter to all medical practitioners in Ireland.[18] The authors confused the distinction between compulsory and voluntary contributors, gave no definition of deposit contributors and made no reference to the many exceptions to compulsory insurance. A figure of 4s capitation was referred to as if it were in the Bill and the provision for the treatment of deposit contributors by dispensary doctors was misquoted as a duty 'to attend and treat *every contributor* resident in his district'.[19] The letter implied that every person earning less than £161 a year, the overwhelming majority of Irish people, would be compelled into insurance and lost to private practice. No reference was made to the exclusion of the self-employed from compulsory insurance or of dependants of insured workers from medical benefit.

This information was hardly designed to encourage Irish doctors to look rationally at the merits of the Bill for the profession as a whole. The doctors who drafted the BMA letter were concerned with the loss of private patients to insurance and capitation fees, and not with the way in which the dispensary medical officers could benefit from a shift to insurance-funded medical treatment. This signalled the way the Irish medical profession would split on the Bill.

The Bill roused the Irish profession. It was clear from meetings of doctors around the country that the profession was divided on whether to reject the Bill entirely or to seek suitable amendments.[20] On 26 June, the medical graduates of Dublin University called for the total rejection of the Bill.[21] They objected to the introduction of contract practice to Ireland. They pointed out that at least one-seventh of the population was already in receipt of medical relief through the dispensary service and the need for medical benefit was therefore small. Their greatest fear was the loss of private patients to insurance.[22] The doctors called instead for a remodelling of the poor law medical system in Ireland.

The graduates of the Dublin University medical school were traditionally the leading hospital physicians and general practitioners and were more susceptible to threats to private practice or their independence than other groups of Irish doctors.

The Irish Medical Association (IMA), representing the interests of dispensary doctors, held a referendum on the Bill, seeking the opinion of the profession on a number of issues, the first five of which were identical with the first five of the BMA's 'six points'. In addition, respondents were asked to indicate their agreement to other demands, the most important of which were for a minimum capitation fee of 8s 6d, extra remuneration for special services, and a mileage payment.

On 30 June, there was a meeting of three hundred doctors in Dublin. The President of the IMA announced his belief that the Bill, if suitably amended, would prove most beneficial to Irish working people. Representatives of the Association had been in contact with Lloyd George, Sir Henry Robinson and John Redmond, and had made their views known to the committee of the Irish Party sitting in Dublin collecting information on the Bill.[23] The meeting then went on to ratify the suggestions which had been submitted to the referendum of the profession. About half the doctors in the country had returned their views and they were almost unanimously in favour of the suggested amendments. The meeting adopted resolutions calling for the Bill to be amended.

The Irish medical profession thereby committed itself to fighting a British battle but demanding more generous terms than their British colleagues. The desired capitation fee of 8s 6d was the rate which the Post Office paid doctors to treat its officials and this demand would be an embarrassment later on. It would have been better tactics to leave negotiation on the fee until a later date, as the BMA had decided and then to insist that the same rate be applied to Ireland. But then Section 59 of the Bill specified that the fees for deposit contributors would be fixed by local committees, appearing to leave no room for negotiation at national level. The assembled doctors pledged themselves not to administer the medical and maternity benefits of the Bill unless their demands were met. The Joint Committee of the IMA and the BMA was charged with protecting the interests of the Irish medical profession in relation to the Bill.

This show of unity hid deep divisions in the profession, even among those at the June meeting. The *Medical Press and Circular* reported that at the meeting a resolution calling for the entire rejection of the medical clauses of the Bill would have been carried if the chairman had not ruled it out of order.[24] Unity and co-ordination also seem to have been lacking in the profession's presentation of their case. The different representative bodies of the profession could not agree on a common strategy. By early July, the Irish Committee of the BMA (responsible for the misleading and inaccurate letter of 30 May) had reached the opinion that the arrangements for medical benefit for Ireland were unworkable.[25] The General Medical Council, on the other hand, in a submission to the Chancellor on 12 July, requested that the amendments sought for Britain be applied to Ireland in particular: deposit contributors should be given a choice of doctor and that the medical service for the insured should be distinct from the dispensary service.[26] Meanwhile, representatives of the IMA were negotiating with the Irish Party's committee on the details of the Bill in Dublin.

A state medical service?

It is surprising that the opportunity afforded by the Insurance Bill to reorganise the dispensary service was not taken by the profession. In June, Lloyd George, in an inspired leak to the *Westminster Gazette*, threatened that if the profession was unreasonable in its demands he would organise a medical service for insured workers.[27] This proposal would have made sense in Ireland. The duties of the employed doctors could then have included treatment of those too poor to be insured as well as the insured themselves and some arrangement could have been made to treat the dependants of insured persons. Patients outside the insurance scheme who could afford it would pay for treatment as before. A share of the state-employed doctor's salary could still have come from local taxation and the remainder from the insurance fund, supplemented by state funds if necessary. The doctors in the scheme could be recruited by competition and enjoy the same conditions of service as civil servants and medical officers in the army and navy. The opposition to such a scheme would have come from doctors with large private practices who feared the loss of paying patients to insurance. But these doctors, while influential, were a minority in the profession and were outnumbered by dispensary medical officers. Such a scheme might be unpopular because it did not offer the patient a choice of doctor, although this demand usually came from doctors rather than patients. It would also be open to the criticism that using the same doctor for the poor and the insured linked poor law relief and insurance benefit, but this was little more than what was being proposed anyway. Perhaps in the interest of solidarity with the profession in Britain, Irish doctors did not further explore the idea of a state service. They let this opportunity for reorganisation slip by. The Irish profession allowed itself to hold out for demands which were substantially British and appropriate to a different type of general practice; they also gave away a tactical advantage in appearing to be greedier on the questions of pay and conditions of service.

On the other hand, no one really tried to persuade the doctors of the merits of insurance or suggested ways of evolving a new system of general practice based on insurance principles. As we have seen, the Irish position was not considered in the Treasury until very late in the preparation of the Bill. The officials of the Treasury were ignorant of Irish conditions. And by his own admission, Lloyd George knew nothing about the problems of Irish doctors; he left it to the Irish to resolve their difficulties with the Bill. He had little choice since he depended on the Irish vote for the government's survival. Sir Henry Robinson and the Local Government Board were hardly likely to promote the notion of an insurance-based medical service. On the contrary, Sir Henry's restrictive drafting of Section 59 was a major impediment to approval of insurance in principle. The members of the Irish Party, whatever they might think personally about the Bill, could not campaign too vigorously for acceptance of a British government measure unless it was Home Rule. Their job was to scrutinise legislation and to badger the government until amendments were accepted to suit Irish conditions. Weak and disorganised, the medical associations in Ireland were not in a position to give enlightened leadership.

The Hierarchy Intervenes

The difficulties of the Irish medical profession with the Bill were overshadowed by the opposition of a more important assembly, the Catholic Hierarchy. In June, the bishops issued a statement opposing the Bill's application to Ireland.[28] They acknowledged the importance of the Bill to the industrial population of England and Wales but considered it inapplicable to Ireland since 'only a mere fraction' of the population were wage earners and 'the immense majority' were workers on their own account who neither received nor paid wages. They criticised the clause which required parents to insure their sons and daughters over sixteen years of age working for them on larger farms or in shops or public houses and considered that these sons and daughters would constitute the majority of those to be insured. The contribution such parents would have to pay would be oppressive and could not justify the medical benefit. The statement assumed that such workers would only be entitled to the same type of medical service as provided by the dispensary system. It made no reference to the maternity, sickness or sanatorium benefit to which all these workers would be entitled or to unemployment insurance which men in the building and engineering trades could claim. The bishops did not seem to be aware of the 800,000 industrial workers and domestic servants in the labour force who stood to benefit from the Bill.

The cost of the insurance scheme would be a heavy burden on small, struggling Irish firms, the bishops argued, and they considered that it was likely to increase unemployment. They therefore requested the Chancellor not to extend the Bill to Ireland but to set aside the state contribution necessary for financing the scheme to the credit of Ireland, either for an insurance scheme specially devised for the needs of the country, or for some other purpose more beneficial to the general welfare of the population. They ended with a request to the Irish Party to urge this policy on the government.

The bishops' statement is interesting for a number of reasons. T.M. Healy MP claimed that it was the first time the Irish Hierarchy had condemned government legislation introduced into the House of Commons, other than a Bill on education.[29] The statement also illustrates the way the bishops viewed the issues raised by the Bill through predominantly rural and capitalist eyes and from the standpoint of the farmer and small trader. No reference was made to the needs of the increasingly desperate working class in the cities. And it seems that the bishops did not fully understand the Bill or the range of benefits offered. This lack of sympathy with the intentions of the Chancellor's Bill, combined with the fear of a financially insolvent Home Rule government, was probably sufficient to convince them of the need to demand Ireland's exclusion from the Bill.[30]

In view of subsequent controversies between the Hierarchy and politicians, it is tempting to speculate that a vested interest lobbied the bishops to issue this unprecedented condemnation of a piece of legislation which raised no issue of faith or morals. It may be that disgruntled members of the Irish Party approached them, or members of the medical profession or representatives of the business community. The reasons given by the bishops for demanding Ireland's exclusion from the Bill are similar to those espoused by the *Irish Independent*, a paper which unashamedly represented the interests of the most conservative sections of Irish society. On the other hand, the influential circles in Ireland were relatively small, and closely knit by matrimonial and professional ties. Active lobbying may not have been necessary since the criticisms raised by the bishops were widely shared. What is significant, in the light of later crises between Church and state over health issues, is that the Hierarchy condemned the Bill on social and economic grounds. Maternity benefit was not seen as a threat to the moral fibre of Irish women nor were insurance benefits seen as undermining the responsibility of the head of the family to provide for his dependants. Thus, the ensuing debate stayed out of the realm of moral theology. Furthermore, the bishops made their views public. Unlike later interventions, they did not rely on the use of influence behind closed doors.

The bishops' pronouncement set the base line for debate on the Bill and complicated the work of the committee of the Irish Party. The Party had publicly committed itself to the principle of Ireland's inclusion in the Bill. Some members, especially Clancy, Devlin and Dillon, were strongly in favour of introducing the insurance provisions to Ireland. The Party now had to strike a deal which would meet the approval of the Hierarchy while still retaining some of the benefits of the Bill. It is not clear if the committee considered the substitution of the dispensary system by a combination of an insurance- and state-funded medical service to include all wage earners, voluntary contributors and their dependants. The Party certainly claimed that it wanted to abolish the dispensary service.[31] But any desire to replace the dispensary system would have run up against the major problem of cost. It was easy to call for state funding of services as long as the imperial Exchequer met any deficit. It was more difficult if an independent Irish government had to foot the bill. The probability of such a government in the near future would have constrained the options open to the committee in providing medical benefit. The committee tried to reconcile insurance-based benefit with the dispensary service but the terms which the doctors sought could not be defrayed by the proposed contributions. Even if they had agreed terms, could the Party have satisfied the bishops that the people would receive much more by way of medical benefit than they were already getting from the dispensary doctor? Despite the wishes of some influential Party members, the medical benefit would have to be dropped.

The Party issued a statement on 12 July setting out the amendments it would be seeking to the Bill.[32] It recommended that the Bill should apply to Ireland but with important exclusions and limitations. The most controversial amendment sought was the exclusion of medical benefit. The reason for this was that 'there is already in Ireland a system of medical relief for the poor which is, generally speaking, efficient, and is paid for chiefly out of the rates'.[33] The demands of the majority of the Irish medical profession were pushed aside with one sweep. At the same time, a major concession was made to the bishops. The Party also sought amendments to meet the other points raised by the bishops and a number of other concessions, the most significant of which was a separate Irish Insurance Commission and Fund.

On the previous day, Redmond, Devlin and two other members of the Party had had breakfast with the Chancellor to inform him of the Party's demands.[34] It is likely that the Irish leaders asked for more time before finalising their amendments because the committee continued to sit during the exceptionally hot summer of 1911. The significance of the Irish Party's decision to exclude medical benefit was not lost on the medical profession. One journal commented that while the Irish medical profession had not really considered whether it would be better if the medical clauses were deleted or amended, the Party had 'cut the Gordian knot'.[35] Nonetheless, branches of the BMA and the IMA passed resolutions calling for the retention of medical benefit.[36] The IMA called a meeting of dispensary medical officers to be held in early October.

On 14 October, the delegates of the dispensary medical officers met in Dublin. They were alarmed at the exclusion of medical benefit from Ireland and the retention of sickness benefit without agreement on the fee for doctors who would have to complete medical certificates. They called on the government not to delete medical benefit. A deputation was appointed to confer with the Joint Committee of the IMA and BMA to settle policy before waiting on the Irish Party and the Chancellor of the Exchequer. The divisions in the Irish medical profession had come to the fore. The medical officers looked to the Insurance Bill and the capitation fees to relieve them of some of their badly paid duties. The removal of medical benefit did nothing to improve the position of the dispensary doctor. The threat of completing medical certificates for little or no reward remained.

Despite the wish of some members of the Irish Party, especially Joseph Devlin, to salvage medical benefit if reasonable terms could be agreed with the doctors, no progress was made in the negotiations with the profession.[37] In early November, the Party submitted its final demands, which differed only in detail from those agreed by the Party meeting in July.[38]

52

Committee Stage — The Irish Clauses

The divisions within the country on the Bill became more apparent during the committee stage debate in mid-October. William O'Brien and T. M. Healy, the maverick Irish nationalists, attacked Redmond for his Party's support for the Bill. They both wanted the complete rejection of the Bill as far as Ireland was concerned and they claimed that every interest group, bar the skilled tradesmen of Belfast and Dublin, supported this view. O'Brien claimed that the government was threatening the Irish Party with resignation if the Bill was not passed.[39] Healy, popularly known as Cardinal Logue's 'tame' politician, attempted to embarrass Redmond by claiming that the bishops were not satisfied with the amendments suggested by the Irish Party.[40] Redmond shook off O'Brien's accusations and repeated his Party's support for the Bill in principle. He said that he would be seeking amendments for which the whole country was asking, and which he took for granted the government would accept.[41]

On 2 November, an important deputation from the Irish Medical Association went to see Lloyd George in the House of Commons to put the case for the retention of medical benefit in Ireland. The Chancellor listened to their arguments but suggested that they consult with members of the Irish Party. A meeting was held that evening with party leaders and the exchange of views was prolonged without, it appears, any effect on the Party's stance.

The position of Irish doctors was made more difficult by the delay in the appearance of the Party's actual amendments to Section 59. They were published by the government less than a week before the debate scheduled for 14 November. Few sections in that much-amended Bill bore as little relationship to the original as the new Section 59. Under the revised clauses, medical benefit would not apply in Ireland. However, some small changes seem to have been incorporated to appease the doctors, including payment of doctors for medical certificates. A separate Irish insurance commission was also to be established.

The debate on the Irish clauses was highly charged. The two main themes of the debate were the Irish Party's defence of its decisions to retain Ireland under much of the Bill and to exclude medical benefit. On the second point they managed to leave the door open for future compromise. Clancy led the debate for the Party. He defended the Bill from 'the exaggeration and misrepresentations and inaccuracies of capitalist newspapers' which had misled public opinion about the true intentions of the Bill from the beginning.[42] Much had been made of the Bill as 'an intolerable tax on Ireland' but it was an abuse of language to call the system of contributions a tax in the ordinary sense of the word. 'It is a tax every penny of which will be spent in Ireland, for ... the preventing and relieving of human suffering and misery'.[43] He said that the government had conceded all the concessions which the Party had sought. Joseph Devlin also defended the application of the Bill to Ireland. Emphasising that as the representative of his constituency, 'no man, be he bishop or layman, has my conscience in his pocket', he politely but firmly suggested that the bishops should not veto what was good for the people.[44]

James Lardner explained the Party's difficulties with medical benefit.[45] The committee wanted to provide medical benefit, particularly in the towns, but was unable to graft the new system onto the dispensary service. It had come to the conclusion that it would be better to wait until the poor law was reformed before introducing medical benefit for the insured.[46] Lardner put the blame for the deletion of medical benefit on the shoulders of the medical profession: 'the demands of the doctors for medical benefit were so extortionate and oppressive, that it was impossible to consider the possibility of working the Bill in Ireland'.[47] The bitterness of the negotiations broke through when he claimed that:

> the real reason for the head-chopping (of medical benefit) is (due to) people who were not friends of this Bill, and who ... considered that the Bill was intended not for the improvement of health, not for the improvement of the working classes, but rather as a doctors' endowment scheme.[48]

There could be no solution unless the medical profession came forward with a reasonable scheme.

John Dillon made it clear that he personally wished that medical benefit could have been retained but that he had yielded to Irish opinion.[49] He thought that the advantage of medical benefit was that it laid the foundation for the complete abolition of pauper medical relief.[50] Even Sir Edward Carson, in a rare show of agreement with his nationalist countrymen, felt it a great pity that the benefit had been removed from the Bill, though he could not blame the government for doing so. He considered that the dispensary doctors had a great deal to gain from medical benefit and asked that the benefit be put back into the Bill.[51] Lloyd George played for touch as usual by saying that he would consider any scheme put to him by the Irish representatives.[52]

The door, while closing, was still ajar. On the 23 and 24 November, the BMA held a special representative meeting to discuss the Bill as amended in committee. Lloyd George had gone a long way to meet the 'six points' of the Association. The only point not conceded was an upper limit for compulsory contributors and the capitation fee had yet to be agreed. These concessions were the result of skilful bargaining by the BMA, led by the secretary, Dr Smith Whittaker. The position of the profession in Ireland was by contrast, a shambles. Far from securing any concessions under the original provisions of the Bill, medical benefit had been removed altogether. A special representative meeting of the BMA endorsed the views put forward by the Irish representatives calling for the reinstatement of medical benefit and instructed its secretary to bring a number of points to the attention of the Chancellor and to write to John Redmond setting out the conditions under which the profession would work the medical benefit.

The letter from Smith Whittaker to Redmond, dated 25 November, sets out at some length the position of the Irish profession.[53] The letter assured Redmond that there was no longer a difference of opinion between the dispensary doctors and the rest of the profession. It threatened 'that the entire force of the medical profession in Great Britain, both pecuniary and in every other way, will be at the disposal of the Irish medical profession for its support in enforcing (its) demands'. The Association demanded that medical benefit should be given to Ireland on the same terms as in Britain. It recognised that some 'adjustment' would be necessary to accommodate the dispensary doctors but the details could be worked out later, provided there was a general provision in the Bill. The letter announced that the Irish profession had withdrawn its demand for an 8s 6d capitation fee and agreed that the fee should be left to subsequent negotiation. It said that the Chancellor would re-introduce the benefit if the Irish Party agreed and that the dispensary service should be replaced. Finally, the Association said it was publishing the letter in the newspapers the following Tuesday. A copy was sent to Lloyd George on 27 November with a general memorandum on the profession's further demands for amendment to the Bill: it claimed that difficulty over benefit in Ireland arose from the attitude of the Irish Party and that 'the members of the Irish (medical) profession are almost, if not entirely, unanimous in demanding that ... medical benefits should apply to that country in the same way as in Great Britain'.[54]

But Redmond was not to be moved by threats of medical solidarity or newspaper revelations. Two days before the BMA special representative meeting, he informed the Chancellor that nothing had occurred to change the opinion of most Irish representatives that medical benefit should be excluded from the Bill.[55] On the 28 November, the Chancellor told a deputation from the BMA that the government would not extend medical benefit to Ireland. It was agreed, however, that if an approved society provided medical benefit as an additional benefit, it would be on the same lines as in Britain, unless the Irish insurance commissioners decided otherwise.

The BMA was seriously divided after 2 December by the Council decision to ratify the appointment of Dr Smith Whittaker to the deputy chairmanship of the English Insurance Commission. This decision seemed like treason to many: 'six points' had not been agreed and the profession had undertaken not to have anything to do with the Bill until all had been conceded. The division was stirred up by what Lloyd George called 'the swell doctors', particularly London consultants who were not affected by the Bill but disliked the policies of the Liberal government and Lloyd George's insurance scheme in particular. It was unlikely that the

BMA at this juncture would rescue the Irish medical profession, even if it could. The Irish doctors conceded defeat. The Bill received the royal assent on 16 December 1911.

The government's resolve to proceed with medical benefit in Britain was strengthened by the Plender Report which examined the books of more than two hundred doctors in England and Scotland.[56] The report revealed that the average capitation fee doctors received from both contract and private patients amounted to not much more than 4s a year, including drugs. The government believed that an attractive capitation rate would break the ranks of the profession. In late October 1912, Lloyd George announced a basic fee of 8s 6d per insured worker to be paid to doctors who participated in the scheme for medical attendance and drugs. A further 6d would be available for doctors from the sanatorium fund for the treatment of tuberculosis at home. The fee included the cost of providing medical certificates and the keeping of records of disease. Notwithstanding this generous offer, a special representative meeting of the BMA on 21 December voted by a majority of over four to one not to accept the fee offered. The government had contingency plans for the establishment of a national medical service but this proved unnecessary. As general practitioners throughout Britain did their sums and realised they could greatly increase their incomes, they had no hesitation in disobeying their Association's instructions, and by early 1913 had applied in their thousands for business under the Act. Irish doctors, however, were never given the opportunity to choose.

None of the conditions existed in Ireland which were critical to Lloyd George's success in persuading British general practitioners to operate the insurance scheme. This success required great political skill and judgement on the part of Lloyd George and his officials and a firm commitment to the scheme. None of this skill, judgement or commitment was apparent in Ireland. The history of the Insurance Bill in Ireland illustrates the pitfalls of British legislation for Ireland, even when devised with the best motives and intended as a measure of reform.

The Debate Re-opens

The passage of the Insurance Act into law opened a new phase in the debate about medical benefit in Ireland. Shortly after the Bill became law, Joseph Devlin raised a scare of the widespread growth of contract practice in Ireland as approved societies offered the option of medical benefit as an additional benefit under the Act.[57] Since there was no agreed procedure for deciding a minimum capitation fee, societies could force doctors to compete against each other for work and the profession feared the results would be a 'revolution in the system of medical practice'.[58]

The issue came to a head over those friendly societies which had provided medical benefit to their members before the Act was introduced, mainly those in the six county boroughs — Dublin, Belfast, Cork, Limerick, Waterford and Londonderry. The societies paid doctors as little as 4s capitation a year and in some cases dependants were included in this fee. In July 1912, the Irish profession, taking advantage of the BMA's decision not to operate the Act in Britain, announced that unless the friendly societies increased the fee to 8s 6d (or 12s 6d if dependants were included), doctors would withdraw their services at the end of the year. By January 1913, many doctors had withdrawn their service.

The friendly societies were in an awkward position. The contributions from workers would not cover the fees demanded, particularly as there was no employer or state contribution. A few succeeded in persuading doctors to take less than the 'official' rate; others reimbursed members in cash for their medical expenses; and some withdrew the benefit altogether. The irony of the Insurance Act for some Irish workers was that they lost a medical benefit which they had previously enjoyed or had to pay much more for the same benefit.

The withdrawal of the doctors from club work, known as 'the doctors' strike', was controversial. It led to the re-opening of discussion about extending medical benefit under the Act to Ireland. On 9 January 1913, the Chancellor, on the initiative of the Irish Party, announced the formation of a committee to examine the application of medical benefit to Ireland. The committee had nine members under the chairmanship of Lord Asby St Ledgers. Joseph Devlin and James Lardner represented the Irish Party, Sir John Bradbury, the Treasury, and Joseph Glynn and Dr William Maguire, the newly formed Irish Insurance Commission.[59]

The committee excluded any examination of extending medical benefit to rural areas and concentrated its attention on the county boroughs. It took evidence from representatives of friendly societies, employers and the medical profession, independent experts and spokesmen of the poor law guardians. The evidence presented and the sometimes fierce interrogation of witnesses by committee members produced fascinating information on medical practice among the 'respectable' working class but no consensus on applying medical benefit to Ireland.

The officials of friendly societies and trades councils were united in demanding medical benefit at as low a rate of contribution as possible. 'Respectable' workers and artisans wanted nothing to do with the dispensary service, despite its comprehensiveness and absence of charges. A leading trade unionist described the dispensary service as 'congested, and the provisions generally for dealing with cases are altogether inadequate, and there is a general air of contamination and poverty about it that is most objectionable to the ordinary worker'.[60] A friendly society representative declared that 'the medical provision made in Ireland was only intended for paupers, and not for the respectable and self-respecting artisan class'.[61] Others put it more strongly. 'A decent working man', one commented, 'objects to go down there to herd with the refuse of society — of humanity'.[62]

Insured workers were prepared to pay regular contributions for medical care for themselves and their families to be independent of the dispensary service. But perhaps because of the safety net provided by the dispensary system or the extent of quasi-charitable work by doctors and hospitals, the issue does not seem to have been a burning one in labour circles in early 1913. The attitudes of working people to doctors and medicine may also account for the relatively low priority accorded to medical benefit. A number of the working class witnesses before the committee proudly claimed that they had never been sick in their lives or been treated by a doctor.

Most of the employer representatives supported the principle of medical benefit for urban workers but felt that the time was not yet ripe for its introduction. With Home Rule around the corner, they saw safety in delay. Ireland's struggling firms, they claimed, could not bear an increase in the employer's insurance contribution. They felt that those who needed medical care and could not afford to pay could go to the dispensary, a service largely financed by the propertied classes through the rates.

The position of the medical profession was difficult to understand. The doctors had reason to fear that they might not get a fair hearing before the Committee. Devlin and Lardner were the presidents of the Ancient Order of Hibernians and the Irish National Foresters respectively; Lardner had bitterly criticised the negotiating methods of the Irish doctors in November 1911; Bradbury was closely identified with the Insurance Act; and there was a strong 'official' presence on the committee. The chairman had an active style of interviewing, described by T.M. Healy as 'clubbing the witnesses who come before him'.[63] The image of a profession which claimed to put the patient's interest first had been badly tarnished by the doctors' action in Britain and the withdrawal of Irish doctors from friendly society work. The Irish doctors' intransigence could be contrasted with the willingness of British doctors to operate the Act. But even making these allowances, the medical witnesses came off much the worst in their encounters with the committee.

The three doctors deputed to represent the profession before the committee were hospital specialists and in the committee's opinion were at one remove from the problems of general practitioners in working class areas.[64] The experience in Britain had shown how out of touch such doctors could be with the mainstream of the profession. The committee's decision to confine its examination of the problem to the cities excluded representations from the dispensary doctors in towns and rural areas who had been most in favour of extending benefit to Ireland. The general practitioners who presented their case were all established practitioners with large private practices. These well-established general practitioners of the cities had least to gain and much to lose from medical benefit.

The official medical position was support for extending medical benefit if the capitation fees were sufficiently high and if the standard safeguards of an income limit and choice of doctor applied. But even here the support was not wholehearted. Dr Maurice Hayes claimed, with disregard for the truth, that 'the profession, as a whole, have not declared either for or against the extension of medical benefits to Ireland'.[65] The capitation fee now demanded by the profession was 21s for each insured worker and dependants. The fee had apparently been calculated by allowing two dependants per insured worker and roughly trebling the basic rate agreed in Britain. Devlin claimed that the profession had only increased the fee from 8s 6d to 21s when the appointment of the committee had been announced.[66]

The medical witnesses were caught off-guard on the question of how much income participating doctors would derive from medical benefit. A number of doctors conceded that the gross income of doctors with a large working class practice was in the region of £500-£800 a year under existing arrangements.[67] There was no definite agreement on the fees doctors charged workers but a number mentioned the sum of 5s a visit. Charity and bad debts reduced income from working class patients. The doctors were slow to see the point that under the insurance scheme they would be paid for every member on their list, whether sick or healthy, and that bad debts and charity work among insured workers would disappear. In addition, they would be paid for persons who had previously gone to the dispensary or to the out-patient departments of voluntary hospitals. When the committee members presented figures showing that such doctors could earn up to £500 a year for insured patients alone under the terms of the British scheme, excluding dependants and income from private patients, the medical witnesses accepted that the doctors would be better off.[68]

Faced with the overwhelming financial advantages of insurance practice to those doctors on the panel at a much lower fee than the profession was seeking, the medical witnesses fell back on what were probably their real reasons for objecting to the insurance scheme. These were largely ideological. The hospital specialists and general practitioners appearing before the committee assumed that the relationship of the doctor to the private patient was the norm for all doctor/patient relationships. Some had experienced contract practice and capitation work in Britain and at home early in their careers and they did not like it. Contract practice could only be tolerated as a necessary evil for young doctors who were struggling to establish their reputation and practice.[69] When a doctor developed a successful private practice, he could afford to drop his club or society work.

Contract practice was a matter of status in the profession. 'He (the contract doctor) does not take the same rank (in medical society) as other leading men', commented a Cork doctor.[70] If medical benefit were provided in Ireland, many people who contributed small fees to established practitioners would be entitled to call upon a panel doctor and the successful doctor was not prepared to demean himself by joining a panel for contract work. 'It is obvious', one Dublin doctor said, '(that) a large number of medical practitioners will not go upon the panel ... because they will not engage in contract work.'[71] For this reason the same doctor, when faced with the figures showing the financial benefits of insurance practice, remarked that doctors were motivated by fear of losing income rather than by desire to increase it.[72]

A second and related objection to the contract system was the kind of doctor/patient relationship it was said to foster. It was compared unfavourably with private practice, because it permitted the intervention of a third party in the doctor/patient relationship.[73] Doctors feared that if they agreed to treat a panel of patients, paid for at a fixed capitation rate, they would be at the mercy of their patients who could demand unlimited service without incurring additional cost. They would have to respond or else lose the patient to another doctor. The prosperous practitioners' fear of losing patients to panel doctors and the general dislike of contract practice were strong enough to overcome the financial advantages that insurance-based medical benefit offered to Irish doctors with large working class practices in the county boroughs.

The committee was deeply divided in its recommendations.[74]

The majority came to the conclusion that the introduction of medical benefit in large urban areas, on the same basis as in England, was impracticable if dependants were to be included. They advised against new legislation giving insured persons and their dependants a statutory right to medical benefit without the fee being agreed with the medical profession beforehand. They thought that legislation would leave too much power in the hands of the doctors to dictate terms. The committee seems not to have drawn a parallel with Britain where the existence of a statutory duty to provide benefit enabled the government to call the BMA's bluff. They recommended instead that each friendly society should be facilitated to come to arrangements with doctors to provide benefit for its members, with the payment of an Exchequer contribution towards the cost. This course of action was recommended as an interim measure pending the establishment of a state medical service. A minority expressed dissatisfaction with the 'interim' proposals for medical benefit in the county boroughs, arguing for the immediate creation of a state medical service.

The Report, published in August 1913, had little impact. The main reason seems to have been the opposition of the Local Government Board to the committee's recommendations, particularly to a state medical service. It took all of Sir Henry Robinson's skill to prevent Joseph Glynn convincing the government to act on the committee's advice. In a letter to Sir Mathew Nathan in March 1915, Robinson admitted that he had 'had a rare fight with (Glynn) on his outrageous schemes for a whole time medical service, but with the assistance of the permanent Treasury officials I crushed it'.[75]

Another reason for the Report's demise was poor timing. It was published on the eve of the great confrontation between employers and trade unionists in Dublin, the Lock Out of 1913. At the end of August, workers, employers and politicians had more important things on their minds than medical benefit. No alliance of interests formed which could overcome the opposition of the Local Government Board, the objections of the medical profession to a new scheme of medical treatment for the working classes or the administrative difficulties in its implementation.

Conclusion

Depending on one's point of view, Ireland was deprived of, or saved from, medical benefit. The country was excluded from the benefit against the official wishes of the profession but to the private satisfaction of the affluent general practitioners and hospital consultants opposed to contract practice. No doctor gained from the affair, but the status quo had been maintained.

The interests of the dispensary doctors, traditionally articulated through the IMA, were over-ruled and an opportunity to improve their position missed. A less emotional and more considered response to the Bill by the Association in the early stages might have led to a different outcome. The tactical errors of the Association were automatically endorsing the BMA's 'six points', demanding a specific capitation fee, and failing to show a united front. Thus their official negotiators played into the hands of those in their own ranks and outside who wanted to have nothing to do with the Bill. In the relatively short space of time between the passage of the Act and the appointment of the committee to examine the extension of medical benefit to Ireland, there was a change in the position of the official negotiators. Medical benefit on the same terms as applied in Britain was no longer the aim of the profession. The medical representatives before the committee (drawn from the ranks of the private practitioners) claimed to want medical benefit but on conditions which they must have known would be impossible to accept.

The Hierarchy's intervention on the Bill was critical because it was unlikely that any agreement reached with the doctors on medical benefit could satisfy the bishops' objections to it, even if the doctors had been prepared to compromise. The Party's handling of the intervention showed that the situation was not a simple one of clerical command and obedience by politicians. The Party avoided the extreme demand of the bishops for exclusion from the whole Bill and with considerable political skill preserved most of the benefits of the Bill for the Irish working classes. That it could pursue a compromise between the government's proposals and the demands of the bishops was due to the support it enjoyed throughout the country. This support would continue as long as it was the most effective means of gaining independent government. In 1911 there was little doubt that the Party was close to its great objective. The efforts of the socially conscious members of the Irish Party were insufficient, however, to overcome the effective veto on medical benefit exercised by the representatives of Irish private practice. It would be a matter of debate in medical circles in years to come whether the affair had been a victory or defeat for the profession and whether the profession or the Party could take the credit or blame for the exclusion of medical benefit.

In summary, it can be said that insurance-based medical benefit was not introduced to Ireland for a combination of reasons among which the most important were the ill-conceived nature of the proposed medical benefit as it affected Ireland, the opposition of the Hierarchy to the Bill, the determined resistance of influential sections of the medical profession, the financial implications of a reorganised system of general practice for a Home Rule government, the poor leadership and organisation of the IMA representatives and the lack of will or ability of the Liberal government to force the benefit on Ireland against the wishes of its representatives. If, as Titmuss argues, the bargains Lloyd George struck 'profoundly affected the structure of our health institutions and the place of the doctor in modern England', the converse proposition, that the bargains Lloyd George failed to strike in Ireland had profound implications for the development of Irish health services, and general practice in particular, is also true.[76] The decision to exclude medical benefit meant that insurance funds would play little part in financing general practice or hospital services in the future and that the remuneration of doctors by capitation fee was never firmly established. No special arrangements were made to meet the medical needs of the working classes and the dispensary system had demonstrated its resilience once again.

The survival of the salaried dispensary officer at least ensured that there would be doctors in the most remote and underpopulated districts of the country, a presence which could not have been guaranteed if capitation had taken root in 1912. Furthermore, eligibility for health services would not now be linked to occupation, unlike most other countries in Western Europe, but would be associated with income and need. Finally, the decision to drop medical benefit affected the future social priorities of an independent Irish government. For its own reasons, Ireland rejected what is considered to be a major foundation of the British welfare state. Irish health services would, in consequence, continue to develop differently from the British.

4
Medical Services in Years of Upheaval
1913~1919

THE 1913-1919 PERIOD was one of profound change and upheaval in Ireland.[1] In 1913, it seemed that the struggle for Home Rule was nearly over and that it was only a matter of a year or two before an Irish parliament was established in Dublin. This expectation was gradually undermined by the revolt in Ulster, the outbreak of world war and the formation of a national government in 1915 in which many of the strongest opponents of Home Rule held office. The failure of constitutional methods to achieve their objective encouraged a small number of militant nationalists to plan an armed insurrection in 1916.

The insurgents enjoyed little popular support initially, but the ruthless suppression of the Rising and the execution of the leaders had a dramatic effect on popular opinion and sympathy grew for the cause in which the men had died. Sinn Fein, a loose alliance of nationalists committed to achieving Irish independence, captured this sympathy and translated it into overwhelming support at the polls in the 1918 general election. The once formidable Irish Party was reduced to six members at Westminster. The elected Sinn Fein deputies refused to take their seats and assembled instead in Dublin where they formed the first Dail of the Irish Republic and appointed a government. In 1919, serious fighting began between the Irish Republican Army, the military wing of Sinn Fein, and the British forces.

Political events dominate these years but much social and economic change also occurred. The war of 1914 – 18 was a mixed economic blessing for the working classes. Recruitment and the demand for labour in war industries reduced unemployment and raised wages. The demand for food brought relative prosperity to Irish farmers and an increase in tillage provided more jobs for agricultural labourers. But a sharp rise in the price of food and the scarcity of fuel reduced the value of wages and brought hardship to those on pensions and fixed incomes. Unemployment returned with the ending of the war and the price of agricultural goods fell. In 1920, a severe economic depression hit Britain and Ireland leading to restrictive economic and social policies in both countries, in contrast to those of the pre-war Liberal government.

The period was an eventful one for the growth of government responsibility for medical services. The provisions of the National Health Insurance Act, 1911 as they applied to Ireland were implemented. Workers and their families were given some protection against destitution due to the illness of the breadwinner and against maternity expenses. The destruction of the First World War brought home to government the need to take positive action to protect the health of the population and of the future generation of young men and women. The war also encouraged thinking about how the administration of government could be improved according to the principles of efficiency and economy. The legacy of British rule, insofar as the health services were concerned, was a radical framework for greater government responsibility for health and for administrative reform.

Implementing the National Health Insurance Act

Despite difficulties, the provisions of the Insurance Act came into operation as scheduled. The Irish Insurance Commission was established in 1912. By April 1913, 700,000 persons, or 15.9 per cent of the population, were insured.[2] In the absence of a medical benefit, sickness benefit accounted for by far the largest charge on the Irish Insurance Fund, amounting to £374,150 in 1914, with maternity benefit costing more than £86,000 in the same year.[3]

The size of the payments gives an indication of their importance to the working population. Medical certification for these benefits gave rise to administrative headaches and it was not until 1915 that doctors agreed to provide certificates for insured patients in return for a modified capitation rate paid by the Insurance Commission.

The administration of sickness, maternity and disability benefits was relatively straightforward once the question of medical certification was out of the way. They were cash benefits paid by the approved societies to members. The sanatorium benefit, on the other hand, took the form of maintenance for the insured worker and dependants in a sanatorium or hospital or payments to a doctor for domiciliary treatment. It was to be administered by the health committee in each county and county borough. To ensure that enough sanatorium beds would be available, the Treasury announced that £1.5 million would be provided for building purposes, of which Ireland's share was £146,000.

Tuberculosis

The government decided to take the opportunity offered by the Insurance Act to clarify policy towards the prevention and treatment of tuberculosis. In 1912 the Treasury appointed a departmental committee under the chairmanship of Waldorf Astor. The Irish representatives were Dr Stafford of the Local Government Board and Dr Maguire of the Insurance Commission.

The committee stressed the need to provide protection against the disease and treatment for the whole population, not just for the poor and the insured.[4] It recommended a two-pronged attack on the disease, based on tuberculosis dispensaries and sanatoria. The dispensaries were to act as centres for the initial diagnosis of the disease and for the co-ordination of treatment. The provision of one sanatorium bed per 5,000 population was suggested as the planning guideline for accommodation. Advanced cases would be treated in hospitals or converted poor law institutions rather than sanatoria.

Referring to Ireland, the Report recommended that pulmonary

tuberculosis should be a compulsorily notifiable disease as it was in Britain, that county councils be entrusted with administrative functions dealing with public health, including the appointment of county medical officers of health and that medical inspection and treatment of school children be undertaken, financed by a government grant. Only the third recommendation was new in the Irish context, the others having been recommended on more than one occasion by official bodies, but without effect. The committee justified its recommendation of medical treatment of school children because of the higher incidence of tuberculosis among Irish children of school-going age.[5]

The government responded quickly to the committee's Report. It accepted the principle that everyone should be entitled to protection against and treatment for the disease. Lloyd George announced that the government would pay county and borough councils about half the cost of treating all non-insured persons; the councils were expected to meet the remaining charges from the rates. By any standards, the government had provided an attractive framework for action.

The main responsibility for implementing the departmental committee's recommendations and for giving practical effect in Ireland to the provisions of the Insurance Act against tuberculosis fell to the Local Government Board and the county and borough councils. Tuberculosis was the major item on the Board's agenda for the years 1912 to 1914. Prior to the Insurance Act sanitary authorities (county borough, urban and rural district councils) had power under the Public Health Acts 1878-1907 to erect and maintain sanatoria but only two sanatoria had been provided in this way, Heatherside in Doneraile, County Cork and Crooksling in County Dublin. The Tuberculosis Prevention (Ireland) Act, 1908 had extended the power to provide sanatoria to county councils, but so far without result. The Insurance Act widened the powers of the county and borough councils by permitting them to provide sanatorium treatment for residents outside their districts and to provide, with the approval of the Board, other forms of treatment such as domiciliary care. Any remaining obstacles restraining the councils' power to act were removed by the

Tuberculosis Prevention (Ireland) Act, 1913. All the legislation on this subject, as with all the Public Health Acts, was permissive – no obligation was placed on a council to act.

Compulsory notification was seen by the Local Government Board as being particularly important to the success of the new tuberculosis dispensaries. The Board attempted to give legislative effect to this recommendation of the departmental committee. But the Irish Party opposed the clause, as they had done in 1908, and it was dropped. The campaign against the disease was weakened from the beginning.

The councils were reluctant to build sanatoria or hospitals, despite the financial incentives and enabling legislation. If it had not been for the Women's National Health Association the health committees would not have been able to fulfil their obligations to insured persons. The Association, despite considerable opposition, had built a large sanatorium at Peamount, County Dublin with 140 beds and a smaller one at Rossclare, County Fermanagh, which were ready in time to receive patients on behalf of the health committees. The Treasury made its first building grants to the Association and the councils then contracted beds in these and other privately run institutions in preference to building their own.

The Local Government Board estimated that an additional three hundred sanatoria beds were needed as well as a large increase in beds for advanced cases but its exhortations seem to have produced little action.[6] At the outbreak of the war, only £41,145 of the £146,000 building grant had been allocated.[7] The Board seems to have met with more success in its efforts to promote a dispensary service for patients suffering from the disease. By March 1913, 25 councils had appointed medical officers to tuberculosis dispensaries.[8] The following year, the number of officers had risen to 28 but does not seem to have increased from that figure.[9] The Board circulated plans for purpose-built dispensaries but few were opened by March 1914. Some councils met local opposition when plans were revealed to build a dispensary. There was a widespread fear that the presence of a tuberculosis institution of any kind would increase the risk of infection in a neighbourhood.

The provision of facilities for treating advanced cases of pulmonary tuberculosis was the most intractable problem and the one about which least was done. Few hospitals or sanatoria accepted such cases because of the risk of infection, yet these were the patients who were most dangerous to their families if left to die at home. At the outbreak of the war there was still a severe shortage of suitable accommodation for this category of patient. Any further progress in the provision of institutional accommodation of any kind for the disease was halted in late 1914 with the suspension by the Treasury of the unused portion of the building grant, the restrictions imposed on local authority borrowing and a steep rise in the cost of building materials and labour. The momentum to control the disease diminished.

Did the financial and legislative provisions of these years have any impact on the incidence of and mortality from the disease? Between 1905 and 1918, the annual number of deaths attributed to the disease had declined by a quarter to about 8,600, with the greatest decrease occurring between 1908 and 1911.[10] This improvement was attributed to a number of factors: better economic conditions, improved housing in rural areas, more efficient sanitary administration, public recognition of the infectiousness of the disease, higher standards of domestic hygiene and more facilities for treatment.[11]

However, since 1912 the rate of decline in mortality had slowed and during the war the number of deaths from the disease began to increase. This may have been due to better diagnosis and more precise death certification but it also suggests that, without compulsory notification and isolation, or the provision of incentives to sufferers to seek medical advice, the effect of 'treatment' facilities on the disease was limited. In these circumstances, economic and social conditions were more significant than intervention. The first world war increased hardship for the poor, especially in the cities and towns, and the disease thrived in the conditions of trench warfare endured by soldiers at the front. With the outbreak of the war, the attention of health administrators switched to protecting soldiers and civilians against the more dramatic epidemics associated with warfare. The fight against tuberculosis was weakened by the withdrawal of Exchequer grants and by the shortage of doctors and nurses. The struggle was not taken up seriously again in Ireland for another thirty years.

The First World War

The outbreak of world war in August 1914 was a watershed in Irish history for many reasons, apart from those directly connected with the hostilities. Home Rule, by this time on the statute book, was postponed until the end of the war; no one suspected just how long the war would last. The threat of civil war over the constitutional position of Ulster receded and the country seemed united behind the government's war effort. Redmond's pledge of loyalty to the government echoed the popular mood and tens of thousands volunteered for service in the armed forces. A significant minority opposed the war for different reasons but only a handful believed that England's adversity was Ireland's opportunity to strike for freedom. As the war continued, disillusionment with the war effort grew and the prospect of Home Rule faded into the distant future. At the same time, the Irish Party lost its power to veto government legislation and action in Ireland.

The war posed major challenges to those responsible for public health. There was a shortage of doctors and nurses as the army and navy medical corps attracted volunteers with the combined appeal of patriotism and higher salaries. A second effect of the war was retrenchment in public expenditure on services not directly connected with the war effort. Local authorities could no longer borrow for capital works and the grants for such purposes from the Exchequer were withdrawn. On the other hand, the war greatly increased the dangers to public health. Attention had to be given to the sanitary conditions in which large numbers of soldiers were accommodated in confined barracks throughout the country. Typhoid was a particular menace in these circumstances. It was also feared that smallpox, typhus, dysentery and other infectious diseases would spread from regions devastated by the war. These fears stimulated a concerted campaign to increase the level of smallpox vaccination which had fallen to a dangerously low level.[12] The high price of food and the scarcity of fuel led to fears that the physical resistance of the urban poor to disease would be weakened and efforts were made to control the price of essential commodities and to provide coal for the most vulnerable. The devastating impact of the influenza epidemic in 1918 may have been partly due to lower resistance in the civilian population. As the war drew to a close and large numbers of soldiers were demobilised, attention switched to controlling venereal disease and tuberculosis among the men as they returned home.

The war also stimulated trends in health provisions which were apparent before 1914 but which might not otherwise have received so much attention. One of these was the phasing out of the general workhouse. The precipitating factor was the army's need for barrack accommodation and some workhouses were commandeered for this purpose. In November 1914, the Chief Secretary introduced a short Bill to enable the Local Government Board to close workhouses by amending or repealing the poor law Acts for any purpose in connection with the war or 'for the better administration of the Poor Relief (Ireland) Acts 1838-1900'.[13] Chief Secretary Birrell thought it 'most desirable to avail ourselves of (the) opportunity for the purpose of making a reform which has been the subject matter of absolute agreement in a Poor Law Report to this House' but English members baulked at the wide powers being given to a government body on the pretext of wartime emergency.[14] The offending words were dropped from the Bill and the clearance of workhouses was confined to the requirements of the army. Six workhouses were cleared under this Act. But the Board had its way in 1916 when an amendment was carried in the Local Government (Emergency Provisions) Bill permitting the Board to carry out changes for the better administration of the poor law.[15] By March 1918, three unions had been dissolved and eleven workhouses closed in whole or in part and there were plans for much more change.[16] In most cases the 'healthy' inmates were transferred from the workhouses while the sick in the infirmary were retained.

The health of mothers and children was another issue which benefited from wartime concern. The deaths of thousands of soldiers at the front and the falling birth rate increased the need to protect the future generation of young men and women. Advocates of better maternal and infant services had to contend with the apathy of the public, long accustomed to the death of infants and mothers in childbirth, and the invidious assumption that infant mortality was nature's way of weeding out the unfit early in life. It was a question of changing attitudes and mobilising resources.

According to the national statistics on infant mortality, Ireland did better than its neighbours. In 1915, 95,583 babies were born, with 8,753 dying before they reached their first birthday, giving a rate of 92 deaths per thousand live births. The corresponding rates in England and Scotland in the same year were 110 and 120 respectively. But the Irish rate was declining more slowly than its neighbours' and the average hid great differences between parts of the country. The rate in Dublin city in 1915, of 160.3 per thousand births, was more than two and half times the rate recorded in the counties with the lowest mortality — Roscommon, Leitrim, Wicklow, Mayo, Tipperary North Riding, Cavan, Galway and Longford.[17] The most common recorded causes of infant deaths in urban areas in the same year were 'wasting' and diarrhoeal diseases, infectious diseases and tuberculosis.[18] It was clear that infection and poor diet were responsible for a great deal of the mortality among infants. Mortality among children of school going age was especially depressing when compared with England. Deaths per 100,000 among children aged 5 to 15 years in the period 1901-1910 were nearly 25 per cent higher in Ireland than in England.[19] Any advantage Irish children enjoyed in infancy was lost as they grew older.

In 1915, 570 women died from disorders associated with childbirth, giving a maternal mortality rate of six per thousand live births. One third of this number died from puerperal septicaemia, a condition associated with unskilled and unhygienic attendance at birth. Irish women faced increased dangers in childbirth because of the late age of marriage and the large size of families.

75

The health of mothers and chidren had received little official attention in Ireland before the war. The Women's National Health Association had done much to raise public awareness of the problem of infant health. A major objective of the Association was to raise the level of knowledge of nutrition and infant care. It opened baby clinics, held classes for mothers and provided milk depots in counties where it was difficult to obtain fresh milk all the year round.

The Notification of Births Act, 1907, to the extent it applied in Ireland, was a first step in the direction of public provision for mothers and children. It enabled urban sanitary authorities to ensure that the medical officer of the district was notified of each birth and to organise health visiting for mothers in the post-partum period. But the Act was permissive, and by 1915 only Dublin and Belfast had adopted it and only in Dublin were special 'sanitary officers' appointed for the purpose of visiting and advising mothers.

The maternity benefit under the Insurance Act was probably the greatest pre-war boon to mothers and infants. The benefit was worth 30s to an insured female worker or the wife of an insured male worker and was paid at the time of confinement. This relatively large sum was to pay for the extra expenses of childbirth and to encourage working mothers to remain at home with the child in the early months. In 1915, benefit was paid in respect of 44,318 mothers, equivalent to just under half the total births in the country.[20] The benefit was usually paid in cash but in Dublin the maternity hospitals and the approved societies agreed that, in return for 5s, each mother entitled to benefit would receive skilled midwifery care at home or in hospital.

The strengthening of birth notification legislation in 1915 was the first war-time initiative of direct benefit to mothers and children in Ireland. There was a certain paradox about the application of the Notification of Births Act's application to Ireland. In one way its provisions were weakened by the restriction of compulsory notification of births to urban areas. But the powers given to Irish sanitary authorities to provide for the needs of mothers and children were much greater than those of the English authorities. During the committee stage of the Bill, the clause giving wide powers to English sanitary authorities to provide for mothers and children was watered down. However, the wide discretionary powers were retained in the Irish clause for both urban and rural authorities.[21] Members of the Irish Party contributed little to the debate. The Bill was the first of a series of legislative measures designed specifically for Britain which were extended to Ireland through the influence of Irish Unionists and which the Irish Party was now powerless to prevent or influence.

The Local Government Board encouraged sanitary authorities to submit schemes for protecting the health of mothers, infants and children. In 1916 it advised local authorities of the services they could provide and issued regulations outlining the basis on which expenditure could be recouped from the Exchequer.[22] The local authorities were empowered but not compelled to appoint health visitors to advise expectant and nursing mothers at home and to provide a wide range of services for women during pregnancy and at childbirth and for infants. The services of a midwife or a doctor, and of hospital treatment at confinement and of food for women and children could be made available to women who could demonstrate need. However, medical supervision and advice, dental care at health centres, hospital treatment for children, convalescent care for nursing mothers and children and the services of health visitors were to be made available to all irrespective of means. In view of the controversy that occurred a generation later on the issue of maternal and child care, it is interesting that these regulations seem not to have aroused any adverse comment from politicians, the Church or the medical profession in 1916. The schemes were slow to get off the ground, partly because of the permissive nature of the legislation and partly because it was not clear to what extent the Exchequer would meet the cost of the salaries of doctors and nurses employed in the schemes. By December 1917, 35 urban and fourteen rural sanitary authorities had been reimbursed only £2,300 for schemes which either they or voluntary organisations had undertaken.[23]

One effect of the wartime preoccupation with the physical welfare of mothers and young children was to interest the philanthropic organisation, the Carnegie Trust, in the problem.

The Trust commissioned research on maternal and child health in each of the three kingdoms. The Irish report was prepared by Dr E. Coey Bigger, recently appointed Medical Commissioner of the Local Government Board and a far-sighted member of the Viceregal Commission on the Poor Laws, 1903-6. These reports influenced the development of policy in the UK. Dr Bigger's report detailed the extent of the problem in Ireland and made radical recommendations to improve the health of mothers and children.[24] He drew attention to the fact that the infant death rate, 90 per 1000 births, was higher than the mortality rate for soldiers at the front: a baby had a greater chance of dying than its father in France. He argued against those who complacently accepted this high level of mortality:

> The process is not the weeding out of the unfit as many believe, leaving the strongest and better to survive, but it is a process by which thousands, both weak and strong are unnecessarily hurried to their graves, and tens of thousands have their constitutions permanently injured ... a burden to their parents, their district, and the state....[25]

He detailed the complex physical, economic and social factors which affected maternal and child mortality. He highlighted the class bias of child mortality, showing that while the death rate per 10,000 population for children aged under 2 years among the professional classes in Dublin was 7, the equivalent rate for the labouring classes was 120.[26]

He suggested that it should be the immediate aim to reduce the rate of infant mortality to 80 per thousand live births in the towns and that the long term goal should be a national rate of 50 deaths. As a first step towards improving the health of mothers and children he recommended that permissive legislation become mandatory. A second group of recommendations concerned the improvement of the environment in which poor families lived: slum clearance, scavenging, better water supply and control of milk, and the provision of playgrounds in working class areas. Thirdly, he recommended specific improvements in health services for mothers and children: more hospital beds for difficult obstetric cases and for childhood diseases; more health visitors, infant and child welfare centres in all towns with more than 5,000 population; maternity benefit to be conditional on attendance by the expectant mother at a maternity centre; better nursing for mothers and children; the scientific examination of diseases of childhood; and the medical inspection of school children. These recommendations built on the arrangements sanctioned by the Local Government Board in 1916 and took them a good deal further.

The Carnegie Report seems to have strengthened the impetus for further improvements in services for mothers and children. In 1918 the Local Government Board announced that it would meet half the expenditure on salaries and expenses of midwives, health visitors and nurses engaged in maternal and child welfare work, hospital treatment for complicated obstetric cases and for children under five, the cost of convalescent care for nursing mothers, research on maternal and child health, contributions to voluntary organisations engaged in maternal and child health schemes, and other aspects of the services approved by the Board in 1916.[27] These financial incentives seem to have been effective. By December 1919, the amount disbursed from the Exchequer to local authorities for maternal and child health services had increased to £8,529.[28]

The problem of untrained midwives or 'handy women' was also tackled. Earlier British legislation regulating the practice of midwifery had not been applied to Ireland. The large number of deaths of women in childbirth from puerperal septicaemia was attributed by doctors to the 'handy women' and their cavalier attitude to, or ignorance of, asepsis. The Royal College of Physicians put pressure on the Local Government Board to act and in 1917 the Midwives (Ireland) Act was passed. The Act prohibited unqualified women from setting up in practice as midwives.[29] A Midwives Board was established with eleven members appointed by the Local Government Board, and the county and county borough councils were made the local supervising authorities. Every 'handy woman' who could show that she was an experienced midwife was permitted to register under the Act as a 'bona fide'. It was not anticipated that the

Act would bring about an immediate improvement in maternal mortality figures. However, the regulation of standards and the training required for all new midwives was expected to improve standards in time.

A framework for the medical inspection and treatment of school children was finally provided. In 1919, a Public Health (Medical Treatment of Children) (Ireland) Bill was introduced which empowered county and county boroughs to undertake medical inspection and treatment of children in national schools. Half the local expenditure would be refunded from the Exchequer. The Bill as originally drafted was permissive in the tradition of Irish public health legislation, but during the debate there was a strong demand from Irish Unionist MPs and the few remaining nationalists that the provision be made mandatory. The government acceded to their wishes, making it the only mandatory public health service on the Irish statute book. Councils were further obliged to charge the cost of the service to the county rate — urban areas with many schools were not to be penalised to the benefit of rural areas with few schools. Although home visiting by medical practitioners was excluded from the scope of the Act, no other limits were placed on the type of medical care which could be provided, and significantly, all children attending national schools, irrespective of means, were entitled to the service.

Nineteen twenty was not a fortuitous year to inaugurate a new public health service among local authorities in Ireland. The authority of the Local Government Board was increasingly questioned by local authorities controlled by Sinn Fein supporters. However, the legislative framework for medical inspection of school children had been laid to be built on in more peaceful times.

The health of soldiers

In 1917, the government extended the medical benefit provisions of the Insurance Act to soldiers invalided in the war or whose health had been impaired during active service, whether or not they were insured contributors. The Irish Insurance Commission was asked to negotiate a scheme of general practitioner treatment for demobilised Irish soldiers and a capitation fee was quickly agreed with the profession. By June 1920, 43,557 men were entitled to treatment by 1,108 general practitioners.[30] Arrangements were also made with voluntary hospitals for the care of wounded or sick soldiers. In a major break with tradition, a portion of the money paid to the hospitals was reserved as fees for the medical staff, the first fees such doctors received for treating patients in the hospitals.

The high incidence of tuberculosis and venereal disease among soldiers also gave rise to concern. It was feared that soldiers on demobilisation would spread these diseases among their families and communities. The government had services to cope with tuberculosis but no provision existed for controlling venereal disease. To fill the gap, the government introduced measures which were applied to Ireland under the Public Health (Prevention and Treatment of Disease) (Ireland) Act, 1917. The Act empowered county and county borough councils to take a wide range of preventive measures, including free medical treatment for venereal disease and testing of specimens at laboratories. In an unprecedented act of generosity, the state agreed to meet 75 per cent of the costs local authorities incurred in providing services under the Act. The government had good reason for concern. In 1918/19 the university laboratories reported a large increase in the incidence of venereal diseases, particularly syphilis.[31] The local authorities along the East coast were most active, since most soldiers came from these counties, but no special service was provided over large parts of the country. One reason for this may have been the attitude towards soldiers returning from the war. Unlike their British comrades, the Irish soldiers were not received as heroes. On the contrary, many experienced open hostility and this may have been a factor restricting local health initiatives on their behalf.

The Minister for Health and the Irish Public Health Council

Shortly after Lloyd George became Prime Minister in 1917, he established a Ministry of Reconstruction to prepare policies for implementation when the war ended. Questions of employment housing and health dominated planning for reconstruction Planning was confined almost exclusively to Britain; Ireland posed the government with problems of a different order. But in spite of the difficult times, there was a 'spill-over' effect from the new policies on Ireland, particularly in the fields of health, education and housing, aided and abetted by the Irish Unionist members of the House who demanded that the principle of union be given practical effect. Underlying the plans of the Ministry of Reconstruction was the theme of greater 'national efficiency', to be achieved by more control and co-ordination of government activity at central and local level.

One of the results of this activity was the creation of a ministry charged with responsibility for the health of the nation. The Ministry of Health Bill, 1919 proposed that most health functions be centralised in one ministry at central government. It provided for the amalgamation of the Local Government Board and the Insurance Commission under a new title, the Ministry of Health and for greater emphasis on protecting the physical welfare of the people.

The Bill as drafted, made no provision for Ireland, because, according to the Minister, 'the system in Ireland in many respects is very different from, and I am afraid, in some respects very far behind, what it is here'.[32] It was a weak excuse which failed to deflect a growing demand that the Bill provide for Ireland. Edward Carson made a strong plea that the neglect of health problems in Ireland be remedied and that the opportunity presented by the Bill be seized.[33] Joseph Devlin agreed with the need for greater attention to health matters but was suspicious of an Irish ministry of health on the English model. He argued instead for an Irish public health board for which, he claimed, the medical profession had already expressed its support.[34]

The government responded by agreeing to include provisions for Ireland in the Bill, as a first step to tackling the ramshackle nature of health administration in Ireland. The Irish clauses of the Bill, as introduced in committee, combined the idea of a Minister of Health for Ireland with that of an Irish public health board.[35] The Chief Secretary became the Minister of Health responsible for promoting the health of the Irish people. His duties were:

> to secure the effective carrying out and co-ordination of measures conducive to health, including measures for the prevention and cure of diseases, the treatment of physical and mental defects, the initiation and direction of research, the collection, preparation, and publication of information and statistics relating thereto, and the training of persons for health services.[36]

This clause gave the new Minister extremely wide powers in relation to the health of the whole population; his remit was not confined to the poor or destitute. But as all the existing services referred to, with the exception of medical research, were already under the formal authority of the Chief Secretary, the Bill involved the minimum of constitutional change in Irish government. The Chief Secretary was empowered by the subsequent clause to establish the Irish Public Health Council to advise and assist him in the exercise of his powers. The Lords made minor amendments to the Irish clauses by including the avoidance of fraud and the care of the blind among the duties of the Minister of Health.

The Bill did not resolve how administrative effect would be given to the new Minister's wide powers over health affairs. This was the task assigned to the Irish Public Health Council appointed in September 1919. The influence of the Local Government Board was evident from the beginning; Dr Coey Bigger, Medical Commissioner, was appointed chairman. The Council was asked to formulate proposals for an Irish public health Bill which would, inter alia, place the public health services in Ireland on a wider and more comprehensive basis and where necessary, make mandatory on the local authorities the various adoptive and permissive health enactments.[37]

The Council's report, which was completed in May 1920, identified the lack of co-ordination in the central control and local administration of public health and medical services as the major problem.[38] At central level, the Local Government Board, the Insurance Commission, the Inspectors of Lunatic Asylums, the

Registrar of Births, Marriages and Deaths and the office of the Chief Secretary dealt more or less independently with health matters and at local level, health administration was now so complicated that only officials understood how it worked. The confusion was exacerbated by the number and variety of Exchequer grants.

The permissive nature of public health legislation was considered by the Council to be a serious defect. The only mandatory requirement, that county and borough councils undertake medical treatment of school children, was rendered much less efficient by the absence of a similar obligation on urban and rural councils to provide maternal and child welfare services. The absence of a legal obligation on councils to act against tuberculosis was identified as a further weakness.

The Council was also concerned that the emergence of a unified hospital service was being hindered by the various ways in which different local authorities managed the hospitals under their control. The dispensary service came in for criticism similar to that made by the Viceregal Commission in 1906 and the absence of a system of medical treatment for insured persons and their dependants was considered to be injurious to the health of the working classes. The Council also drew attention to the financial plight of the voluntary hospitals, some of which would be forced to close if assistance was not forthcoming.

The Council, in making its recommendations, hoped to bring about the co-ordination of all health services, the reorganisation of local health administration on a county basis and the reform of the medical services to secure 'the best possible medical and surgical treatment, including hospital and specialist treatment for all who are in need of it'.[39] All members agreed about the need for a strong central health authority to achieve these aims, but the question was what form it should take. They considered whether it would be possible to create a central body solely concerned with public health and medical services but decided that it could not be done because it would be impossible to separate the health functions from the engineering functions of the Local Government Board.[40] The Council went on to recommend the concentration of health functions under the Local Government

Board which would change its name to the Ministry of Health for Ireland. The Board would retain control in practice, if not in name, of the system proposed.

The members disagreed about how the Ministry ought to be structured; the majority favoured an organisation which would have meant the least possible change in the existing administration of the Board. All agreed that the activities of the Ministry concerning health should be 'subject to the general control and direction of a Health Council comprising representatives of the local authorities, of the medical and allied professions, and of other organisations concerned with medical and health services'.[41] The Council gave explicit recognition to the principle of involving the interests affected by health policy and warned that 'no comprehensive scheme of health reform can be successfully instituted or carried out, without the support of the medical profession'.[42]

The Council's recommendations for local administration involved more radical changes. It recommended that the local unit for all matters pertaining to health and medical services should be the county or county borough councils and that in each case, the council should establish a board of health which would be the health authority for the area. The Report repeated the constantly expressed need for county medical officers of health and for the separation of health administration from association with the poor law. One consequence of these recommendations, barely treated in the Report, was the abolition of a large number of local bodies.

The Report strongly advocated a national medical service to provide general practitioner and hospital treatment for insured persons and for those who were, in a subtle change from the terminology of the poor law, 'unable to contribute towards the cost of such treatment'.[43] The structure of the service proposed had many of the features of the state medical service recommended by the Viceregal Commission. The Council referred to the difficulty of introducing salaried medical officers to treat insured persons in the larger urban areas, and suggested that these areas be excluded temporarily from the scheme. The salaried medical officers, with

85

the exception of the county medical officers, were to be permitted private practice. The Council recommended that half the cost of the service after deducting receipts from paying patients, insurance contributions, etc, should be met by the rates and the other half by Exchequer grants.

The Council could hardly recommend that the voluntary hospitals form part of the state medical service but it proposed that all grants to these hospitals be administered by the Ministry of Health. It strongly advocated increased financial assistance 'if suitable and adequate hospital treatment is to be available for all classes of the community who are in need of it'.[44]

The Council's report could hardly have been published at a less auspicious time in the history of government in Ireland. In a year when the conflict over who should govern the country was at its height, the problem of administering the health services was a minor detail. But the analysis and recommendations of the Report were not swept aside with the ending of British rule: they deeply influenced those who had other reasons for planning an overhaul of the local government system. It is ironic that many of the Council's proposals were implemented by a new independent government which would have dismissed the Council as a tool of an alien administration. The Council's achievement was to devise a structure for the health service which was independent of the poor law, building on the recommendations of the Viceregal and Royal Poor Law Commissions and applying the principles of 'efficient' government which had become popular during and after the war. Furthermore, its recommendations rested on the relatively new assumptions that government had a positive duty to protect the health of the people, that access to medical services should be based on medical need, not destitution, and that the state had a duty to assist those who could not contribute to the cost of treatment. The Council, in this way, provided an underlying rationale for the development of the Irish health service.

Conclusion

Government involvement in medical services greatly expanded between 1913 and 1922. In some cases it was a strengthening of previously accepted responsibilities, as with tuberculosis; in others, responsibility was extended to new services, such as medical inspection of school children, maternal and child health, the treatment of soldiers and the control of venereal disease. By 1922 there is a striking consensus among officials about the importance of health services in themselves and the need to separate them from the poor law. The recommendations of the Irish Public Health Council for a unified health authority at central and local level represents the culmination of this trend. The problem was no longer what to do about the poor law but how to co-ordinate and develop medical services. The emphasis had shifted from providing medical treatment to the poor to providing medical services for all those who needed them. The precipitating factor in bringing about this change was the experience of the First World War. Wartime dangers gave those who had been calling for more health measures an opportunity to put their ideas into practice, highlighted the need for efficient administration and stimulated government into taking greater steps to protect the health of the population.

It was increasingly obvious that the expansion of health activity had outgrown administrative structures. New services were allocated to local authorities on an ad hoc basis, although the county and borough were recognised more and more as the most appropriate administrative units at local level. The war had drawn attention to the need for a more efficient 'machinery' of government. By 1919, co-ordination and control were major themes of administrative reform, apparent in the Ministry of Health Act and the recommendations of the Public Health Council. They were to receive a renewed impetus during the reorganisation of government that took place during and after the war of independence.

The years 1913 to 1919 were dominated by the struggle for independence and histories of the period usually concentrate on political and military events. It would be misleading to think that every facet of Irish life was equally affected by these events and that nothing much else of consequence happened during the period. As this chapter shows, these years were seminal for the future direction and administration of the health services. The sense of continuity between the periods before and after independence for the development of the Irish health services cannot be over emphasised.

5
Efficiency, Economy and the New State
1919-1932

THE LEGITIMACY OF the British administration in Ireland was coming under increasing attack from militant nationalists in the years 1913-19. The execution of the leaders of the Easter Rising in 1916 caused a leadership vacuum which the discredited Irish Party was unable to fill. The people and ideas associated with Sinn Fein filled the gap, providing a national programme for the achievement of independence.

Sinn Fein's economic and social outlook was deeply influenced by the thinking of the journalist and writer, Arthur Griffith. He believed in economic self-sufficiency, protection of Irish industry, and the reduction of government spending to a minimum, and shared the general belief that the Irish administration under British rule was extravagant and inefficient. He had opposed the application of the National Health Insurance Act, 1911 and the other social measures of the Liberal government because they imposed a burden on struggling native industries and had taken the employers' side during the Dublin lock-out of 1913 for similar reasons. He and his followers argued for protectionist policies to encourage industrial and agricultural capitalism.[1] Given their dislike of the Irish administration and their wish to curtail government expenditure, Sinn Fein was unlikely to see much to admire in the expansion of government responsibility for medical services.

Apart from Griffith's ideas, the new generation of nationalist

89

leaders had few thoughts about policy after independence. The Sinn Fein coalition saw independence as a precondition for progress on other fronts; many believed it to be a panacea for social and economic ills. As Joseph Devlin lamented in 1919, 'so many of our vast social interests have been forgotten in the perfervid character of the political controversies in which we have been engaged'.[2]

The Sinn Fein leaders did, however, have views on the conduct of government: views inspired by idealism, probity and a commitment to national regeneration. Tom Garvin has commented that the pre-1922 Sinn Fein leaders were 'puritanical, idealistic and austere and were adherents of the politics of national redemption rather than of the politics of compromise, bargaining and pay-offs'.[3] They wanted honest, efficient and streamlined government, divorced from 'politics' and 'politicians'. This concern with the form of government brought Sinn Fein, by a circuitous route, to similar conclusions about the organisation of health services to those of the Public Health Council and its predecessors, the Viceregal and Royal Commissions on the Poor Law. The new leaders did not, however, attach the same priority to improving the health of the population.

The County Schemes

In October 1917, at the Sinn Fein Ardfheis (conference) in Dublin, delegates adopted a constitution committing them to the formation of a constituent assembly to 'devise and formulate measures for the welfare of the whole people of Ireland'.[4] These measures included a pledge to introduce a competitive examination for appointment of local officials and the replacement of the poor law with increased outdoor relief for the aged and infirm.[5] Sinn Fein won a landslide victory in the 1918 election. The newly elected members refused to take their seats at Westminster and in January 1919 formed themselves into the first Dail (Parliament) of the Irish Republic in Dublin. Few of the elected members had any previous political or government experience; only ten per cent had previously been members of local authorities.[6] One-third were under 35 years of age and three-quarters were aged 45 or less.[7] Many were to dominate Irish political life until the 1960s.

The first Dail adopted a provisional constitution, appointed government ministers and approved a radical statement of intent on social matters known as the 'Democratic Programme'. This document, among other things, committed the new Republic to abolishing 'the present odious, degrading and foreign poor-law system' and replacing it with a 'sympathetic native scheme for the care of the nation's aged and infirm', who, it declared optimistically, 'shall no longer be regarded as a burden but rather entitled to the nation's gratitude and consideration'.[8] A duty was imposed on the new government to take measures to safeguard the health of the people and 'ensure the physical as well as the moral well-being of the nation'.[9]

The Dail appointed William T. Cosgrave as Minister for Local Government. Unusual among his colleagues, Cosgrave had extensive experience of local government. He was assisted by Kevin O'Higgins, a young deputy with exceptional drive and determination. Together they set about weaning the allegiance of the population from the established system of local government. Their small staff included Thomas McArdle, a former official with the Local Government Board who had resigned in 1916 rather than take the oath of allegiance to the crown required of all officials following the insurrection. An active but not original thinker, McArdle provided the new Minister and his assistant with an essential element of official expertise and was no doubt familiar with the many current proposals for reform of the poor law.

The objective of the subterranean department was to persuade local representatives, officials and ratepayers to ignore the authority of the Local Government Board and to transfer loyalty to the new Dail. To succeed, the department had to overcome the enormous financial power and legal authority of the Local Government Board. In 1920, the Local Government Board seemed to hold the trump card: Exchequer grants. Without these grants, local authorities would not be able to finance the services which they were legally bound to provide. The Dail lacked anything to match these 'dazzling bribes'.[10] But by injudicious moves, the British government threw away its hand. Most serious of all was the legal authority given to the Board in August 1920 to retain Exchequer grants and put them towards unsatisfied claims against local authorities for criminal injuries to individuals or property as a result of military activities.[11] This greatly simplified the choices facing local authorities. By 1921, the demands for compensation amounted to claims for more than £10 million while the annual value of the Exchequer grants was only £1.5 million.[12]

Cosgrave and O'Higgins, foreseeing that the British government would withhold grants for local services, set about planning for that eventuality. In June 1920, the Dail agreed to establish a Commission on Local Government to examine reforms and economies should local authorities 'break' with the Local Government Board.[13] The report of the Commission recommended substantial economies in the operation of local authorities.[14] Among the savings proposed were a reduction of £25,000 in services for venereal disease and child welfare schemes, £50,000 from the abolition and amalgamation of workhouses and £10,000 from a reduction in the number of patients with tuberculosis undergoing hospital treatment and the amalgamation of hospitals. These accounted for about one-quarter of the total savings the Commission proposed be made by local authorities.

There was a lively debate in the Dail on the Report in September 1920.[15] Sean MacEntee successfully opposed the inclusion of child welfare services in the list of economies;[16] the sum of £25,000 was now to be saved by further cuts in the venereal disease services. Joseph McGrath objected to the proposed closure of tuberculosis hospitals, with no effect.[17] The Report was approved by the Dail. The Minister for Local Government was given authority to amend local government legislation without further reference to the assembly.[18]

The Report gave only an outline of the economies proposed although its recommendations were firm. The Local Government Department was desperate for ideas which would lead to economies but still preserve the fabric of local government. It fell back on proposals of the Viceregal and Royal Commissions and the Public Health Council for reform of the poor law system. Since economy was the overriding goal, Cosgrave and O'Higgins were only interested in recommendations which promised to save money.

On 30 September 1920, the Minister wrote to the local authorities outlining his ideas for what became known as 'amalgamation' or the 'county schemes'.[19] Unions were to be amalgamated and boards of guardians abolished, and administration and institutional relief were to be centralised under the county councils. Workhouses were to be replaced by a central 'county home' providing accommodation for the aged and infirm poor and a county hospital with a number of supporting district hospitals for the acutely ill. The rating system would be based on the county for all purposes. Interestingly, no change was proposed in the dispensary system apart from any which would result from the transfer to county administration.

The Minister dispatched envoys around the country to spread the new gospel of amalgamation. The young Dr James Ryan, later Minister for Health, was one of these.[20] The level of enthusiasm varied from county to county and initial progress was slow. By mid-1921, however, many local authorities were forced to take action owing to the Local Government Board's withholding of grants. In County Galway, to take an extreme example, ten workhouses and the county infirmary were closed in 1921, while the Galway city workhouse was adapted to accommodate a new county hospital. David Fitzpatrick has described how the County Clare scheme was adopted.[21] Although the county council approved amalgamation in principle in October 1920, it was not until June 1921 that a scheme was drafted by a Sinn Fein organiser, Fr Patrick Gaynor. Two of the seven workhouses were to close, another converted to a sanatorium and parts of the remaining four reconstituted as district hospitals. The aged and infirm, chronic sufferers, sane epileptics and harmless lunatics were to be concentrated in a county home in Ennis. These proposals gave rise to much controversy. In addition to the closure and reclassification, the county council proposed to dismiss, without compensation, superfluous employees, to the intense annoyance of the council's solicitor and district clerks. The chairman of a board of guardians, which was to be abolished and lose its

93

workhouse and officials, resigned from the county council in protest, warning that loyalty to the Dail had its limits. By mid October 1921, the amalgamation scheme was provisionally accepted.

Clare illustrates the general policy of the Department which in pressing for schemes of amalgamation formed an alliance with the county councils, stressing their role in supervising the entire local administration of the county. The Department complained that when confronted with schemes for amalgamation of workhouses:

> *Boards of Guardians not infrequently show themselves susceptible to purely parochial influences and interests which prevent them giving whole hearted cooperation to schemes of reform and economy which are undoubtedly conceived in the best interests of the County as a whole.*[22]

Kevin O'Higgins later explained that the main reason for local opposition to the closure of workhouses was the removal of what was considered as a local industry, the only one in some places.[23] The Department found the moral pressure exercised by county councils in these circumstances 'invaluable'.[24] If the worst came to the worst, the Minister would instruct the council not to pay the guardians any monies. The objectives of the Department were helped by the destruction of some workhouses and by the occupation of many others by soldiers and guerrillas.[25]

By April 1921, the Department's policy of persuading local authorities to transfer their allegiance was succeeding. Some 289 out of 362 local authorities in 26 of the counties refused to recognise the authority of the Local Government Board and 40 more were described as 'doubtful'.[26] As pressure on local government finance mounted in May and June 1921, the republican government may have felt the need of a further gesture to persuade wavering authorities. This may be why it was decided to carry out the most symbolic attack yet on the authority of the old regime. The headquarters of the Local Government Board, the Custom House, was attacked and burned on 25 May. The caretaker who resisted was fatally shot and some attackers also lost their lives. Vital records

94

and files were destroyed and leading officials left the country to ensure their own safety. The assault achieved its purpose: the Local Government Board, the most important branch of British civil government in Ireland, was reduced to impotence.

By the summer of 1921, political and military considerations on both sides of the conflict pointed to the need for a negotiated settlement of the war. A truce was agreed on 11 July and by the end of the year a treaty had been signed which established the Irish Free State, excluding six counties of Ulster. The clandestine Local Government Department and the demoralised Local Government Board were integrated as a new department under control of the Dail on 1 April 1922. The combined staff of the new department was 288, of which about 70 belonged to the former Dail department.[27]

The Ministers and Secretaries Act, 1924 formally established the departments of the new state under the Free State Constitution. It brought a number of health-related functions under the control of the Minister for Local Government, such as lunatic asylums, health insurance and the registration of births, marriages and deaths, and the Department was renamed the Department of Local Government and Public Health. By bringing responsibility for health services at national level together under one Department, the Act gave effect to one of the principal recommendations of the Public Health Council. A call for a separate minister for health from Thomas Johnson, the leader of the Labour Party was, however, rejected.[28]

The first task of the new Department was to bring some order to the conduct of local government and to assist the new government under the control of the Cumann na nGaedheal party, in asserting its authority to govern. This was complicated by the outbreak of civil war which brought administration to a standstill in some counties in 1922 and early 1923. The rebels were defeated and order restored by the summer of 1923, but not before more workhouses had been destroyed. Delays in payment of Exchequer grants, the difficulty in collecting rates and land annuities and the general lawlessness made it extremely difficult for local authorities to carry out their statutory responsibilities.

County schemes of some sort were put into effect in all but four counties and Dublin and Cork county boroughs by 1923.[29] But each scheme was different and their legality was doubtful. The Local Government Act, 1925, the most important piece of legislation affecting medical relief and public health of the decade, formally abolished the boards of guardians, with the exception of Dublin, and legalised the county rate.

The next step was to bring some uniformity to the various schemes and to persuade the laggard counties and county boroughs to overhaul their poor law arrangements. By 1925, the functions of boards of guardians everywhere except in Dublin were being carried out by boards of health and public assistance — specialised committees of the county councils dealing with health and poor relief similar to those recommended by the majority report of the Royal Commission on the Poor Laws. The finances of each board were raised by a rate levied throughout the county. The result was that by the mid-1920s, 33 workhouses had been converted into county homes (19 of which were also used in part as hospitals); 9 had been converted into county hospitals and 32 into district or fever hospitals. Fifty former workhouses, some of which had been destroyed during hostilities, were no longer in use for any poor law purpose.[30] All counties except Louth had provided a county home; county hospitals were designated in all but Counties Carlow, Louth, Tipperary North and South Ridings, and South Cork County District and one or more district hospitals had been selected in eighteen counties.[31]

Commission on the Relief of the Sick and Destitute Poor

The sick and the poor suffered a good deal as a result of these reforms, according to the Commission on the Relief of the Sick and Destitute Poor, appointed in 1925.[32] The Commission went behind the complacent claim of the government and the Department that the poor law and workhouses had been abolished and looked at the reality of the services available to those in need.

The Commission, chaired by Charles H. O'Connor, consisted of a majority of public representatives and persons with an interest in the poor. Its secretary was John Collins who later became an outstanding civil servant in the Department of Local Government and Public Health.

Appointed in response to mounting criticism, particularly from the Labour Party, of the inhumanity of the amalgamation schemes in some counties and the pressure from the Department for economies in every aspect of local authority activity, the Commission had no nostalgia for the old poor law. While accepting the necessity for reform, it found that between 1920 and 1924 'it was difficult if not impossible for either the poor or those interested on their behalf to know what law, if any, was being administered' and the poor law services became 'to a large extent disorganised and chaotic'.[33]

The Commission found that the policy of one county hospital per county had in practice been subject to considerable modification. In some counties there was no county hospital; in others there was a county hospital only. In a few counties, there was a county hospital supplemented by district or cottage hospitals as envisaged in official policy. The Commission had difficulty reconciling the policy of the Department towards county hospitals with what it found on the ground. Dr Stephenson, principal medical advisor to the Department, explained in his evidence to the Commission that the aim was to dissociate the treatment of the sick from other forms of poor relief and to turn the county hospital into a well equipped institution in which medical and surgical treatment for all forms of disease would be available.[34] The Commission agreed with the policy but found little evidence that it was being implemented. In some cases it reported that the new hospital arrangement 'instead of being an improvement on what existed before is rather the reverse'.[35] The Commission had no sympathy with those who advocated the retention of a hospital in each small town but informed policy makers that 'what the poor look for and desire is competent and skilled treatment in a hospital which has established for itself a record of efficient and sympathetic administration' and that they are admitted 'in priority to those who are able to pay'.[36]

In some areas medical treatment had not been separated from

poor relief: medical cases were being treated in the county home in Sligo. The Commission felt strongly that county hospitals should be institutions which catered for both surgical and medical cases. It was particularly critical of the situation in Kerry, where the medical and surgical hospitals were a mile apart and administered separately, declaring that it had 'not seen worse accommodation styled a County Hospital'.[37] In other hospitals, presumably the third or so of former county infirmaries which had been absorbed into the county hospital system, paying patients were more readily received than the poor for whom the accommodation was primarily intended. Praise was reserved for some county hospitals which were meeting the criteria for medical and surgical treatment, particularly the hospitals in Galway, Meath, Wexford, Offaly, Monaghan and Limerick.

The abolition of the boards of guardians and the transfer of their functions to boards of health and public assistance had reduced the number of elected representatives involved in poor relief in any county from about 150 to about 10. Many boards found it impossible to carry out all their functions properly. The Commission drew the conclusion that the boards should be abolished and that their poor relief functions be handed over to paid county council officials who would be in charge of the poor relief service under the direction of the council in the same manner 'as a general manager of a company under the control of a board of directors'.[38]

Finally, on the question of who should pay for improving the relief and medical services for the poor, the Commission nailed its flag firmly to the mast:

> The relief of the poor is a social service of a national character and it is only equitable that the state should give substantial aid in its administration.[39]

In particular it recommended a free grant of a portion of the capital sums required to improve the county and district institutions and the balance to be in loans at low rates of interest with generous periods of repayment.

The improvement of poor relief was low on the list of

government concerns and this highly critical report does not seem to have caused it much embarrassment. The government's priority was to maintain law and order and to establish its authority throughout the country. The collection of rates and land annuities was a major problem in the state's early years as property owners took advantage of the political unrest to avoid paying tax. Public bodies had no wish to increase the difficulty of rate collection by adding to what was already considered a heavy burden. The government's second concern was to promote agriculture which, as the country's chief export earner, was crucial to prosperity and development. The dependence of Irish farmers on the British market and the competition from efficient producers in Denmark and New Zealand meant that Irish products had to become more competitive. Farmers' costs had to be kept low, particularly rates which affected the farming community more than any other sector.[40] Given this policy, the government was unlikely to be sympathetic to improvements in local services which would add to the level of taxation. The interests of the farming community were further assured when, after the general election of 1927, Cumann na nGaedheal could only form a government with the help of the Farmers' Party.

Nor would the government increase the Exchequer's contribution to the cost of improving hospital and medical services. The strength of the recession which began in 1920 made the new government nervous that it would not be able to pay its way. It was a matter of pride that the new state could manage its affairs according to the principles of fiscal rectitude current at the time: economy was pursued with 'almost penitential zeal'.[41] Government expenditure was cut to a minimum and the social provisions of the Liberal era were severely pruned. The numbers employed in government departments were cut and the salaries and wages of local authority employees reduced. The Department of Local Government and Public Health campaigned to curb the increasing tendency of local authorities to send patients to voluntary hospitals, describing it as an 'avoidable expense'.[42] Only housing was exempted from the Irish 'Geddes axe'.[43] The result of these and other economies was that Exchequer expenditure in Ireland fell dramatically from £28.7 million in 1923 to £18.9 million in 1927.[44] The government was able to reduce the rate of income tax from 5s to 3s in the pound. The fact that the Minister for Local Government and Public Health was not a member of the Cabinet between 1923 and 1927 must have made the local government sector more vulnerable to cuts than might otherwise have been the case.

Reforming Local Government

The new government set out to achieve greater efficiency, economy and honesty in local government in conformity with Sinn Fein ideas about how local authorities ought to conduct their affairs and with the demands of a prudent fiscal policy. The Department of Local Government and Public Health pursued a dual approach of rationalisation and centralisation. The poor law unions were formally abolished in 1923 and the rural district councils in 1925; the councils' functions (mainly sanitation and housing) were transferred to the boards of health and public assistance of the county councils.[45] Referring to the abolition of the rural district councils, the Minister, Seamus Burke, put the issue starkly:

> it is a clear choice between the reform of local administration, between the more efficient and more economic operation of local administration, and the rural councils. You cannot make omelettes without breaking eggs.[46]

At the same time the Department extended its statutory powers to control the operation of local authorities in the belief that local authorities were primarily executive agencies of central government. The strict powers which the former Local Government Board exercised over the poor law authorities were extended to the affairs of county and urban councils. The Minister was given powers to dissolve a council if it failed to carry out its duties to his satisfaction and to appoint commissioners in its place.[47] The Minister saw the relationship between the local authorities and the public as:

*a business rather than a political relationship and those who administer
local government should be judged rather by the principles by which
commercial concerns are judged than by the principles which should
guide statesmen or politicians.*[48]

The success of the commissioners in carrying out the functions
of the dissolved authorities and in controlling expenditure, the
belief in the essentially business nature of local government and
the widespread admiration for the management system of American
cities, persuaded the Department to remodel the relationship
between elected representatives and officials of local authorities.
The first city manager was appointed in Cork in 1929, with power
to exercise all the functions of the city borough not reserved by
law to the elected representatives. The new system proved
successful and was gradually extended to other cities and eventually
to the counties.

The Local Authorities (Officers and Employees) Act, 1926
brought about radical changes in the appointment and promotion
of local authority staff with the objective of establishing 'a national
service which should be recruited on the principle of merit alone'
in accordance with Sinn Fein beliefs.[49] The need for action was
underlined in 1924 when two members of Roscommon County
Council were convicted of attempted bribery in the filling of a
dispensary vacancy.) Candidates for posts of chief executive officer
of a local authority and for professional posts, such as dispensary
officers and district nurses, were required to compete for selection
through competitions organised by a Local Appointments
Commission, modelled on the Civil Service Commission.

The Act put an end to the political favouritism, nepotism and
bribery which characterised appointment by local representatives.
This had major implications for the dispensary service. It introduced
appointment and recruitment on merit by competitive examination,
as advocated by the Viceregal Commission in 1906 and by the
Public Health Council. A new generation of dispensary doctors
would enjoy much greater independence from local politicians.
An added bonus was that the Act opened up promotion possibilities
for serving doctors who wished to improve their income. A young

doctor could take a job in a poor district to gain experience and then compete for a post in a more prosperous area. The introduction of pensions based on continuous service in any area further increased mobility. The reform was popular with the majority of the profession. Competition for the fifty odd posts each year was keen and many doctors sought post-graduate qualifications to improve their chances of appointment.[50]

County Medical Officers of Health

The appointment of county medical officers (CMOs) had long been identified as an urgent priority in public health but it was a native government which finally acted. The appointment of dispensary officers as medical officers of health had clearly failed. In its Report for 1925-27, the Department of Local Government and Public Health admitted that the dispensary officer was 'individualistic rather than communal in outlook, and his public duties conflict with his interest as a private practitioner and often bring him into collision with his fellow practitioners'.[51] The Local Government Act, 1925 provided for the appointment of medical officers of health to each county and county borough and assistant medical officers where necessary. Their duties were strictly defined as 'public health' and they had no function in regard to the district hospitals or the dispensary service which were governed by the separate code of 'public assistance'. The CMO was responsible for supervising the implementation of the sanitary laws, the operation of the maternity and child welfare services, the medical inspection of school children, the inspection of midwives, the operation of the tuberculosis service and the welfare of the blind but was not allowed to engage in private practice.[52] A veterinary surgeon was also appointed to each county to ensure the implementation of meat and milk regulations. The same Act made most of the permissive Public Health Acts relating to infectious diseases and tuberculosis mandatory on local authorities but schemes for the welfare of mothers and children under the Birth Notification Act, 1915 were not included.

The Minister justified the expense of appointing CMOs on the grounds of protecting agricultural exports rather than on the need to reduce the incidence of disease: to compete in international markets, food products required greater control of sanitation.[53] The Minister included a clause in the Local Government Act, taken from the Ministry of Health Act, 1919, which gave the Minister wide powers to take measures conducive to the health of the people. The Minister's reasoning was that it might be useful, in the event of an outbreak of disease affecting agricultural exports, to demonstrate to English medical opinion that someone in Ireland was charged by law with protecting the nation's health.[54]

The first CMOs were appointed in Cork, Carlow, Kildare and Offaly in 1927. But the Department's refusal to contribute to the CMO's salary made many counties reluctant to employ them. Only 18 counties had appointed officers by March 1932.[55] In those counties where CMOs were appointed, they soon began to make their presence felt. Perhaps their most important contribution was in school medical inspections. Irish sanitary authorities had been obliged since 1919 to organise the medical inspection of children in national schools but the Act was a dead letter over much of the country. As CMOs were appointed, a service began to develop. In 1931, 85,513 out of an estimated 331,087 eligible children were examined.[56] The main defects found were conditions of the nose, throat and teeth. A significant minority of children were suffering from the effects of malnutrition: 8.5 per cent of those inspected in 1931.[57] The majority of children were verminous. Some 26,000 children were treated in 1931 as a result of defects found at school inspections.[58] Children of parents eligible for public assistance were treated free of charge but otherwise parents had to pay general practitioners or hospital specialists for treatment. Such free treatment as existed was mostly confined to common defects of the eyes, ears and teeth and enlarged tonsils and adenoids. A problem faced by most CMOs and the public health nurses appointed to assist them was the reluctance of parents to have their children medically examined. A mixture of shame, pride and ignorance motivated parents to keep their children at home on inspection day.

The expansion of school medical services suited the ethos of economy and efficiency preached by the Department. It maintained that:

> *no other activity on the preventive side of public health gives a more direct return than the early diagnosis and correction of children's ailments. The cost per child is inconsiderable, it purchases an increase of health, happiness and efficiency for the individual, and cumulatively for the community at large.*[59]

The same logic was not, however, applied to services for mothers and infants. The Notification of Births Act, 1915 had given local authorities wide powers to provide a maternity and child welfare service but the legislation was permissive, not mandatory. The Department's policy was to encourage voluntary organisations to provide the service.[60] The level of the grant paid from central funds was only £13,210 in 1924.[61] Most expenditure was incurred by health visitors employed by voluntary district nursing associations. The comprehensive maternity and child service for needy persons envisaged before independence barely existed. Although the Department claimed that accommodation was available for mothers requiring hospital confinement (in the county and district hospitals and the county homes), the Commission on the Relief of the Sick and Destitute Poor found that in many cases such accommodation did not exist, and where it did it was often below acceptable standards.[62] The maternal mortality rate, at about 5 deaths per 1,000 births, was only slightly better than during the war years and the infant mortality rate in 1928, while an improvement on previous years, remained high at 68 deaths per 1,000 births.[63]

The Department was aware of fashionable thinking about pregnancy, particularly the importance of ante-natal care for all expectant mothers and a wholesome diet.[64] But words of encouragement to local authorities to act on their responsibility for maternal welfare fell on deaf ears. In 1930, ante-natal clinics were available only in the four county boroughs.[65] The Department wrung its hands and lamented that 'the problem of ensuring safety in child birth remains unsolved' but refrained from taking the positive action for which the situation called.[66] Only

Dublin County Borough could point to considerable progress. Thanks to a grant from the Carnegie Trust, a model child welfare centre was opened in Lord Edward Street and in 1928 a full-time medical officer was appointed to direct a maternity and child welfare service.

Apart from Dublin, and to a lesser extent the other county boroughs, the appointment of county medical officers seems to have resulted in few improvements in the maternity services for lower income women. The improvement of these services seems not to have been a priority of Irish women, local authorities or the Department. There was development on one front, however. With the enthusiastic support of the Midwives Board chaired by Dr Coey Bigger, the CMOs, in their capacity as inspectors of midwives, began to campaign against unregistered handywomen and through successful prosecutions put many out of business. The Midwives Act, 1931 closed loopholes in earlier legislation; by 1933, the Department was able to report that only in Mayo was the practice of midwifery by unqualified women still widespread.[67]

Tuberculosis

The amalgamation schemes and the drive for economies in the early 1920s curtailed the already inadequate services for the treatment of tuberculosis. Subsequent reform was concerned almost exclusively with administrative matters. Significantly, the Local Government Act, 1925 made notification of the disease mandatory, thus succeeding where the former British administration had failed. The same Act transferred responsibility for providing sanatorium benefit from the health committees to the county boards of health and public assistance, but no obligation was placed on local authorities to provide sanatorium accommodation. When the CMOs were appointed, they were given overall responsibility for the development of tuberculosis schemes in their county. Notification was half-heartedly put into operation in those counties with CMOs; in 1928-29 there were only 799 cases notified but over 3,500 deaths.[68] The Department estimated that for every death from the disease, there were eight sufferers.[69]

This administrative rationalisation was not accompanied by serious attempts to expand facilities for treatment of the disease. There was a particular shortage of accommodation for advanced cases. Inertia seems to have prevented the spending of the remains of Lloyd George's sanatorium grant, transferred to the Irish account on independence.[70] The efforts made to contain the disease before the First World War were not maintained in the 1920s. The rate of decrease in deaths from the disease began to slow down and to fall far behind the rates of other countries at a comparable level of economic development.[71] Controlling tuberculosis was not a priority among the people, their politicians or administrators. In 1929, Limerick County Borough and five counties were still refusing to put approved schemes into operation.[72]

National Health Insurance

The national insurance system did not escape the scrutiny of ministers bent on economies. The National Insurance Act, 1924 reduced the state's contribution to insurance funds and lowered the fees paid to doctors for medical certification.[73] On the future of insurance, the government was more cautious. The Labour Party, though small, was vociferous in its demand that insurance be retained and expanded to include medical benefit. The interests of over 400,000 insured workers were not to be put aside lightly. The Minister for Finance, Ernest Blythe, decided in 1924 to set up an inter-departmental committee on insurance with some outside experts to review the issue. It was chaired by Professor W. Magennis, TD.

In its terms of reference, the committee was charged with inquiring into 'the advisability of the continued maintenance of the system of National Health Insurance in its present form', the desirability of introducing medical benefit and examining whether 'the medical services at present assisted or maintained out of State or local funds can be improved as respects efficiency and economy'.[74] The committee in its interim report came out strongly in favour of the retention of national insurance, although it recommended major changes in its organisation, particularly the unification of the eighty or so friendly societies.[75]

The committee spent the next two years discussing the question of medical benefit. In their final report, the members agreed on the desirability of a comprehensive scheme of medical treatment for the working classes and their dependants but because of its cost could not unanimously recommend it.[76] Only Dr Rowlette, a member of the Public Health Council of 1919, argued for the implementation of a national medical service to cover insured persons, their dependants and those entitled to public assistance services.[77] This solution also had the support of the Irish Medical Committee which presented evidence before the committee. Their witnesses advocated medical benefit under the Insurance Acts and claimed that medical benefit was dropped from the 1911 Act 'at the expense of and in opposition to the wishes of the Irish Medical profession'.[78] They were prepared to accept a national service with panels of doctors providing a choice to patients in urban areas and salaried dispensary doctors in rural areas.[79]

The majority of the committee opted for the less than perfect solution of medical benefit for insured persons only. As far as the dispensary and public hospital doctors were concerned, they recommended that they be reorganised into a national medical service, with appointments, promotion and dismissals under central control and with standard salaries and superannuation. They recommended that the state should meet half the cost of the reorganised service and of providing new buildings to replace the estimated two-thirds of buildings which were considered below standard.

The majority's proposals met the predictable opposition of the representatives of the Departments of Local Government and Public Health and Finance. Dr Stephenson, although he signed the majority report, thought that medical benefit was 'unnecessary and superfluous' and that there was no evidence that insured persons were suffering for lack of medical care.[80] His civil service colleagues, Mr Hurson and Mr McElligott, agreed and argued against the transformation of the dispensary and public hospital system into a service controlled by a state department as this would 'weaken local responsibility and would be accompanied by grave administrative risks'.[81] In their view recent legislation setting up the Local Appointments Commission had removed most of the objections against the dispensary service. They expressed their firm opposition to any recommendations which would put additional burdens on employers or the state, in particular the suggestion that the state should help finance the reconstruction of dispensaries.[82]

The opposition of the Departments effectively killed any suggestion of providing medical services for the insured. The National Health Insurance Act, 1929 implemented those parts of the committee's report which promised greater economy and efficiency and ignored those which advocated increased expenditure. Once again, the existence of the dispensary system was used to prevent the emergence of a less stigmatising system of medical treatment for those on low incomes. The obstinate position of the departmental representatives was highlighted in 1929 when the Northern Irish government introduced a scheme of medical benefit for insured workers with dispensary doctors retaining their salaries but receiving 7s 6d for each insured person.

The Hospitals Sweepstakes

By the late 1920s, the voluntary hospitals in Dublin were in a desperate way. The value of their endowment funds was reduced by inflation during and after the First World War and income from new charitable sources fell away. At the same time, costs rose as advances in radiology, pathology and surgery required new facilities and staff. The hospitals were increasingly dependent on income from paying patients and organised collections. The income from paying patients in six voluntary hospitals in Dublin averaged £2,000 a year before the war; in the 1920s the income had risen to an average of £24,000.[83] As the financial position of the hospitals worsened, there was increasing criticism from public representatives that paying patients were being treated in preference to the poor for whom the hospitals were intended. The hospitals had their own defence. They were not obliged by their charters to provide unlimited accommodation for poor patients, only as much as their legacies and charitable income would finance. As these funds dwindled, so did their commitment to the sick poor.

A number of hospitals ran sweepstakes to raise money. Although this was illegal, the government, both before and after independence, turned a blind eye provided no irregularities occurred. Several attempts were made in the early 1920s to legalise sweepstakes for hospital purposes but each failed mainly due to the opposition of the Minister for Justice, Kevin O'Higgins, who did not think it was possible to run sweepstakes without fraud. Neither was the government prepared to come to the aid of the hospitals by increasing the level of parliamentary grants last fixed in the 1850s.

The issue came to a head in 1929 when the National Maternity Hospital, Holles Street, unable to raise money to carry out essential repairs and threatening to close its doors, organised a group of hospitals to promote a private members Bill to legalise hospital sweepstakes. The government accepted the option of a legalised sweepstake as preferable to a direct grant or closure of the hospital. The Public Charitable Hospitals Act, 1930 authorised a monopoly in the promotion of sweepstakes on horse races for hospital purposes. Hospitals wishing to participate in a sweepstake had to show that they reserved at least a quarter of their beds for non-paying patients. The Minister for Justice was made responsible for the operation of the Act, which was to run until 1934.

Six hospitals participated in the first sweepstake on the Manchester November Handicap in 1930; the hospitals' share of the proceeds, £131,671, surprised even the sweepstake's most enthusiastic supporters. By the summer of 1931, £1 million had been raised, with about 90 per cent of the money coming from overseas.[84] It was an enormous sum by comparison with an income for 52 voluntary hospitals in 1933 of less than £400,000 and an annual expenditure by boards of public health and assistance of less than £3 million.[85]

The manner in which the hospitals divided out the proceeds of the sweepstakes was not edifying. Hospital boards scrambled to secure as large a share of the bonanza as they could without any consideration of the overall medical needs of the city or country. In 1931, the government stepped in and half-heartedly attempted to establish some order in the distribution of funds.[86] A Committee of Reference was established to decide in what proportion hospitals should share in the proceeds of each sweepstake, subject to the approval of the Minister for Justice. More significantly, it was decided that one quarter of the proceeds would go towards development of the county hospitals, under the direction of the Minister for Local Government and Public Health. The Committee of Reference had little success in bringing order to the distribution of funds among voluntary hospitals. In its Report for 1931, it noted that:

> The main features of the majority of the claims were variously related to a single anxiety, namely, to obtain the largest possible , award from sweepstake funds.[87]

The Cumann na nGaedheal government fell from office before it had an opportunity to bring about more fundamental changes. The problem of rationally distributing the proceeds of the sweepstakes was one of the priorities of the incoming Fianna Fail administration which had radical ideas about how the money ought to be spent.

Conclusion

The health services gained and lost during the struggle for independence and the establishment of the new state. The Dail Department of Local Government, caught between the necessity of maintaining a responsible system of local government and breaking the connection with the Local Government Board, devised a radical plan of reform to reorganise relief to the poor. The ideas behind the plan can be traced back to the Viceregal and Royal Commissions and the Public Health Council. But the Dail Department had the advantage of being able to put reform into effect. It would have been well nigh impossible to overcome the local and vested interests which had grown up around the poor law without the incentive of a war of independence.[88] The amalgamation schemes achieved an administrative reform of the poor law that was only being discussed in Britain. The unusual circumstances of 1920-21 encouraged the forces for political, economic and social reform of local government and the poor law system. For the first time, the machinery of local government was successfully subjected to the exigencies of a national goal. It anticipated the movement towards much greater central control of local government under the Free State.

The long term benefits of the amalgamation schemes were to establish the county and county borough as the primary unit of local administration and to begin the separation of public medical services from the relief of the poor. The county and district hospitals were intended, at least in theory, to provide medical treatment for the sick in their area, irrespective of income. The county plans involved rationalisation on a geographical basis and specialisation of care.

The changes did not benefit the sick poor in the short term, firstly because of the conditions under which the amalgamation of workhouses took place and secondly because the finance required to bring the new system up to modern standards was not forthcoming. It was unfortunate for the health services that as the new state came into being, a long and severe depression in agricultural prices began. The cheese-paring approach of the government was matched only by the determination of many local authorities not to engage in any activity which raised by one penny the burden of the rates. The important changes which were put into effect, especially the appointment of county medical officers and the selection of dispensary officers on merit, were primarily motivated by a wish to increase the economy, efficiency or honesty of local administration. Cost was the excuse for the refusal to contemplate a national medical service or even the extension of medical benefit to insured workers.

In the late 1920s the problem of financing the voluntary hospitals finally impinged on the consciousness of government. The first step towards much greater involvement by public authorities in the affairs of the hospitals was the authorisation and supervision of the hospitals sweepstakes. As unprecedented amounts of money became available for hospital development, the state, in its role of guardian of the common good, was challenged to develop a hospital policy for the whole country and for both voluntary and public hospitals.

As far as the health services are concerned, the achievements of the first decade of the new state could be summarised as the laying of radical foundations for a building to be completed at a later stage. The events of these years certainly bear out Oliver MacDonagh's contention that Cumann na nGaedheal acted with 'a single-mindedness which Irish administrations had lacked almost since the Act of Union' even if he underestimates the innovative nature of much of this change.[89]

6
Hospitals for the People
1932~1942

FIANNA FAIL'S ACCESSION to power in 1932 under the leadership of Eamon de Valera began a new era in Irish politics. The young party offered a radical alternative to the conservatism of the Cumann na nGaedheal government. Fianna Fail's economic policies aimed to make Ireland economically independent of Britain. To a lesser extent they were a response to growing protectionism in the rest of the world. The new government's social policies were governed by the ideal of creating a society in which there would be neither poverty nor great wealth and in which the poorest would enjoy the dignity of a good house, clean water, a hospital bed when ill, a job or at least a minimum income. The maintenance of Irish agricultural prices at competitive levels, thus excluding any increase in taxation for social purposes, was no longer the dominant aim of the government. Fianna Fail were prepared to increase the rates if the common good required. Their victory in 1932 was a victory of the small farmer and farm labourer of the west and the Dublin worker over the comfortable farmers, business people and professionals represented by Cumann na nGaedheal.

The achievements of the first Fianna Fail governments in the social sphere, in housing assistance for the unemployed and pensions, were considerable. The health services benefited from measures to ameliorate social conditions. In 1933, the government initiated a free milk scheme for poor children and pregnant

113

women.[1] The large grants made available by the government each year to encourage employment were spent mainly on laying a modern public health infrastructure of sewers and clean water. The bonanza of the hospitals sweepstakes enabled the Minister for Local Government and Public Health to improve the hospital service in most counties. Finally, the health insurance system was radically overhauled, and strenuous measures were taken to ensure compliance with the law by employers. The scale of the government's activity is all the more impressive as it took place against a background of severe world economic depression and a fierce trade war with Britain which reduced Ireland's export earnings.[3]

Fianna Fail shared some of its predecessor's attitudes to local government. Local authorities were accused of being inefficient and wasteful of the ratepayers' money. In the first ten years of Fianna Fail government, 31 local authorities were abolished and replaced by commissioners appointed by the Minister.[4] The salaries of local officials, in common with other public servants, were considered too high and in 1934 were compulsorily reduced to achieve economies. Dispensary doctors were reprieved from the cuts only at the last minute. The government gave serious consideration to a memorandum from the Department of Local Government and Public Health proposing the abolition of elected local authorities and the substitution of permanent commissioners.[5] But the proposal was rejected on the grounds that it would be too unpopular to put into effect.[6] The Minister and his parliamentary secretary then turned their attention to ensuring that the local authorities danced to the tune of the Custom House. Cumann na nGaedheal had greatly increased central control over local government but was conservative in its views of what local authorities should do. Fianna Fail had ideas and was prepared to back its proposals with cash and put great pressure on local authorities to carry out government policy. It increased its control by fighting local elections on a strict party ticket and by insisting that local representatives put party before local or vested interest in the council chamber. It also removed the bias in the local government franchise in favour of the propertied classes and against

114

those with little or no property who supported Fianna Fail.

Fianna Fail's search for economy in government contradicted its ambitious plans to improve and initiate services. Its policies at local level soon led to a sharp increase in the rates; receipts from rates in county health districts rose from £2.4 million in the year to March 1932 to £3.5 million in the year to March 1942.[7] The expenditure of the Department of Local Government and Public Health rose nearly threefold in the same period.[8] The number of local officials and civil servants, having fallen up to 1932, began to rise. The staff of the Department doubled in size from 236 in 1932 to 467 in 1946, with more than half the increase occurring by 1936.[9] If the increasing size of the public service embarrassed Fianna Fail, it did not unduly worry them in the 1930s and early 1940s in the absence of a strong challenge to their leadership. Public expectation of greater government involvement in economic and social life seemed to confirm the validity of their approach to the country's problems.

Hospital Policy

Mr de Valera appointed Sean T. O Ceallaigh Minister for Local Government and Public Health and Dr F. C. Ward as his parliamentary secretary. Mr. O Ceallaigh's main interest was housing and he quickly assigned Dr Ward responsibility for public health and public assistance. This was a fortunate arrangement as far as the development of the health services was concerned. Dr Ward was a dispensary doctor from County Monaghan with a private interest in a bacon curing company. A highly intelligent man, Dr Ward's ambition was matched by great energy and toughness but his rough and abrasive personality won him few friends. Unlike the senior members of the Party, he had not participated in the 1916 Rising, then a serious handicap to achieving full ministerial office, although he did play an active part in the war of independence. He was feared and respected by his officials rather than liked. A good judge of ability, he refused to work with or support the promotion of officers who he considered to be incompetent. He also earned the bitter dislike of the medical

115

profession which was to play a part in his dramatic downfall more than a decade later.

It was Dr Ward's good fortune that he should come to office just as the unexpected bonanza of the sweepstakes made it possible to overhaul the Irish hospital system. The principle that the state should benefit from the sweeps windfall was established by the Public Charitable Hospitals Act, 1931. Negotiations were under way with local authorities as to which hospitals were to be rebuilt or repaired when Fianna Fail came into office. The Act had done little, however, to improve the methods by which the voluntary hospitals divided their share of the proceeds.

In opposition, Fianna Fail had signalled its support for a more rational method of distributing sweepstake funds. Mr de Valera thought there was a need for a 'controlling committee' to examine hospital needs and 'to make certain that the money is being allocated in accordance with the needs and the services of the hospitals in general'.[10] He thought that all the funds should be allocated on the same criteria rather than the arbitrary division of the funds between the voluntary hospitals and public hospitals under the control of the Minister.[11] Shortly after taking up office, Dr Ward visited Scandinavia with officials to see the latest developments in hospital treatment. The Public Hospitals Bill, introduced soon afterwards, indicates a clear idea of the direction of hospital treatment.

Introducing the Bill, Dr Ward went to some trouble to outline his view of hospital development.[12] The country, he said, had a unique opportunity to tackle the question of hospital organisation in a comprehensive way. He admitted that there was no general hospital system in the strict sense and that the government could no longer allow millions of pounds to be poured into 'a system obviously unorganised and insufficient'.[13] The imperative behind the Bill was clear:

> Too many institutions must not be allowed to specialise along the same lines to the neglect of other less popular branches of curative medicine. The central specialised hospitals must be made available for all, and the poor must get the use of them free. The local hospitals

must be developed to afford the maximum of utility without a high
degree of specialisation and their geographical organisation must
be carefully planned.[14]

Voluntary hospitals would be expected to work in harmony
with the overall plan for hospital reorganistion so that 'the sick
poor throughout the country shall be given every facility of
treatment and nursing that their richer brethren can afford to
obtain'.[15] Dr Ward spoke of 'the essential unity of the
institutional problem ... both as regards the voluntary hospitals
and the poor law hospitals' and of the Minister's responsibility
to supervise and control the reorganised system.[16] Ireland had to
follow the experience of other countries and plan its hospital services
to take advantage of the advances in medicine. For the first time,
the Minister was asserting the right to direct the development
of hospital services in the public interest.

The Public Hospitals Act, 1933 abolished the Committee of
Reference and the fixed share of 25 per cent reserved for public
hospitals under the control of the Minister. The Minister now
assumed responsibility for the distribution of the entire fund. A
Hospitals Commission was established and charged with the task
of surveying hospital facilities in each area, reporting on applications
from voluntary hospitals for grants from the sweepstake funds
and with power to inspect any hospital and examine receipts and
expenditures. The only restriction on the participation of voluntary
hospitals was that they should not exist solely for private profit.
Proceeds from the sweepstakes would no longer be distributed
immediately after each draw but would be paid into a new
Hospitals Trust Fund which would invest what was not
immediately needed. It was a source of controversy that the
Minister could allocate sweepstake funds to public hospitals without
consulting the Commission. Although he did have to seek the
views of the Commission before allocating funds to voluntary
hospitals, he was not bound by its recommendations.[17] The new
Fund was not subject to the normal controls of public finance:
the Minister did not have to seek the approval of the Minister
for Finance before spending money from the Fund and expenditure

was not audited by the Comptroller and Auditor General.

The opposition denounced the Act as 'the death knell of all voluntary hospitals in this country'.[18] The voluntary hospitals viewed the measure as an act of piracy by the government. The hospitals sweepstakes was something which they had initiated when in dire financial distress and they alone should be allowed to benefit from the gravy train. They had little sympathy with the parliamentary secretary's wish to improve hospital services in each county and were mostly opposed to any suggestion of rationalising services in Dublin. Their medical staffs were nervous about the development of county hospitals with surgeons who might reduce the volume of business referred to the voluntary hospitals.

In one sense, the hospitals were victims of the very success of the sweepstakes. If the proceeds of the venture had been modest, the state might have simply devised a system for allocating the proceeds among the hospitals. But the sheer size of the funds available was bound to excite any government's interest in the possibility of funding a modern hospital system, especially that of a Fianna Fail administration committed to transforming many aspects of Irish life. Contemporaries were also aware that the sweepstakes, while bringing some controls on voluntary hospital independence, had averted or postponed a demand for the state financing and perhaps complete takeover of the hospitals. As it was, many hospitals in the 1920s were faced with the choice of closing, becoming wholly private or throwing themselves on the mercy of the government. There was nothing peculiar to Ireland about the changing role of the voluntary hospital. The same was happening in Britain and the United States. In the latter country, many small and inefficient hospitals closed while others began to be run as business concerns with a great emphasis on hospital administration. In Britain, lack of money made the voluntary hospitals more receptive to proposals for a national health service in the 1940s than they might have otherwise have been.[19] In Ireland, the sweepstakes permitted voluntary hospitals, particularly in Dublin, to postpone the evil day of rationalisation. It allowed smaller hospitals which might otherwise have been closed or amalgamated to survive. The hospitals remained independent of the state but it was an uneasy independence. A reduction of sweepstake funds or an ill-disposed Minister could bring about a radical change in fortune; and it is understandable that their attitude to the state should have become somewhat paranoid.

It is understandable too that a government with a social conscience should wish to ensure fair access to hospital treatment. By the 1930s, medical advances had made the hospital the pivot of modern medicine. The decision of the working and middle classes to seek hospital treatment, which had been a trickle in the pre-war period, became a flood by the 1930s. This trend raised important issues for both voluntary and local authority hospitals. Before the First World War, voluntary hospital consultants received no fees for any patients under their care in the hospital wards. But as the hospitals began charging patients with means the full or partial cost of their stay, the medical staff followed suit by charging them fees for treatment. The rising demand for hospital accommodation, the reluctance of the voluntary hospitals in Dublin and Cork to expand to meet this demand and the pecuniary interest to consultants and hard-pressed hospitals in treating private patients, led to increasing criticism in the 1930s that the poor in both cities were being discriminated against in favour of those who could pay. By 1935, the proportion of patients treated free in voluntary hospitals had fallen to 40 per cent.[20] This trend had the effect of underlining the need for a planned approach to hospital provision for the whole population. It drew attention to the cost of the latest medical treatment to those on small incomes and raised the issue of whether or not they were to be protected from large hospital and specialist bills. Finally, it gave consultants a much greater financial stake in the treatment of the working and middle classes than they had ever had before. The question which perplexed Dr Ward and his advisers was how to ensure that the poor benefited from medical progress to the same extent as those who could afford to pay. The response was an assault on privilege to match Fianna Fail's campaign to remove constitutional and economic privileges.

The demand by private patients for hospital treatment created problems of a different order for local authority hospitals. Those hospitals were obliged by law to give priority of admission to the poor and most county surgeons were forbidden by the terms of their contracts to charge fees for attendance in hospital. Local authorities could, however, charge patients who did not qualify for public assistance, a contribution towards the cost of their stay. County surgeons increasingly felt a sense of grievance that they could not charge fees to private patients.

The Hospitals Commission began its work in September 1933, under the full time chairmanship of Michael Doran, an engineer. The Commission lost no time in enquiring into the hospital needs of the community. In the period of its first report, 1933-36, it found just over 14,000 acute hospital beds, of which 63 per cent were in publicly owned hospitals and the remaining 37 per cent in voluntary hospitals.[21] It was critical of the county hospitals, both in the accommodation and services provided and of their location.[22] The Commission was not in favour of developing each county hospital but advised the grouping of hospitals in suitable geographical centres 'irrespective of county boundaries'.[23] The Commission argued that such a policy:

> would enable not only better and more up-to-date central and special services to be provided but would enable a more complete hospital medical staff to be employed, at less cost to the rate-payers of such grouped counties.[24]

The Commission submitted a scheme to the Minister which provided for the development of twelve main hospital centres, which included regional centres in Dublin, Cork, Galway, Limerick and Sligo and county hospitals catering for acute medical and surgical cases in counties remote from regional centres. A network of district hospitals in the principal towns was recommended to cater for acute medical, minor surgical and maternity cases.

The Commission was even more critical of the situation among the voluntary hospitals in Dublin.[25] There were too many small hospitals; facilities were out of date; co-operation between specialists was lacking; patients were treated indiscriminately in the wards; and medical teaching was falling behind international standards.[26] It examined the possibility of a federation or amalgamation of hospitals and came down in favour of amalgamation, recommending two general hospitals in south Dublin and two in the north of the city.[27] In a clear warning to the voluntary hospitals, it suggested that St Kevin's, the former workhouse for south Dublin be developed as the chief hospital and clinical teaching centre in Dublin, if the voluntary hospitals failed to respond to the challenge of providing sufficient accommodation for the poor.

This first report of the Hospitals Commission was a major advance in thinking about hospitals in Ireland and echoed the ideas outlined by Dr Ward in his speech on the Public Hospitals Bill. In an important change of emphasis, the Commission was charged with the task of enquiring into the hospital needs of the community rather than the needs of individual hospitals. Looked at from this angle, the situation required rationalisation and co-ordination of voluntary hospitals and investment in hospital accommodation outside the cities where no voluntary hospitals existed. The Commission proposed a plan in which voluntary and local authority hospitals would complement each other, rather than inhabit different worlds. If the voluntary hospitals felt uncomfortable with this new order, it was because they were reluctant to see themselves as part of any system.

The Commission was obviously alarmed at the extent to which the voluntary hospitals had come to cater for the new class of paying patient at the expense of the poor.[28] The Commission opposed this tendency not so much on the grounds of social justice as on medical grounds:

> *The maintenance of separate middle-class hospitals, as distinct from middle-class accommodation in a General Hospital, is opposed to the principles of all modern hospital development.*[29]

A good hospital system catered for the entire population: the alternative, of a local authority service for the poor and a voluntary system for the rich, was a second-rate system. The Commission argued that private hospitals should not receive public funds at the expense of those hospitals providing a comprehensive service. In recommending the conditions to be attached to grants from the Hospitals Trust Fund, the Commission emphasised that hospitals should be run as charitable institutions, that they trea a certain proportion of patients without charge and that th Minister, by supervision and inspection, should insist that thes conditions were met.[30] The main objective of the conditions 'wa to ensure the ready admission of the poor to hospital beds anc to secure that Local Authority patients sent to Voluntary Hospital will be admitted with a minimum of delay'.[31] The Commissior warned the voluntary hospitals that it was in their interests 'tc remove any impression – however unfounded – that exists in the public mind that these important categories of patients are in any way discriminated against'.[32]

The continuing inability of the voluntary hospitals to meet the demand for hospital accommodation among the poor persuadec the Dublin public assistance authority in the late 1930s of the neec to develop St Kevin's, the former workhouse, as a major hospital. Plans to reconstruct a large part of the hospital, interrupted by the war, gathered momentum in the late 1940s.

The Commission's views on the relationship between private and public hospital medicine were important since they guided the Minister in decisions to allocate money from the Hospitals Trust Fund. In this way they helped to ensure that Irish hospitals, as they entered a crucial phase of development, were developed to meet the needs of the whole population. The combination of public ward accommodation for the poor and 'middle class' accommodation for the better off in hospitals, and the same medical, nursing, diagnostic and other facilities, was a good compromise between the need to provide first class hospital treatment for all and the attractions of private medicine for the medical profession and those who could pay.

The Commission's recommendations on the development of provincial and Dublin hospitals did not meet such ready acceptance. By the time the Commission had been set up, many of the key decisions about the development of provincial hospitals had been taken. As soon as the Public Charitable Hospitals Act, 1931 had assigned 25 per cent of the proceeds of the sweepstakes to the Minister, the Department entered 'prolonged negotiations' on the size and nature of the hospitals to be provided.[33] By March 1933, it had been agreed to build new county hospitals in Clare, North Cork, South Cork, Kilkenny, Laois, Mayo, Monaghan, Offaly, Roscommon, Tipperary North, Tipperary South and Westmeath and plans for other major works had been approved.[34] The former workhouse buildings in Tralee and Dublin were to be reconstructed and a number of district and cottage hospitals were to be built.[35]

The Department had no difficulty in persuading local authorities to provide new hospital accommodation, in contrast to their continuing reluctance to appoint county medical officers of health. The financial arrangements offered by the Department were attractive. The bulk of the money would be advanced from the Hospitals Trust Fund and the remainder would be advanced to the local authority at a low rate of interest. The financial incentives were compounded by the increased employment a larger institution would give the designated town and the added prestige of having a new modern hospital. Little thought, on the other hand, was given to the cost of maintaining the new hospitals, the full cost of which would fall on the rates. Sean T. O Ceallaigh, defending the Department's decisions on hospital development in 1939 when the full cost of maintenance was becoming apparent, explained that:

> there is not a board of health that has ever come to me on deputations ... that did not want the largest county hospital they could get, several district hospitals in addition and the usual sanatorium and fever hospitals. The fight was always to get them to see reason over the number of beds they wanted to provide in their county.[36]

Once the decision to develop a relatively large number of county hospitals was taken, it would have been politically impossible for the government to do an about-turn and renege on its commitments by implementing the Hospitals Commission plan for twelve hospital centres, even if it agreed with the Commission's radical blueprint. On the contrary, the pressure to sanction new county hospitals grew. However, the Minister seems to have accepted the Commission's recommendations for the development of regional hospital centres, not as an alternative to the proliferation of county hospitals but in addition to them.[37]

The scale of county, district and fever hospital building in the

123

1930s was impressive by any standards, even if some of it was unnecessary by the criteria of the Hospitals Commission. By 1942, when shortages of building materials postponed further construction, thirteen new county hospitals, seventeen district hospitals and eight fever hospitals had been completed.[38] By 1944, the amount of Hospitals Trust Funds paid in respect of local authority hospitals was £1.2 million, out of a total of over £14 million received for all hospitals up to 31 December 1944.[39]

Contemporaries were quick to compare the progress made by local authorities with the inertia of the voluntary sector. Hospitals in Dublin were slow to accept the new arrangements established by the Public Hospitals Act, 1933. Each hospital continued to submit claims to the Commission without regard to wider needs. The Commission's position vis-a-vis the hospitals was weakened by the delay in the Minister's acceptance of its recommendations for Dublin until 1939.[40] But neither the Minister nor the Commission could do much to bring about rationalisation of Dublin hospitals in the short term. The Hospitals Commission pointed out that while the principle of ministerial intervention had been accepted by the voluntary hospitals, in practice it had met considerable opposition from some of the hospitals. It blamed the refusal to co-operate on 'the tenacity with which those hospitals cling to their time-honoured claim for complete individual independence'.[41]

Hospital deficits

Relations between hospitals and government were not helped by the problem of the hospital deficits. In 1933, 28 hospitals had deficits amounting to £54,868; by 1941, some 40 hospitals had deficits totalling £222,466.[42] The advent of the sweepstakes was partly blamed for the increase. The hospitals' income from charitable sources fell off sharply as the funds raised by the sweepstakes rose and after years of penny-pinching, the hospitals may have become a little less careful of economy, knowing that the sweepstakes would provide.

However, the main reason for hospital deficits was probably

the greater demand upon hospital services. 'There appears to be no end to the demand for more and more hospital accommodation' said the Hospitals Commission in 1938.[43] Out-patient attendances at Dublin hospitals, for example, grew from 627,236 in 1933 to 874,749 in 1938.[44] The increasing success of surgical treatment and the impact of a new generation of dispensary doctors and county surgeons appointed on merit contributed to the rising number of referrals for specialist treatment. The growing confidence of the people in hospitals is well illustrated by the changes in the pattern of hospital confinements for maternity. In 1933, there were 4,900 births in the three Dublin maternity hospitals; in 1941, the number had nearly doubled to 8,188.[45] Voluntary hospitals received no payment from local authorities for the treatment of poor patients, but were obliged to maintain beds for non-paying patients if they wished to benefit from the sweepstake funds. Therefore, it is not surprising that they should have accumulated deficits.

It had originally been intended that sweepstakes funds should pay for capital items of expenditure and not for the running costs of hospitals. The Minister was careful never to allow any breach in the principle that the funds at his disposal were for capital purposes when dealing with local authorities. But with the voluntary hospitals it was accepted early on that the Hospital Trust Fund should pay their deficits, and a special reserve was accumulated to ensure their solvency for a number of years ahead. As the years went by, more and more of the voluntary hospitals' share of the Fund was going to meet current debts with a corresponding drop in the amount available for building purposes.

The rise in deficits was the occasion for greater government involvement in hospital management. Payments from the Hospitals Trust Fund were only approved on the basis of accounts submitted and hospitals were asked to send in quarterly statements of expenditure. The Commission was dissatisfied with the running of the hospitals for the same reasons the Cumann na nGaedheal and Fianna Fail governments criticised local authorities: 'hospitals should be looked upon as business establishments as far as their management is concerned'.[46]

125

The tensions generated by the hospitals' deficits damaged relations between the state and the hospitals. The hospitals, on the one hand, could point to the fact that they were responding to the increasing demand for hospitalisation without due recompense from the state. They resented demands that they should improve their management, instead of being paid for the job they were doing. All the major hospitals had been established long before the new state was set up. The Protestant hospitals were suspicious of the overwhelmingly Catholic ethos of the state and its government; the Catholic hospitals jealously guarded their special position against state interference. By maintaining a policy of minimal co-operation with the Hospitals Commission, the hospitals made clear their determination to retain their independence of the state. Their medical staff, who had most to lose from any change in the status quo, and who were dismayed by the rapid development of a modern public hospital network outside of Dublin, became increasingly anxious about state interference with the voluntary hospitals.[47]

Health Insurance

The Fianna Fail governments of the 1930s carried out a major overhaul of the system of national insurance and took the first halting steps towards protecting the working class against the cost of hospital treatment. The National Health Insurance Act, 1929 had provided for the unification of societies but it had had little effect. About 65 friendly societies, ranging in membership from 90 to 90,000, continued to provide sickness, maternity and other benefits for their members, and some were in financial difficulty.[48] As far as the new government was concerned, the system was inefficient and uneconomic. The National Health Insurance Act, 1933 provided for the unification of all the societies over a three-year period into one national society, and the abolition of the National Health Insurance Commission. The National Insurance Commission was replaced in 1936 by the Unified Health Insurance Society under the chairmanship of the Bishop of Clonfert, Dr John Dignan. The Bishop, not noted for his views on social affairs, had been on good terms with the leaders of Fianna Fail since the days of the civil war.[49] As a result of increased employment and better enforcement of the Insurance Acts, membership of the Society rose rapidly, reaching 580,000 in 1937.[50]

Although Sean T. O Ceallaigh had supported medical benefit when in opposition, he did not introduce it as Minister in this Act. His strategy was to get the new society on a firm administrative and financial footing and then give consideration to the question of extending benefits. In 1938 he admitted that the government had been examining the possibility of paying medical benefit but he could not see how it could operate 'as long as we have the present poor law medical system in operation in the country'.[51] The old argument against medical benefit for the insured was still compelling. However, the Minister was continuing to examine a possible system of medical benefit, and in addition, a variety of other benefits.

The result of this examination was the National Health Insurance Act, 1941. This changed the actuarial basis of insurance from one based on reserve values, whereby a fund is built up to finance payment, to one based on 'pay-as-you-go' principles. The effect of this measure was to release about £175,000 annually for five years, for additional benefits. Dr Ward wanted the Society to extend *hospital* benefits, rather than what was traditionally understood as medical benefit. In his judgement, the 'fundamental defect ... in our national health insurance system, is the lack of (hospital) treatment.'[52] Many workers and their families were already entitled to medical benefit and there would be a net loss if dependants were not included in a national scheme. There was no strong demand for general practitioner medical benefit among the opposition.[53]

The removal of medical benefit as an issue reflects the very different concerns of the government thirty years after the introduction of health insurance. The problem now was to ensure that workers benefited from the newly extended hospital system. The government could have fallen back on the argument that had been used so effectively against the introduction of medical benefit, that if a worker needed hospital treatment he or she could apply for public assistance. That the government accepted the worker's right to have hospital benefit but not the right to general practitioner treatment can probably be explained by acceptance of the necessity of hospital treatment and of the desirability of encouraging those who could contribute towards the cost to do so through insurance. In Dublin, the insured worker requiring specialist treatment had no choice but to seek admission to a voluntary hospital and face what could be substantial bills. There were good political and social reasons why such workers should be encouraged to help themselves.

In 1942, the National Health Society announced that benefits would be extended to cover hospital treatment of insured persons, to operate from 1943.[54] The scheme was readily accepted by the local authority hospitals but a number of voluntary hospitals initially refused to accept patients under the scheme until the issue of fees to specialists was resolved.[55] The scheme suffered from serious defects. The most objectionable was that the benefit applied only so long as the Society had not exhausted its annual allowance for the benefit. Entitlement ceased as soon as the funds had been used. Secondly, the benefit covered the insured person only, not his family. There was a consensus that the scheme was unsatisfactory but no agreement on how hospital services ought to be provided for the insured population. The problem was linked to a wider one: how to provide hospital services for the large proportion of the population who were self employed — farmers, shopkeepers, tradesmen — and outside the insurance system, and who found the cost of hospital treatment an increasing burden.

Public Health

The government, in the guise of Dr Ward, was equally determined to improve the standard of public health. Thanks to the government's wish to create employment, considerable progress was made in providing modern water and sewerage schemes. The ten county councils who had refused to appoint county medical officers of health under the previous government were persuaded one by one to change their minds. In 1936, Clare, the last bastion of resistance, fell. There was now a network of trained public health doctors to implement the various public health schemes which previously had existed only in name. The Notification of Births Act, 1907, for example, was finally extended to the whole country, though not the more far-reaching provisions of the 1915 Act of the same name. New legislation on the sale of food and drugs and the slaughter of animals outlawed some of the worst abuses in food production and made the CMOs responsible for its implementation.[56] The number of children inspected at school medical examinations grew steadily from 85,500 in 1931 to 135,400 in 1939; this still represented less than 30 per cent of children attending national schools.[57] The reports of the CMOs highlighted the insanitary condition of many national schools, the problem of ensuring specialist treatment for defects found on examination and the extent of childhood problems associated with malnutrition and imbalanced diets.[58] The free milk scheme, which was supervised by the CMOs, was an important benefit to those families with young children who could not afford to buy adequate amounts of good milk. By 1940, the Department of Local Government and Public Health could point to a decline in the incidence of, and deaths from, most infectious diseases, although the rate of decline was not even and under war conditions threatened to rise again.[59] While this improvement was encouraging, other health problems showed little sign of diminishing, namely, tuberculosis and maternal and infant mortality.

Tuberculosis

By comparison with its active approach to other health issues, the government's attitude to tuberculosis in the 1930s was a mixture of complacency and despair. The death rate from tuberculosis in 1940, 1.25 per 1,000, was almost exactly the same as it had been in 1933.[60] From 1937 onwards, the death rate from the disease began to show an upward trend, isolating Ireland from most European countries where the rates were falling rapidly.[61]

The annual reports of the Department of Local Government and

Public Health in the early 1930s hid behind the official figures for the number of approved schemes, dispensaries and beds set aside for tuberculosis patients. The cosy picture was broken when the Hospitals Commission surveyed the beds actually in use: there were 3,164 beds officially approved for tuberculosis, but only 2,686 available.[62] On the basis of guidelines issued by the League of Nations which recommended as many beds as there were deaths from the disease, some 3,510 beds were required, making a shortfall of more than 1,000 beds.[63] The Commission pointed out that the Danes, with a death rate from tuberculosis that was half the Irish rate, had 1,000 beds more than their actual number of deaths. There were few hospital beds for non-pulmonary cases in the Free State.[64] Tuberculosis dispensaries, although charged with the task of diagnosing the disease, did not have x-ray equipment.[65] Most of the sanatoria could not treat the disease as they lacked modern surgical facilities and some buildings were most unsuitable. 'Rest, food and fresh air alone will not cure all tuberculosis', the Commission warned.[66] The sanatoria, designed for patients in the early stages of the disease, were filled with advanced, incurable cases.

The Commission proposed a plan to fight the disease, applying the yardstick of modern hospital planning to the problem. It recommended the provision of four regional sanatoria with a total of 2,181 beds and linked to chest hospitals.[67] But there was still no communal will to tackle the disease in a serious way and nothing came of the Commission's recommendations in the short term. The emphasis on hospital building in the 1930s, with the full support of the Commission, was on the provision of general hospitals with little attention to the need for special hospitals. The government's lack of activity was matched by a public who continued to view the disease as a matter to be concealed.[68] The Irish reluctance to notify the disease contrasted sharply with the English experience where in 1938 only nine per cent of deaths from the disease were not previously known to the medical officers of health.[69] James Dillon, a persistent campaigner in the Dail for improved tuberculosis services, put his finger on the cause of the government's impotence before the disease:

*it is one of these problems in respect of which a sort of universal
lethargy descends on us, not for the want of good will, but because
there does not seem to be anybody to kick up a row about it.*[70]

Maternal and Infant Mortality

More attention was paid during the 1930s to preventing avoidable
deaths of women in childbirth and of young children than in the
previous decade but action still fell short of what was required.
The strengthening of the legislation on midwives gave women
some protection from untrained handy women.[71] The
Registration of Maternity Homes Act, 1934 was introduced to
bring all homes under proper control and to ensure that the patients
received skilled treatment and that the health of babies was
protected. The maternal mortality rate showed a slight decline
from 4.44 deaths per thousand births in 1933 to 3.39 deaths in
1939.[72]

Dublin, however, experienced a lower death rate. In 1933, while
the national rate was 4.44, the rate in Dublin was only 0.86 per
thousand births.[73] The reason was that Dublin had three
maternity hospitals and the only extensive maternity and child
welfare scheme in the country. In Dublin many women used the
services provided by the hospitals and the local authorities, which
testified to women's willingness to seek medical advice during
pregnancy when available. Births in the three maternity hospitals,
as a percentage of total births in Dublin city and county, rose
from 39 to 48 per cent between 1933 and 1938.[74] Out-patient
attendances almost doubled from 32,000 to 60,400 in the same
period.[75]

The maternal and child welfare services outside Dublin were
far from satisfactory. Schemes had been put into effect in only
26 cities and towns and 5 county health districts.[76] Apart from
Dublin, the schemes consisted of little more than health visiting
before and after the birth. Few general practitioners at the time
had any training in antenatal care and hospital facilities throughout
the country for maternity were inadequate. The Minister accepted
the shortcomings of the maternity service and committed the local

authorities to provide accommodation for maternity cases in all new hospitals but in other respects official thinking still lagged behind that of Dr Coey Bigger's report for the Carnegie Trust in 1917.[77]

While the maternal mortality rate was falling slowly, infant mortality rates showed no improvement. At 66 deaths per thousand births in 1939, the rate was about the same as in 1930 and was 16 deaths higher than that for England and Wales.[78] The incidence of infant mortality showed a different pattern from that of maternal mortality, with the relative positions of town and country being reversed. Cities and towns continued to experience a much higher fatality than rural areas. The problem was particularly serious in Dublin. In 1941, 1,293 infants died in Dublin County Borough from a severe epidemic of gastroenteritis.[79] The death rate among infants would rise to 79 per 1,000 births in 1944 before anyone 'kicked up a row about it'.[80]

Administration

Two Acts introduced in 1939 and 1940 changed the administration of health services. The first, the Public Assistance Act, 1939, consolidated some 34 poor law statutes and transferred the public assistance functions of the boards of health and public assistance to the county councils. The Act codified the poor laws, a task left unfinished by earlier legislation. In this respect, it proposed no new ideas. The transfer of public assistance to the direct control of county councils was more far-reaching. It arose out of the government's increasing dissatisfaction with the committee system of local authorities. The slow deliberations of many boards of health and public assistance were contrasted unfavourably with the efficiency of the city management system. The County Management Act, 1940 transferred the remaining functions of the boards of health and all other subsidiary bodies to the county council and introduced the institution of county managers to Irish local government.

The passage of the County Management Act aroused the anger of opposition deputies because of a perceived threat to local democracy; more than one speaker compared the government proposals with the recent undermining of democracy in Germany and Italy. Deputy McGovern warned that 'it is only one step from county manager to national manager'.[81] Deputy Esmonde considered that the trend of legislation since he had come into the House had been towards a dictatorship by the executive of the county and the liberties of individual citizens were being undermined.[82] The proposed county managers were perceived as agents of the Minister and the Department, whose appointment would deprive local representatives of their traditional powers and local communities of personal attention.

The debate on the second stage revealed a fundamental difference of views between Fianna Fail and the opposition about the role of local government. Erskine Childers of Fianna Fail voiced an extreme view. He thought the local government machinery 'totally ineffective from a purely business like standard' and drew an unfavourable comparison between it and the management of a chain store with branches throughout the country.[83] For Deputy Broderick, on the other hand, local government was an essential ingredient of democracy where 'Public men learned restraint, moderation, and respect for one another's point of view. They learned what is really essential in the building up of a nation — how to administer their own affairs'.[84] He saw local authorities 'as in somewhat the position of the family life, which is the basis of spiritual life', and believed that the opinions formed there were the basis of the national opinion.[85] This clash, between the purely functional view of the role of the state which justified increasing central control and the view which emphasised the value of local autonomy and individual liberty over concern with efficiency and economy, foreshadowed a much more serious debate in the 1940s and early 1950s.

The Public Assistance Act, 1939 introduced important changes in the medical staffing of the county hospitals. From 1942 onwards, the county and borough councils were required to appoint a physician and resident medical officer to a county hospital in addition to the traditional surgeon.

133

The Dispensary Service

The dispensary service received little or no attention during the 1930s. Dispensaries were not included in the wide definition of 'hospital' in the Public Hospitals Act, 1933 and as a result could not be built or improved with sweepstake funds. The condition of many dispensaries remained primitive. If these conditions were tolerated in the days when the county hospital was little more than a workhouse, they were unacceptable by the standards of accommodation provided in the new county hospitals. In Dublin the dispensary system was breaking down. The city was expanding rapidly, but no more dispensary doctors were appointed nor were the districts reorganised to correspond with the movement of people to the new housing estates of Crumlin, Kimmage and Ballyfermot. Dublin dispensary doctors were responsible for the treatment of approximately 6,220 persons each.[86]

The Medical Profession

Relations between the medical profession and Dr Ward deteriorated throughout the 1930s and early 1940s. An active parliamentary secretary with egalitarian views and an abrasive personality was likely to antagonise the main interest group in the field. The medical staffs of the voluntary hospitals were alarmed at the increasing state interference in their affairs and the development of a hospital system outside Dublin which seemed to threaten their private practice. The dispensary doctors were aggrieved by the neglect of the dispensary service and in particular by the refusal to increase dispensary salaries. Many were annoyed by Dr Ward's handling of disciplinary cases. Dr Ward refused to turn the traditional blind eye to abuses by dispensary doctors and during his term of office a number were removed from office. A long running dispute with the Medical Association about fees for diphtheria immunisation caused much bad feeling on both sides. The county surgeons were riled by attempts by Dr Ward to limit their private practice and in some cases to remove it altogether. Nor was he averse to removing a county surgeon who abused his position.[87]

Dr Ward seems to have dealt with the medical profession in the same way as he and the Minister dealt with local authorities. He insisted on economy and value for money and if doctors did not live up to their responsibilities they were removed. His rough manner increased the profession's anger. It is significant that during the 1930s the profession dropped its earlier demand for a state medical service. In the days of unreformed local government, a state medical service offered doctors in public employment release from the tyranny of local representatives. In the 1930s a state medical service became less attractive because of the gains made during the 1920s in appointment, promotion and pension rights. Some doctors saw the appointment of full-time county medical officers as an encroachment on the work of private practitioners and perhaps as a model which the state might use to organise other areas of medicine.[88] Hospital doctors resented the claim by the Hospitals Commission that the state had a right to protect 'the people's hospital rights'.[89] A state-controlled medical service began to look decidedly menacing as the implications of an all-powerful Custom House became apparent. The profession began to look at ways to protect itself from any further state encroachment.

Conclusion

The main achievement of the years 1932-42 was the development of a modern general hospital service throughout much of the country. At the same time, the principles were established that the Minister had overall responsibility for the development of all hospital services and that if a hospital were to benefit from public funds, it had to cater for all classes. There were still many inadequacies in the county hospitals and little had been done to rationalise hospitals in Dublin but nonetheless it is possible to speak of a modern hospital system developing in these years. This progress was made possible by the proceeds of the Hospitals Sweepstakes and a commitment to provide hospital services for all on the part of the Fianna Fail government, the Department and the Hospitals Commission. The extension of hospital services raised vividly the

135

question of how those above the level of public assistance entitlement but unable to pay for hospital care for themselves and their dependants were to benefit from the new developments. The preoccupation with hospitals during these years, however, contrasts with the relative neglect of the dispensary service, tuberculosis and the health of mothers and children. By the early 1940s, these health problems demanded attention.

The improvements in health services achieved during this period were gained at the price of greatly increased control of local government activities, a large increase in central and local government expenditure and the resentment of powerful interest groups, most notably the voluntary hospitals and the medical profession. The concern expressed by Fine Gael deputies about increasing state interference and centralisation reflected a wider questioning of whether the price required for improved services was too high. The interest of principle and pocket overlapped in much of the criticism of government activity. The debate was to take on a wider ideological significance as Catholic social teaching began to permeate Irish society in the 1940s.

7
Towards a
National Health Service
1942~1945

IT IS A PARADOX that war-time should be a stimulant to the development of health services. Like the Great War and the War of Independence, 'the Emergency' during the Second World War was a dividing line in the development of health services. Firstly, there was a recognition that access to the health services would have to be widened and that the old code of medical relief was no longer adequate. Secondly, there was a great burst of administrative zeal directed at eliminating the black spots on the nation's health, tuberculosis, other infectious diseases and infant mortality, and at planning a comprehensive health service. The thrust of thinking and action on health services met opposition from predictable and unpredictable quarters, an opposition which would grow in significance by the end of the 1940s.

Ireland's neutrality in the Second World War protected the country from the worst effects of aggression but it did not prevent the population from experiencing shortages of fuel, raw materials, medical supplies and foodstuffs.[1] By 1942, there was acute deprivation among certain sections of the population. Rationing, food allowances and a cheap fuel scheme ensured fairer distribution of vital commodities. The hospital building programme was interrupted by the closure of the Hospitals Sweepstakes for the duration of the war and a scarcity of steel, timber, cement, mechanical appliances and fittings for sanitary and electrical plant.

Shortage of fuel had a serious effect on the public health service. County tuberculosis officers were only permitted to use as much petrol in a month as they had previously used in two days. The rationing of petrol to county medical officers and dispensary doctors was equally strict. District health nurses were forbidden to use motor cars, and the medical inspectors of the Department ceased to travel outside Dublin. As a result, there were reductions in the already inadequate tuberculosis service, medical inspection of school children and home visiting of pregnant women and mothers of young children. In 1943, one county medical officer said that the machinery for coping with tuberculosis had been immobilised for the previous four years.[2]

As the war lengthened and deprivation increased, the Department of Local Government and Public Health concentrated its efforts on controlling outbreaks of infectious diseases. While deaths from the main notifiable infectious diseases had declined from 687 in 1936 to 268 in 1941, the continuing residues of typhus, typhoid, diphtheria and other infections gave cause for alarm that epidemics would occur under war-time conditions.[3] Drastic powers to control such outbreaks of disease were considered necessary. Under the Emergency Powers (no.26) Order 1940, the Minister was given power to issue a warrant for the detection and isolation of any person considered to be a probable source of infection by a county medical officer. The Public Health (Infectious Diseases) Regulations, 1941 increased the number of notifiable infectious diseases and greatly strengthened the powers of medical officers dealing with infectious persons. In an outbreak of typhus, the medical officer was empowered to destroy lice on persons, their clothing and premises and to segregate and disinfect contacts. If a medical officer suspected that a person was a carrier of typhoid, diphtheria or dysentery, he could medically examine the person and prohibit his or her employment in any job dealing with food or drink. These were far-reaching powers but their introduction scarcely raised a murmur of opposition at the time, as the country became accustomed to the regimentation associated with the Emergency. The need for increased control could be justified by the sharp rise in the incidence of some infectious diseases and an increased number of deaths from 1942 onwards.[4]

138

The increase in deaths from tuberculosis was even more alarming. It was still not classified as an infectious disease and only notifiable in the advanced stage. Deaths from the disease had risen from 1.23 per thousand population in 1937, to 1.25 in 1940 and 1.46 in 1942.[5] The Department's chief adviser on tuberculosis, Dr E.J.T. McWeeney, put the blame on deficient nutrition, particularly among the working classes, the curtailment of services for sufferers of the disease, and lack of financial support for patients undergoing treatment.[6]

The movement of people in the other direction, from Ireland to Britain, gave rise to problems of a different sort. In 1943 the British government insisted that every immigrant from Ireland undergo a health inspection before being allowed to enter the country. The object was to control the body louse, indigenous to emigrants from the west of Ireland, and to prevent the spread of the two diseases associated with the louse: impetigo and typhus. The Irish government was given the choice of delousing the prospective emigrants before leaving Ireland or allowing the British do the job at the other side. Reluctantly, the government set up a health embarkation scheme whereby emigrants were examined and certified before leaving for Britain. Between 1943 and 1947, some 55,000 persons were examined in the special depots established in Dublin for the purpose.[7]

The examinations were carried out with little regard to individual dignity. An inspection of one of the depots left an abiding impression on Dr James Deeny.[8] He, Mr J. Hurson, the Secretary of the Department of Local Government and Public Health, Mr J. J. McElligott, the Secretary of the Department of Finance, and Mr R.C. Ferguson, the Secretary of the Department of Industry and Commerce, were invited to visit the Iveagh Baths where the male inspections were carried out. Sherry casks, half filled with water, occupied the emptied baths. In and around the sherry casks stood 100 to 150 naked men having their heads, under-arms and pubic areas washed, shaved and painted with a noxious blue dye by disinfectors in rubber aprons and wellington boots. In another part of the building, the men's hats and braces were ironed to ensure that no larvae survived. The sight and smell were so upsetting that one of the visiting party fainted and had to be carried from the building. It was a dehumanising experience for those who underwent the delousing and those who carried it out.

The embarkation inspections had at least two beneficial results. Blood samples taken from many of the emigrants showed that a large proportion had some previous contact with typhus and that it was therefore more common in the west of Ireland than had been suspected. Secondly, the visit to the Iveagh Baths made such an impression on the Secretary of the Department of Finance that the Department of Local Government and Public Health experienced little difficulty in securing approval to spend money on public health measures, including the manufacture and distribution of the chemical DDT, which destroyed lice, when its formula became known in 1945.[9]

Administration

During the war years, the centralisation policy of the Department of Local Government and Public Health quickened in pace. The appointment of county managers in 1942, the reduction in the size of county councils by a third and the introduction of new codes of procedure governing the activities of local authorities might have been expected to lead to heightened confidence by the Department in local authorities. But, as Desmond Roche comments, there was 'a substantial increase in the already formidable powers of central authorities in relation to local authorities, their staffs and services'.[10] The defensive attitude of some of the new managers to their responsibilities confirmed the suspicions of many local representatives that the new officers were agents of the Custom House.[11]

The appointment of Sean MacEntee, previously Minister for Finance, as Minister for Local Government and Public Health in 1942 signalled an intensification of the tough policy towards laggard local bodies. Mr MacEntee was a veteran of the war of independence, a founder member of Fianna Fail and had long experience of local government. A highly cultivated man, his skill in debate was legendary. He gave no quarter to opponents of government policy. When a deputy criticised him for his ruthless abolition of public bodies, he remarked: 'They (the local authorities) are getting their warning now. They will either do their job or get out.'[12] As far as Mr MacEntee was concerned a local authority existed 'for the purpose of ensuring that the affairs of the local community are administered with efficiency and integrity.'[13] During these years the Department came under increasing criticism in the Dail for its dictatorial methods, unhelpfulness and slowness to reach decisions. One diagnosis of the problem was that the Department was trying to carry out too many responsibilities, and there were calls for the establishment of a separate department of public health and social services.[14]

The Beveridge Report

It is difficult to judge the extent to which developments in Britain after independence influenced the direction of Irish affairs. There seems little doubt, however, that the report, *Social Insurance and Allied Services,* prepared by Sir William Beveridge and published in late 1942, had considerable influence on Irish public opinion.[15] Sir William's blend of radical proposals for comprehensive social insurance and a universal health service, with conservative views on the role of the state and the need for individual initiative and responsibility, appealed to Irish reformers and the report was widely read and discussed in Ireland.[16] Beveridge believed that comprehensive social insurance could only provide against loss of income, one of 'five giants on the road of reconstruction — the others are Disease, Ignorance, Squalor and Idleness'.[17] To combat disease he recommended a 'health service providing full preventive and curative treatment of every kind to every citizen without exceptions, without remuneration limit and without an economic barrier at any point to delay recourse to it'.[18] This health service could not be organised on insurance principles because medical need, not contribution conditions, should be the primary consideration in treatment, he believed. He also recommended that the health service be administered by a separate department. The report and the subsequent British White Paper, *A National Health*

Service, stimulated thinking about the health services in Ireland and made an impression on many influential people, including the Minister, Mr MacEntee.[19]

The Debate Opens

Sean MacEntee's conservative role in later Fianna Fail governments has overshadowed his radical contribution to the reorganisation of the health services in the 1940s. Convinced by Dr Ward's arguments for reform, influenced by the Beveridge Report and no doubt by his medical friends and aware of the political popularity of better health services, Mr MacEntee decided sometime in 1943 that the services should be improved as a matter of urgency, that a separate ministry was necessary and that the public health functions of local authorities should be divorced from their other activities. Mr MacEntee later claimed that the establishment of the Department of Health, against considerable opposition, was the achievement of his ministerial career of which he was most proud.[20]

The first step towards the establishment of a new ministry was taken on 4 January 1944 when the Cabinet agreed to delegate, by order, the functions of the Minister relating to health, public assistance and national insurance to Dr Ward, his parliamentary secretary. High on the list of the problems which the Minister proposed to tackle were better control of infectious diseases, infestation, venereal disease and tuberculosis; improved services for mothers and children; the provision of medical treatment of insured persons and their dependants; the building of new hospitals and improvement of St Kevin's Hospital, Dublin and the development of a good preventive health service.[21]

In June 1944, the government agreed to the introduction of a Public Health Bill which proposed stringent control of infectious persons, brought the treatment of tuberculosis and venereal disease under the same legislation as other infectious diseases and made the medical inspection of school children compulsory for every child.[22] The Bill was a tidying up exercise, designed to remedy the inadequacies in services highlighted by the war. The

Department did not expect the Bill to involve any charge on state funds 'beyond the cost of incidental printing'.[23] By November 1944, the Department had found 27 other items to include in the Bill, the most important being sections to incorporate and extend the maternity and child welfare provisions of the Notification of Births Act, 1915.[24] While the Bill itself contained little that was new, the delegation of health responsibilities to Dr Ward and the apparent zeal to tackle health problems on a wider front were both a response to general dissatisfaction with the health services and a stimulus to wider debate on the organisation of the services.

Catholic Social Teaching

Intellectual currents were stirring at this time which were to have great significance for the development of the health services. Chief among these was the growth in popularity in Ireland of Catholic social teaching. The lack of an informed social outlook among Irish Catholics in the early years of the century made this country unique among Catholic nations in Europe.[25] In the 1930s, however, an indigenous Catholic social movement took root in Ireland, a movement which attempted to apply the teachings of papal encyclicals to contemporary social and economic problems. The movement was part of a wider awakening in the society to the evils and injustices of poverty which received its political expression in the welfare policies of the first Fianna Fail government.

The Catholic movement in Ireland drew its inspiration from the papal encyclical, *Quadragesimo Anno,* published in 1931, written to advise Catholics how to order social priorities in a period of great economic upheaval in industrial societies and a loss of faith in democracy.[26] The encyclical advocated the organisation of society in vocational groups or corporations in which employers and workers would collaborate to further their common interest. Such an arrangement would provide an alternative to class conflict and allow the state to carry out its necessary tasks. The task of the state, as far as the Church was concerned, was to facilitate activity by other groups and persons within the community but

143

not to supersede these if they were working with reasonable effectiveness. This became known as the principle of subsidiarity.

In an encyclical of 1930 on Christian marriage, *Casti Connubii*, Pope Pius XI warned Catholics against divorce, contraception and abortion and outlined the Church's view on the role of the state vis a vis the family, teachings which were to receive powerful support in Ireland in the late 1940s and early 1950s.[27] The family, the Church taught, was the foundation of moral and social order. The state had an obligation to protect chastity, the indissolubility of marriage and promote an economic and social environment which would enable every head of a family to support his wife and children. If private resources were insufficient for the purpose, the state had an obligation to provide for the maintenance of the family. The encyclical underlined the duty of religious authorities to intervene to ensure that the moral order was preserved. The Church's teaching was humanitarian in conception and noble in objective. Few in Ireland would have disagreed with it in principle because the teaching coincided with Irish views on the minimalist role of the state in matters affecting the individual and the family. The problems arose when the principles were applied in practice to the problems of Irish society.

During the 1930s and 1940s, committed Catholics attempted to put the Church's views into practice. In 1933, the Minister for Local Government and Public Health, Mr S. T. O Ceallaigh, announced in Geneva that 'in no country was this inspiring pronouncement *(Quadragesimo Anno)* read and studied with greater eagerness than in Ireland'. He pledged that in 'the development of (the government's) programme of economic and political reform its work is founded on the same Catholic principles'.[28] Following representations from the Hierarchy, the government passed the Criminal Law (Amendment) Act, 1935 which banned the importation and sale of contraceptives. Similar concerns on the part of the bishops led to the Dance Hall Act, 1935, which was designed to protect the morals of young people by controlling the conduct of public dancing. More significantly, the Constitution of 1937, the creation of Eamon de Valera, reflected closely the Church's teaching on the role of the state, the family and Christian marriage and recognised the special position of the Catholic Church as the church of the majority. It eschewed, however, any fundamental reorganisation of society on the basis of vocational groupings. Mr de Valera, a devout Catholic and a man who equated Irishness with Catholicism, had a republican's suspicion of the influence of corporate interests, including the Church, in the political sphere. In drafting the new Constitution, he resisted the demands of some bishops and lay people to declare a confessional, Catholic state and by careful wording, skilfully avoided a political crisis between Church and state.[29] As far as the political and administrative organisation of society was concerned, he continued to adhere to the requirements of democratic centralism while aware of the dangers of over-centralisation.[30] He did, however, reluctantly agree to set up a commission to enquire into the application of vocational principles to Ireland.

The Catholic Hierarchy was enthusiastic about the new ideas.[31] By the early 1940s, a number of new and able bishops had been appointed who were deeply committed to restructuring Irish society according to Catholic principles. John Charles McQuaid was appointed Archbishop of Dublin in 1940. His appointment was out of the ordinary as he was not a member of the diocesan clergy but of a religious order. Dr McQuaid set about his new responsibilities with great energy and from the beginning showed his concern for the material as well as spiritual welfare of his diocese. He encouraged voluntary and communal organisations to help the poor and the sick, giving effect to the principles of Christian charity and reducing the need for state intervention. In 1942, he took the initiative to persuade some Catholic Dublin voluntary hospitals to open clinics for sufferers of venereal disease. He provided a site and organised the building of Our Lady's Hospital for Sick Children in Crumlin. A major achievement was the initiation of the Catholic Social Service Conference in April 1941. The Conference co-ordinated what had up to then been disparate activities by a number of groups into a relatively efficient organisation providing food and clothing for those in need. He considered the level of infant mortality in the city a reproach and by 1943 the Conference was catering for up to 900 mothers in

27 food and 14 pre-natal centres.[32] Doctors and nurses in some
voluntary hospitals responded to the Archbishop's concern by
giving lectures and talks to expectant mothers on maternal and
child health.[33] In 1942, he established the Catholic Social Welfare
Bureau to assist emigrants.

The son of a dispensary doctor, Dr McQuaid had close links
with the medical profession and, through a common association
with Blackrock College, was on good terms with Mr de Valera.
The Taoiseach had openly favoured Dr McQuaid's candidacy for
the post because of his social concern and leadership qualities.[34]
Because of the importance of the See of Dublin, and the strength
of his own personality and convictions, Dr McQuaid exercised
great influence over his fellow bishops. Concerned always to protect
his flock from influences which might undermine their faith, he
regarded the Protestant Trinity College with deep suspicion and
under his influence, the Hierarchy forbade Catholics to study there.
For the same reason, he opposed changes in society which would
interfere with the primacy of the family, the responsibilities of
parents, or the education of children in a Catholic ethos.

Dr Michael Browne was appointed Bishop of Galway in 1937.
An outspoken man of strong views, he had a pathological dislike
of civil servants and bureaucracy, matched only by his deep respect
for the professions, particularly the medical profession.[35] Dr
Browne was also on good terms with Mr de Valera and when
in 1939, he appointed the Commission to examine vocational
organisation, Dr Browne was offered the chairmanship.

The Commission devised the most comprehensive blueprint for
the re-ordering of society along Catholic principles.[36] Its massive
300,000-word report analysed the faults of Irish government and
recommended sweeping changes in the organisation of economic
and social life. The Commission expressed most concern about
the dangers of bureaucracy, a bureaucracy:

> which would control all spheres of social life and which is in danger
> of ignoring the subtler developments and needs of professional
> technique and service.[37]

The Commission was careful not to condemn state intervention when it was necessary for the good of the people, but reserved its censure for state control merely for administrative convenience or for its own sake. It pointed to the Department of Local Government and Public Health's refusal to meet deputations from the Irish Medical Association as evidence of bureaucratic attitudes in government.[38] It rejected civil service planning as both undemocratic and inefficient and warned of the danger of excessive centralisation and bureaucracy in the county management system. The members were also alarmed at the discretion given to ministers and departments to make legislation by statutory orders and regulations, and were of the opinion that politicians, bound to vote according to party loyalties, were unable to judge issues on their merits.

As an alternative to a highly centralised and bureaucratic society, the Commission recommended the setting up of a vocational assembly with a lower tier of vocational councils representing all the major interest groups to advise government on policy. They envisaged such councils for industry, agriculture, education, law, health and other sectors. The functions recommended for the Council of Health were to act as a consultative body to the Minister, examine and report to the Oireachtas on public health legislation, co-ordinate all agencies interested in health, plan for the long term development of the health services and examine how far existing services were provided at reasonable cost to persons of small or moderate means. It was to have its own secretariat and a director who would not be a civil servant.

The Commission drew its inspiration for vocational councils from the organisation of the professions, which were described as 'outstanding examples of self-regulation by a vocational body effected without expense to the taxpayer and yet safeguarding the rights of the state'.[39] The professions, unlike politicians, could discuss issues in a non-partisan way and in an atmosphere of 'objective knowledge and science'.[40] The Commission was particularly impressed by the organisation of the medical profession and by its role in society:

On the competence, skill and public spirit of doctors, the efficiency

147

of the service, and consequently the health and physical well-being of the community, largely depend.[41]

This admiration of the medical profession seems to have been the peculiar contribution of Dr Browne. He believed that medical doctors placed public above private interest, commenting at one stage that:

the medical profession has wonderful advantages in regard to wide social questions. They are in closer contact with life than many other professions. They have the confidence of the public, of the workers and of the employers. They are men of integrity and education ... and why should not these non-medical values be utilised in the service of the community?[42]

Given the Commission's deprecation of politicians and civil servants and its elevation of the role of what many might call vested interests, it is hardly surprising that the report received a frosty reception in government circles in 1943. Fianna Fail had just won their sixth general election in a row and were not inclined to hand over power to a vocational council, no matter how public spirited or attuned to Catholic social teaching. The report received a warmer welcome from the chief opposition party, Fine Gael which, since its flirtation with corporatist political ideas in the early 1930s, was sympathetic to proposals for vocational organisation. The Commission's recommendations also provided useful ammunition with which to attack an apparently impregnable government. The report was widely referred to in debates on social policy and used in arguments against further encroachments of the state in the sphere of family or individual liberty. The common interest, identified in the Report, between the medical profession and the Church in vocational organisation and limits on the power of bureaucracy and politicians, laid the foundations for an alliance which by the end of the 1940s challenged the efforts of politicians and civil servants to provide a comprehensive health service for the whole population.

There were other reasons why the Hierarchy might see an alliance with the medical profession as important. The bishops cannot have been unaware of the growing support amongst the members of the medical profession in Britain for contraception and even abortion in certain circumstances. In 1938, for example, in a celebrated case, a Dr Bourne terminated a pregnancy after rape in a fourteen-year-old girl and openly invited prosecution. Censorship of publications would protect the Irish public from knowing about such moral dangers but the best bulwark of defence in the long term was a medical profession imbued with Catholic values which would have nothing to do with such practices. The extent of the Hierarchy's fears of contraception is illustrated by one example. During the Easter meeting of the Hierarchy in 1944, the use of the new sanitary tampons, called 'Tampax', had been discussed and the bishops had strongly disapproved. The Archbishop of Dublin was instructed to contact Dr Ward to explain their misgivings that the tampons could harmfully stimulate girls at an impressionable age and lead to the use of contraceptives and whether he would take action to prohibit their sale. Dr Ward, sharing the bishops' misgivings, acceded to the request.[43] The revelations at the end of the war of medical experiments in Nazi Germany probably strengthened the belief in a firm ethical basis in medical training and practice. While some doctors shared the Hierarchy's views, others used the bishops' fears in later debates to argue that certain health proposals threatened the Church's teaching on sexuality and contraception and their influence over medical education.

The Dignan plan

The influence of Catholic social teaching and the Beveridge Report were evident in a report by Bishop John Dignan, the chairman of the National Health Insurance Society, which put the case for an overhaul of the existing health services.[44] These services were 'not noted for their Christian spirit, as they were materialistic in their conception and merely palliative in their results'.[45] In a Catholic country, the social services should be consonant with the Church's social principles, 'built on the strong foundations of Christianity and not on the shifting sands of "economics" '

149

and should not undermine a father's obligation to support his family.[46] The health services were unsatisfactory and inefficient and the standard of treatment provided for the public unacceptable in a Christian country in the twentieth century. He was particularly critical of the dispensary service which he described as 'the core, the hub and heart of the degrading Poor Law system' and considered that no lasting improvement could be made so long as a large proportion of the population depended on the dispensary doctor for medical relief.[47]

Dr Dignan's recommendations applied some old and some new ideas to the problems of the 1940s, expressed in the moral language of Catholic sociology. He proposed the removal of health services from the purview of local government altogether and the transfer of responsibility for the health of the people to a governing body under the National Health Insurance Society. Each member of the Society would be entitled to a full range of health benefits, with access based on right not on charity. A special minister for social services would represent the interest of the governing body at Cabinet but would have little scope for intervening with the autonomous powers of the governing body. All the hospitals in the country would be transferred to the extended insurance society, the dispensaries closed and replaced by health centres attached to each hospital.

Hospitals would be the 'central agency of cure and ... the axis around which the whole range of medical care must revolve'.[48] General practitioners employed in the health centres would be paid a salary or a combination of salary and fee or capitation with private practice 'maintained insofar as freedom of choice of doctor and hospital remains'.[49] With an enthusiasm which would have surprised his ecclesiastical predecessors, Dr Dignan advocated the extension of insurance to finance the new system. Insurance, in his view, fitted in best with Catholic teaching on the family's duty to look after its own needs and on the residual role of the state. His plan was an explicit alternative to a state-organised medical service.[50] Because of the Church's role as 'the greatest force in the country for the social uplifting of the people, and as its teaching of the Social Encyclicals is the foundation on which our social services should be built', he believed that the Church should be represented on the central and regional committees which would supervise the service.[51]

The government's response to Dr Dignan's plan was unreasonably hostile and tinged with the arrogance of thirteen uninterrupted years of political power. In a speech to a Fianna Fail meeting on 13 March 1945, the Minister, Sean MacEntee refused to argue on the issues raised in the plan but instead condemned Dr Dignan for publishing it without submitting it to him first and for exceeding his terms of reference as chairman of the Insurance Society.[52] When in August 1945, his term as chairman was up, Dr Dignan was replaced by a civil servant, D.J. O'Donovan. While the discomfiture of Dr Dignan at the hands of the Fianna Fail government may not have upset his fellow bishops unduly, the heavy-handed way in which his proposals were dismissed could be construed as a sign of the bureaucratic mentality and arrogance of central government.

It would not have been difficult to argue against the Dignan plan on its own terms. It provided no costings to show that the scheme was financially solvent. It avoided the question of how to deal with those who could not pay contributions by assuming that they would amount to only five per cent of the population. Nor did it pay more than passing reference to the problem of those who refused to pay contributions and whether they would be denied access to treatment. The plan preferred to assume a level of public-spiritedness which was not borne out by the operation of national health insurance in practice. By limiting the role of the Minister and excluding local representatives from the organisation of the new service, Dr Dignan may have been putting vocational principles into practice but he could be accused of being anti-democratic. Nor did he seem to be aware of the danger of creating a new bureaucracy around his central and regional committees.

Both the report of the Commission on Vocational Organisation and the Dignan plan could be criticised for a rather simplistic application of Catholic moral precepts to the Irish social situation. This lack of sophistication in thinking about social problems was partly a result of the novelty of any thought about social problems among Irish Catholics.[53] Their approach was characterised by another feature which was to have profound implications for the future debate on health services. The problem stemmed partly from a misunderstanding of the nature of moral principles. If the Church was bitterly opposed to the philosophies of scientism and marxist materialism, some of its Irish defenders made the same claims for the moral law as its opponents made for the laws of nature and of history. One of the characteristics of Irish Catholic moralists in the 1940s and 1950s was their assumption that the moral law was there for all to see and that it could be applied in only one way. On this assumption, the Hierarchy's claim to be the guardian of moral law in society was easily translated into a claim to be the arbiter of which social policy was acceptable by the criterion of the moral or social teaching of the Church. The overwhelmingly Catholic ethos of Irish life and the absence of competing native ideas on social issues meant that the Hierarchy's assumptions and claims went almost unchallenged.

Even if the Dignan plan seems naive, both in retrospect and by comparison with Beveridge's proposals, it was an important contribution to the debate on the future shape of the Irish health services. That such an influential person as Dr Dignan could condemn existing arrangements as inefficient, degrading and un-Christian made wider criticism of the health services legitimate. This dislike of criticism probably lay behind Mr MacEntee's sharp reprimand to the bishop to keep to his place. Secondly, the bishop articulated a new view of the health services, divorced from public assistance, with access by right not by charity, and first class treatment available to all in hospitals and closely associated health centres staffed by medical doctors who would be more employees than entrepreneurs. Finally, the Dignan plan helped stimulate thought in official circles as politicians responded to the growing desire for a different kind of health service.

The Shanley and Irish Medical Association Plans

The medical profession, aware of the demands for better health services, of the impact of the Beveridge report, and of the

152

preoccupation of their British colleagues with reform at this time, had also begun thinking of plans for reform. At the time that Dr Dignan was preparing his plan, Dr John Shanley, president of the Irish Medical Association between 1942 and 1944, was preparing a scheme on behalf of the profession. With initial experience as a poor law medical officer in Dublin, Dr Shanley had subsequently become one of the first doctors in the country to specialise in children's diseases and was in a position to see at first hand the damage caused to children by deprivation and poor health services. He had been closely associated with the Hospitals Sweepstakes and with the amalgamation of the former Irish Medical Association and the branches of the British Medical Association in Ireland into a single Irish-based Association in 1936. As an added bonus, Dr Shanley, an influential member of Fianna Fail, was on good terms with Mr MacEntee and Dr Ward.[54]

During his terms as president, Dr Shanley stressed the urgent need for the profession to recognise the social changes that were taking place in society and to plan for the future. He believed that the comprehensive health service advocated in the Beveridge Report was impracticable in Ireland for financial reasons but was convinced of the need to provide free medical attendance for all those 'for whom serious and prolonged illness carried not alone jeopardy to life but also a load of debt which may take years to liquidate or lead to bankruptcy'.[55] During his presidency a committee was appointed to inquire into the reorganisation of medical services but could not agree to Dr Shanley's proposals for reform. Going over the heads of the committee, Dr Shanley published his plan in the Association's *Journal* in April 1944.[56] He recommended the appointment of a Minister for Health assisted by a medical council, which would have wide executive powers over the services and be subject only to the overriding control of the Minister in matters of major policy. All association with local government and public assistance at local level would be broken and the country divided into four regions for health purposes to be administered by regional councils. Most radical of all was his proposal that all persons with incomes below £550 and their dependants should be entitled to 'a complete and efficient medical service, including consultant, specialist and hospital treatment free of at least direct payment'.[57] The service would be financed from a combination of central funds, local rates, and insurance contributions. The dispensary system would continue but with much improved facilities, working conditions and salaries. Doctors would be paid a capitation rate of £1 for treating persons with incomes below £550. He advocated group practice, health clinics, a choice of doctor and the continuing independence of the voluntary hospitals. Finally, he called for improved services to fight tuberculosis and for the development of child welfare and school medical services.

Dr Shanley's plan aroused considerable reaction in the profession. He was criticised by dispensary doctors for advocating the continuation of the dispensary system and by private practitioners for suggesting a panel system which they claimed was 'inherently bad for the patient and the doctor' and 'not suitable to this country'.[58] The private practitioners were particularly insistent that maternity could not be included in the services for persons with incomes up to £550.[59]

The 'official' scheme produced by the Medical Association in December 1944 showed all the signs of a compromise between different medical interests at the expense of a workable scheme.[60] The scheme adopted Dr Shanley's proposals for a ministry of health and executive medical council and regional councils but rejected his notion of a comprehensive medical service without charge to persons ineligible for medical relief but with incomes below £550. In its place, the Association proposed a system based on the dispensary system and insurance for those with incomes not exceeding £400. Insurance for those in employment would be compulsory. In Dublin, where the dispensary system had broken down, the contributions of the unemployed would be paid 'by the city purse'.[61] It recommended substantial increases in dispensary salaries and a capitation rate of 50s for each insured patient on the doctor's list, to cover all aspects of the patient's care including the payment of specialists. Maternity services were specifically excluded from the scope of the proposed service.

The Medical Association scheme did not get a good press. The

154

Irish Press thought that the proposals were 'likely to be regarded as claims put forward on behalf of the profession rather than as a scheme for the reorganisation of the medical services'.[62] A medical correspondent in *The Irish Times* described the proposals as being of a 'very definitely pre-Beveridge vintage'.[63] The proposals were compared unfavourably with the radical alternatives of Beveridge and Dignan.[64] If Dr Dignan sought to overhaul the system, it seems that the profession was building defences against any radical change. Irish doctors, no less than their British and American counterparts at this time, were more eager 'to insure doctors against patients' inability to pay rather than insure patients against the high cost of medical services'.[65]

The two schemes had similarities. Both were critical of the bureaucratic nature of the health services and expressed a profound distrust of the role of the Minister, the Department and the local authorities. Both advocated reorganisation along vocational lines. They agreed that insurance was an inherently better way of financing health services than the rates or taxation.

Official Proposals

By late 1944, there were three schemes for overhauling the health services on the table, legal responsibility for health policy had been assigned to the parliamentary secretary and a Health Bill had been drafted as the first stage in a still undefined official commitment to reorganise the health services. It was at this auspicious moment that the Department recruited a new chief medical officer, Dr James Deeny, whose ideas were to make a fundamental contribution to the future direction of health policy. Dr Deeny's appointment was out of the ordinary. The post of chief medical officer normally passed to the most senior medical officer in the Department but when the vacancy arose on this occasion, Dr Ward refused to appoint any of the serving officers and decided that the post should be filled by open competition. Dr Deeny, a general practitioner in Lurgan, Northern Ireland, applied for the post. With several higher degrees to his credit, an impressive record of research and publications on socio-medical problems including infant mortality and tuberculosis, he had also made discoveries in nutrition, in particular about the effects of vitamin C deficiency. His clinical and research experience marked him out from all other candidates for the job, and the interview board, chaired by Dr Shanley, had no hesitation in recommending him for appointment, even though he had no administrative experience. He took up duty in September 1944.

Dr Deeny had, by all accounts, an electrifying effect on the Department, throwing out ideas in the way a generating plant discharges current.[66] Aged 38, he was full of energy and zeal for reform. He soon established a close working relationship with Dr Ward, who in later years described him as a genius and the decision to employ him as one of the best things the government ever did.[67] Like all men of ideas, not all of his suggestions were equally practical. Dr Deeny was lucky in his early years as medical adviser to enjoy the support of seasoned civil servants, such as Thomas McArdle and John Garvin, who were prepared to sift the practical from the impractical and translate raw ideas into administrative and legal formulae.

Shortly after his appointment, Mr MacEntee and Dr Ward took the important step of setting up a departmental committee to examine the public medical services, report on trends in other countries, assess the Dignan plan and the Medical Association scheme and put forward official proposals for reform. The members of the committee were James Deeny, John Collins, an authority on local government, John Garvin, principal officer in charge of public assistance services, P.J. Keady, the Department's expert on insurance, and Desmond Roche, a young officer of the Department, was appointed the secretary. All were outstanding civil servants and their report reflects the calibre of its authors.[68]

It is worthwhile examining the *Report of the Departmental Committee on Health Services,* which has never been discussed in public, because of the far-reaching influence of its recommendations and because its proposals are at the root of later controversies. The committee first examined medical services in other countries, emphasising that in each country examined the medical services were undergoing change. This was followed by a lengthy and devastating analysis of the Dignan and Medical Association plans.[69] A major objection raised to the Dignan plan was that while it was described as a scheme of national health insurance, only half the population would be compulsorily insured. If insurance principles were to operate, those who refused to insure voluntarily would have to be denied medical attention as a right. There would have to be some form of means test to establish whether the person was one of the poor and destitute which Dr Dignan proposed could be treated free under the plan. Yet Dr Dignan's plan was supposed to avoid means tests of this kind. And if some people received medical treatment according to need and not contributions, the insurance structure, the committee argued, fell to the ground and the contributions became a form of income tax. They could see no good reason 'for forcing the greater part of the citizens of the State into a tax collecting association independent of the State'.[70]

The committee pointed out that the doctors' scheme proposed a system of health insurance for a large section of the population, without any reference to how it would link into existing insurance arrangements. They suggested that it was about changes in the way general practitioners were paid for work they were already doing.

The core of the report is the committee's own ideas for a reorganised medical service, which was written by Dr Deeny.[71] The committee's proposals were based on the premises that the health services required reorganisation and that changes must be suited to the particular conditions of the country. An uprooting of existing services was rejected as 'wholly unnecessary and almost unthinkable'.[72] Four objectives were identified; the integration of all medical services; the promotion of the health of the individual, the family and the community; the encouragement of the idea of the 'family doctor'; and the availability of specialist and hospital services to the ordinary public.

These objectives were to be achieved by the reorganisation of services into county and regional services. The distinction between public assistance and public health services would be removed. The county would be responsible for the family medical services, while hospitals and specialist services would be organised in three region based in Dublin, Cork and Galway. The family medical service would be provided in each county by district medical officers assisted by a nurse and a midwife, who would look after 700 t 1,000 households. High on the list of the duties of the medica officers would be the provision of ante-natal and maternity services the welfare of infants and children under school age, schoo inspections, an annual medical survey of the members of eacl family, health education and the investigation of matters relating to health within their areas. The effect would be to integrate 'general practitioner, maternity, child health, and public healtl ... into a unified machine providing complete local family care with special emphasis on child health, maternal care, the contro of social and environmental causes of illness and the promotior of good health', while at the same time preserving 'a maximum amount of decentralisation'.[73] The CMOs would cease to carry out clinical work but would instead supervise the work of the district medical officers.

The committee accepted that different arrangements would have to be made for Dublin, where the doctor/patient relationship did not exist to the same extent as elsewhere in Ireland. They proposed a series of health centres around the city which would provide medical services comparable to those provided in hospital out-patient departments but which would also accommodate the tuberculosis, school, maternity and child services. The clinics would be staffed by public health officers, general practitioners and junior staff from the voluntary hospitals. Each clinic would be closely linked to a parent hospital. It recommended that the three maternity hospitals be responsible for ante-natal care of mothers and the care of infants for the first nine months, sessions being held in the health centres.

On eligibility for the services, the group was equally radical: 'the proposed free and extended medical services should be available to the whole population':[74]

> The ideal to be aimed at is a national health service embracing all classes within its scope, recognising no limitation of effectiveness on mere economic grounds, and treating the people, from the health point of view, as a unit.[75]

They thought such a scheme would attract public support, despite its high cost. The committee did not recommend an immediate provision of a free service because of the problem of integrating national health insurance into the new scheme and the cost. It therefore proposed the introduction of a free service on a phased basis. In the first phase, the services would be provided for an enlarged insurance class, farmers on land below a certain valuation and persons currently eligible for medical relief, giving a total of about two million people. During the second phase, eligibility would be extended to specially designated classes, such as children and tuberculosis sufferers. Finally, the service would be opened to the whole population.

The committee estimated that about 1,000 general practitioners would be required as district medical officers to provide the family doctor service for the whole population. The first phase would require about 750 doctors or 100 more than the existing complement of dispensary doctors. The cost of the entire programme was estimated at £7.5 million, a doubling of the cost of services in 1944, with the initial extension of services costing £1.75 million. The expenditure would be met from state grants, insurance contributions and rates, with the bulk of the increased expenditure coming from general taxation.

The departmental committee's recommendations were radical by any standards. They are all the more surprising given the status of their authors. Deeny, Garvin, Collins and Keady were not in the position of Beveridge, independent of the system and free to toss ideas into the political and administrative court. The latter three were senior civil servants, cautious by training and working in an environment suspicious of new ideas. The fact that they agreed with Dr Deeny's prescription for the future direction of the services indicates the logic of those proposals and their apparent feasibility. All were practising Catholics and did not at any time view their proposals as contravening Catholic social teaching or as akin to socialised medicine.[76] On the contrary, Dr Deeny's model for the relationship of district and county medical officers had been inspired by the role played in ecclesiastical organisation by priests and bishops.[77] From the official vantage point, the

159

committee's recommendations seemed to be the best means of meeting the demand for improved health services in a way that built on existing structures. They submitted their report in September 1945.

The implications of the recommendations for the medical profession were far-reaching. The majority of all general practitioners would eventually be employed as district medical officers and specialists would be employed by public or voluntary hospitals, and private fees would be eliminated. The district medical officer would be paid a salary or a mixture of salary and capitation. As the public health officer for the district, his or her work would be supervised by the county medical officer of health. The work of the voluntary hospitals would be co-ordinated through the regional authorities and 'the entire machinery, regional and local, will be under the control of a Minister for Public Health'.[78] No concessions were made to the profession's demand for much greater say in the running of the services. In short, the proposals of the departmental committee posed a more fundamental threat to the profession than Lloyd George's insurance scheme in 1911. The Department's intentions took some time to percolate through to the profession but when they did, the reaction was intense.

Dr Ward, who had taken a close interest in the work of the committee, was very pleased with its report. It gave him a blueprint for the way forward and a means of realising his political ambitions.[79] The impact of the report was reinforced by long discussions with Dr Deeny about his ideas for reform.[80] As a parliamentary secretary, Dr Ward could not win the support of the Cabinet for his plans directly. He had to work through Mr MacEntee who, to judge from the memoranda prepared at this time, agreed with the report's recommendations.[81] Less discreetly, Dr Ward maintained pressure for change by briefing journalists about proposed developments in the health services, a habit which alarmed Mr de Valera and which in retrospect may have weakened his confidence in the parliamentary secretary and his proposals for reform. Within the Department, John Garvin was most closely associated with the translation of the departmental committee's recommendations into memoranda and legislative proposals for decision by government.

Dr Ward's wish to publish the committee's report was thwarted by the Department of Finance, on the grounds of its financial implications.[82] It was agreed instead that the Department of Local Government and Public Health would submit proposals for the reform of the health services in the form of a draft White Paper. Drafting began immediately.

Tuberculosis

A campaign to combat tuberculosis gradually gathered momentum in the early 1940s. Professor Theo Dillon highlighted Ireland's poor performance in combating the disease by international standards; and he identified manual workers, the unemployed and their dependants as the main victims of the disease. He outlined the main steps required to control the disease and quantified the sanatoria and dispensary facilities necessary for effective diagnosis and treatment. James Dillon, Professor Dillon's brother, used his position to challenge the apathy of government on the issue. The Royal Irish Academy of Medicine, the most respected medical body in the country, formulated a plan to combat the disease in 1942.[83]

A number of influential people, among whom were Dr Robert Rowlette, Dr W.R.F. Collis, Dr Dorothy Price, Judge W.E. Wiley and Professor Dillon, felt that it was necessary to mobilise public opinion if the disease was to be fought successfully. In November 1942, the formation of the National Anti-Tuberculosis League was announced. The object of the League was to unite all classes of society in a nation-wide campaign against the disease and to enlist the support of other social service agencies. Membership would be open to all citizens, medical and lay.

Efforts to form the League met, however, with opposition from an unexpected quarter. A public meeting to inaugurate it was held on 15 February 1943 with Dr Rowlette in the chair. Before the proceedings had gone very far, Monsignor Daniel Moloney, a priest of the Dublin diocese, stood up and read a letter from Dr McQuaid, Archbishop of Dublin, in which he gave it as his 'definite' opinion that the campaign should be carried out not by the proposed League but by the Irish Red Cross.[84] This was followed by interjections from Dr Conor Maguire and Dr Shanley, the Chairman and Secretary of the Red Cross, respectively, supporting the Archbishop's position.[85] The organisers of the meeting, who had not been informed of the Archbishop's views in advance, were dismayed and the meeting ended in uncertainty. The Archbishop's intervention made it extremely difficult for Catholics to participate in the League and a few weeks later it was announced that the still-born League would merge with the Irish Red Cross Society.

This episode illustrates the kind of power the Archbishop could exercise on issues not directly related to his spiritual responsibilities, the way in which he chose to exercise that power and the ready compliance with his wishes. Why, one might well ask, should the Archbishop be suspicious of the efforts of well intentioned people to fight tuberculosis? In an interview with John Whyte many years later, Archbishop McQuaid disclaimed any wish to put pressure on anyone and maintained that he merely wished to express his objections to what was proposed.[86] Dr John Shanley informed this writer that Dr McQuaid had approached the Red Cross prior to the meeting asking for their support. Dr Shanley suggested that Dr McQuaid was motivated by a desire to control social initiatives in Dublin and was alarmed by the Protestant flavour of the leadership of the proposed league. The Archbishop clearly thought that such a crusade would be safer in the predominantly Catholic hands of the Red Cross.

By the end of 1944, the universal lethargy towards the disease, of which James Dillon had complained in 1942, seemed to be lifting. The government had before it proposals from the Royal Irish Academy of Medicine, the Hospitals Commission and the Irish Red Cross which differed only in detail in their prescriptions for reform. Common themes were the need for early detection, segregation of infectious patients, large sanatoria with up-to-date surgical facilities, and financial assistance for patients while undergoing treatment for the disease. But these ideas had not yet been translated into a programme backed by government authority and finance.

It was Dr Deeny's arrival in the Department that precipitated a break-through. At a meeting with a deputation of concerned doctors in early 1945, Dr Deeny publicly committed the government to producing a plan to combat the disease.[87] Within a short space of time Dr Deeny had drafted a plan for the parliamentary secretary's approval. Dr Ward, however he might deplore his chief medical adviser stealing the initiative, was sensitive to the need for action. The plan was quickly approved by the government and facilitating legislation introduced by March 1945. The plan was published in 1946 as the White Paper, *Tuberculosis*.[88]

The White Paper set out the aims of the proposed reorganisation of the tuberculosis service: to apply modern methods of detection and to ensure that every person who developed the disease would receive first class treatment in a sanatorium. Three new sanatoria would be provided, one with 1,000 beds in Dublin, one with 700 beds in Cork and one with 400 beds in Galway, each providing a service for the surrounding counties. Each sanatorium would have a surgical hospital staffed by thoracic surgeons and provide advanced radiotherapy, physiotherapy and treatment for tubercular infections of eye, ear, nose and throat. Patients with tuberculosis would no longer be treated in general hospitals. Patients referred to a sanatorium would receive an allowance towards the cost of maintaining themselves and their families while undergoing treatment. A mass radiographic unit was to be set up in Dublin to screen vulnerable groups; and tuberculosis dispensaries around the country were to be equipped with up-to-date diagnostic facilities.

The Tuberculosis (Establishment of Sanatoria) Act, 1945 gave the Minister power to acquire land and build new sanatoria directly, that is without waiting for local authorities to act. The cost of the new sanatoria, estimated at £2 million, was to be met from the Hospitals Trust Fund and when completed, the institutions would be transferred to local authorities who would be responsible for their maintenance and management. A special section was set up within the Department to plan and build the sanatoria. County medical and tuberculosis officers were sent to Scandinavia, the United States, Canada and Britain to study the latest methods of detection and treatment. Significantly, the Minister and Dr Ward

163

accepted the recommendation of the Departmental Committee on Health Services that treatment in the new sanatoria should be free to everyone, irrespective of income.[89]

This rigorous approach to the problem, committing the political and administrative will to a well defined programme of action, laid the foundations for the comprehensive and successful attack on the disease of the next few years. The decision to invest so heavily in sanatoria was criticised later as misguided, since chemotherapy would soon make prolonged institutional care for most forms of tuberculosis unnecessary. At the time these plans were made, however, it was not known that drugs would soon revolutionise the treatment of the disease. In October 1946, the United States government, through the good offices of a member of the embassy staff in Dublin, made a limited amount of streptomycin available to the Irish authorities. The drug was extremely expensive because it was not yet artificially produced. Still at the experimental stage, it was not clear that the drug would remove the need for a large increase in sanatorium accommodation. On the contrary, the group of patients who were in most danger and who posed the greatest threat to their relatives, those in the advanced stage of pulmonary tuberculosis, would benefit least from the new drug. It was as urgent as ever to segregate those patients to prevent infection spreading and to offer chest surgery to improve their chances of survival. Whether the sanatoria needed to be of such imposing and durable structure is, of course, another matter.

Conclusion

The Emergency years have been described as a watershed in the social and cultural development of the country.[90] The war helped to loosen old bonds and ways of thinking. The widespread rejection of rural life and high levels of emigration, particularly among young women, which became very noticeable during the early 1940s, are signs of a loosening of social ties and loyalties. One reason suggested for this movement is a rejection of the rural ideal to which so many Irish leaders subscribed and a dissatisfaction with the lack of material progress since independence. There was, as this chapter has indicated, widespread dissatisfaction with the health services during this period and a willingness to contemplate different and better ways of doing things. The principles of Catholic social teaching, the ideas of Sir William Beveridge and a more scientific analysis of health problems generated ideas for reform. The result was a rush of proposals for a reorganised health service, comparable only to the outburst of ideas for reforming medical relief between 1906 and 1911.

The *Report of the Departmental Committee on Health Services*, probably the most radical document ever produced on the Irish health services, put forward the goal of a free national health service for all those who wished to avail of it. The link between health services and public assistance would be broken, emphasis would be placed on the maintenance of health, and public expenditure on health services would be doubled in real terms. The proposals would have required a fundamental change in the relationship of the medical profession to the state; private medicine would have become a peripheral activity. Such proposals were bound to be resisted. It remained to be seen whether the Cabinet would agree in detail to the Department's blueprint for reform.

The same rigorous approach characterised the Department's response to the growing demand for measures to counteract the ravages of tuberculosis. The plan of action, the result of a consensus which had been maturing for a number of years, did not disturb any vested interests but simply required the political will to put it into action. Although some might protest that free treatment in sanatoria without regard to means infringed the principle that the state should only support the family where necessary, the argument carried little weight since most sufferers were needy.[91]

If the attempt to apply Catholic social teaching to Irish conditions stimulated thought on social issues and led to demands for more humane services, it also served to emphasise the rights of the individual, the family and the Church in society as against the right of the state to act in the common good. These rights would increasingly be used as yardsticks to judge proposals from the Custom House and to condemn them as contrary to Catholic social, and even moral, teaching. The attempt to form the Anti-Tuberculosis League demonstrated how defensive the Archbishop of Dublin could be on an issue which barely touched on matters of faith and morals. One of the other significant effects of the growth of Catholic social thinking and of changing attitudes to reproduction and abortion in other countries was the opening it gave to an alliance of interests between the Church and the Irish medical profession. The bishops and the profession shared other grounds for common cause. Both feared autocratic bureaucracy, meddlesome politicians and ambitious civil service planners.

8
Drawing the Battle Lines
1945~1948

THE DEPARTMENT OF Local Government and Public Health had a coherent and radical blueprint for the reform of the health services by the end of 1945. This included a long term strategy to provide a free health service and short term priorities to improve the treatment of tuberculosis and other specialist conditions and to protect the health of mothers and children. The challenge was to persuade the government and the medical profession to follow the road charted by the Department.

Mr MacEntee and Dr Ward pursued the campaign on two fronts. At Cabinet level, the Minister pushed for a government decision on the proposals of the Departmental Committee on Health Services.[1] He won agreement to the publication of a White Paper. In a major breakthrough in January 1946, Mr de Valera committed the government to the establishment of two new and separate departments of health and social welfare in response to 'a very strong public demand'.[2] Meanwhile, Dr Ward proceeded with the Public Health Bill which had been lying around the Department since 1944. What had originally been intended as a Bill to tighten up the law on infectious diseases had by late 1945 become a catch-all measure of over a hundred sections. Since the Bill aroused intense controversy, it is worth examining in some detail what it proposed.

167

Public Health Bill, 1945

The core of the Bill remained the measures to deal with infectious diseases which strengthened and consolidated the Public Health Acts, 1878-1931.[3] This code for controlling infectious diseases in Part IV of the Bill proved to be the most contentious. Unlike earlier legislation, a means was provided for the enforcement of sanitary laws by calling in the Garda Siochana (police) if necessary. Tuberculosis and venereal disease, which had not been previously classified as infectious diseases, were included in the new code. Responsibility for dealing with all infectious diseases was transferred from the sanitary authorities to the county and county boroughs. New measures were introduced to prevent the spread of infectious diseases: a person who was infectious or in charge of an infectious person was obliged to take precautions to prevent others from being infected; parents of infectious or verminous children were required to keep them away from schools, places of public worship, theatres, concert halls and cinemas; and doctors treating infectious children were obliged to notify the district medical officer. The power to arrest and detain a person who was a probable source of infection, which had been exercised under the Emergency Powers Order, 1940, was incorporated in the Bill. A person who caught an infectious disease from the failure of another person to take precautions was given the right to take an action for damages in court. More positively, the Bill provided for the payment by local authorities of maintenance allowances to persons undergoing treatment for an infectious disease if they were unable to maintain themselves or their dependants. The sections on food and drink were designed to prevent manufacturers making nutritive claims for products which were not true and to improve the general nutritive value of food.

A number of significant proposals on mothers and children were included in the miscellaneous sections of the Bill. The Bill as introduced repealed previous legislation on the welfare of mothers and children and medical inspection of school children. County and county boroughs were empowered to provide maternity and child health services and to inspect medically all school children up to sixteen years. The services would be provided free of charge. Mothers were given a choice whether or not to use the local authority services but parents were obliged to submit their children for medical inspection at school. The aim was to:

> coordinate the maternity and child welfare schemes into a unified free service, which will give continuous care to the mother and child during the ante-natal period, during birth, and until the child reaches the age of 16 years.[4]

Local authorities were given explicit power to educate mothers and children in matters relating to health, a function implicit in the maternity and child welfare provisions of the Notification of Births Act, 1915. At the committee stage, the parliamentary secretary moved an amendment to give local authorities wide powers to provide services for expectant mothers, including health education. Furthermore, the Minister took power to ensure that county authorities carried out their responsibilities.

John Whyte's assessment of the Bill is that in it the 'bureaucratic, centralising traditions of the Department of Local Government and Public Health had passed all bounds'.[5] He could not find in the literature on comparative health services any comparable provisions in which compulsion was stressed so much as in the Public Health Bill, 1945. The measures were certainly severe but the Department could argue that the situation warranted them. Most European countries had passed the stage when compulsory detention of infectious persons or inspection of school children were necessary. Ireland was the last country in Western Europe where louse-born typhus was endemic; it was at this time known as 'the Irish disease'. The health embarkation scheme had shown that lice infestation was common among adults and the school medical inspectors' reports said that infestation was the norm among national-school children. A serious outbreak of typhus was a constant fear among health officials. A memorandum to the government in 1944 expressed alarm at the rise in venereal disease, particularly among married people and called for much more radical measures to deal with the situation.[6] Many prostitutes refused to accept treatment for venereal disease and continued to spread infection. The powers of arrest and detention in the Bill were primarily aimed at such women and at tinkers, who were suspected of being primary sources of typhus infection. It is perhaps significant that the Irish Medical Association approved of these measures and the Bill in general, though they had not been consulted.[7] And contemporaneously, the same parliamentary secretary and Department had been responsible for one of the most enlightened mental treatment measures of its time, the Mental Treatment Act, 1945. The Act made it much more difficult to detain a mental patient for treatment against his or her will and made it possible for patients to seek treatment voluntarily in district mental hospitals.

The opposition the Bill aroused can perhaps be better understood by taking a longer view of Irish health legislation. When the Public Health Act was passed in 1878, Irish parliamentary representatives were not in a position to influence it one way or another. When attempts were made in 1908 and 1913 to make tuberculosis a notifiable disease, Irish members of parliament were able to prevent the legislation being given any teeth. The Public Health Bill, 1945 was the first attempt under the new state to tackle the legal basis for preventing disease. Many of Fine Gael's objections to the measure were similar to those raised by the Irish Party to attempts to make tuberculosis a notifiable disease a generation before. What was different about the 1940s was that the dimension of Catholic social teaching had been added to the cultural dislike of regimentation and a native government which accepted the Catholic Hierarchy's authority to pronounce on the direction of social policies. Furthermore, the Department, after twenty years of tightening control over local authorities and fired by a new enthusiasm to improve the health of the nation, was vulnerable to charges of excessive centralisation and bureaucratic zeal. The ending of the war brought a reaction against the strict regime of the Emergency and revulsion at totalitarian Nazi government as its excesses became public.

It could also be argued that the draconian powers over infective persons proposed in the Bill were obsolete. Isolation and detention were the tried and trusted means of protecting the public health in the days before antibiotics and DDT. It was the parliamentary secretary's bad luck that he was pushing measures conceived during the nineteenth century and refined during the Emergency at a time when new forms of treatment were becoming available which would make isolation and detention unnecessary for the vast majority of cases. But this is to argue with the benefit of hindsight since the effectiveness of DDT and antibiotics at the end of 1945 was not guaranteed and most antibiotics were prohibitively expensive.

Dr Ward's second-stage speech on the Bill in November reflected the new ideas sweeping through the Department. Since good health meant 'much more than mere freedom of disease', it was necessary to use new methods to 'improve the general well-being of the people and their power of resistance to disease' and promote an 'equable (sic) balance between the spiritual and material aspects of life'.[8] He considered that the most important measure in the large Bill was the provision for maternity and child health services. The service for mothers and infants would be provided by the family doctor, who outside Dublin would be the dispensary doctor, retitled the district medical officer, assisted by the dispensary midwife.[9] A consultant obstetrical service would gradually be made available to all women. He defended compulsory school medical examinations on the grounds that the clean, healthy child should not be subject to 'the constant risk and danger of disease because of the carelessness and prejudices of the inconsiderate few'.[10] District medical officers would undertake medical inspection of school children and trained nurses would follow up cases and educate children in a healthy way of life. Specialist medical services would be eventually provided for all children.

The Fine Gael opposition to the Bill was immediate and violent. General Mulcahy accused the parliamentary secretary of introducing a kind of 'medical constabulary' and an 'unprecedented series of attacks on public liberty, (and) on local authorities'.[11] At this stage, the proposed mother and child services were not a point of contention. Fine Gael speakers objected to the sections on infectious diseases, especially those which forbade parents sending infectious or verminous children to school or church. General

Mulcahy could not understand how the Minister could pass a law
'that a child should not be allowed to go to Mass because it has
nits in its hair'.[12] He thought Dr Ward was presumptuous in
referring to a balance between the spiritual and material aspects
of life when the spiritual authorities had not even been consulted
on the Bill. Furthermore, the sections of the Bill dealing with
compulsory medical inspection of school children interfered with
the fundamental rights of parents and was an intrusion in the
rightful sphere of the family. Other deputies criticised the
regimentation and increased state control in the Bill, with Deputy
Hughes suggesting it was 'not only unconstitutional but
unchristian as well' and commenting that he would be surprised
if those responsible for the moral welfare of the people let the
measure go unchallenged.[13]

It was not long before the guardians of moral welfare responded
to the challenge. On 23 January 1946, before the committee stage
of the Bill had begun, the Conference of Superiors of Convent
Secondary Schools in Ireland (one of the most influential religious
bodies in education) wrote to the Taoiseach objecting to
compulsory medical inspection. They described it as 'a serious
infringement of the natural rights of parents and of the liberty
both of the family and School' and considered the medical
inspection of adolescent girls as altogether undesirable.[14] On 24
January, Archbishop McQuaid contacted the Taoiseach to voice
his apprehension on the same issue.[15] The Taoiseach arranged that
Dr Ward call on Dr McQuaid on 7 February.[16] At that meeting,
Dr Ward outlined the background to the Bill and explained that
there was little new in the provisions on infectious diseases.[17] The
Archbishop said that the Bill was excellent in many respects but
there was uneasiness about the state's powers of interference
particularly in regard to compulsory inspection of school children.
Dr Ward replied that he intended to introduce an amendment
at committee stage to allow exemptions from medical inspection
for children with a certificate from their family doctor and to
exclude secondary schools from inspection where adequate provision
for medical supervision was made. The interview ended after a
wide ranging discussion, leaving Dr Ward with the impression

that the Archbishop was fully satisfied with all aspects of the measure.[18] Dr Ward sent the Archbishop a list of the proposed amendments and Dr McQuaid replied that they were quite satisfactory.[19] There is no suggestion that the Archbishop raised problems on the other maternity and child welfare proposals.

The committee stage of the Bill, which began in March 1946, was extraordinarily acrimonious. Some 640 amendments were tabled, the largest number put down on any Bill up to then, with the Fine Gael party responsible for 516 of the total.[20] Fine Gael deputies equated the proposed measures to control infectious diseases with totalitarianism, the horrors of concentration camps, sterilisation and 'socialistic tendencies'.[21] Dr Ward raised the temperature by his lack of tolerance for the rhetoric of the opposition and his refusal to accept their amendments. He argued in vain that the Bill was largely a consolidatory measure, updating rather than extending the powers already enjoyed by the Minister under the Public Health Act, 1878. He could not understand how any reasonable person could oppose measures to control persons infected with venereal disease, typhoid carriers and verminous children. In later years, the parliamentary secretary described the opposition to his Bill as 'political' and there is little doubt that the Fine Gael stance was sharpened by fourteen frustrating years in opposition.[22] But it is clear from the debate that a significant number of opposition speakers were genuinely concerned about increasing state control over citizens' lives and the affairs of local authorities and a fear that the liberty of the individual and the rights of families were under attack.

While the opposition to the Bill was largely confined to the infectious diseases provisions and compulsory school inspection, deputies were also critical of the proposed mother and child services. They objected to the association of the scheme with the dispensary system which would allow no choice of doctor in many areas. They did not see how the stigma associated with the dispensary doctor could be removed and objected to the idea of a state-controlled system. Some queried whether it was practicable for the dispensary doctor to look after all the women and children in an area and suggested that it would not be good medicine if the mother and child were treated by a doctor different from the father's.[23] But if they were critical of the details, there was a wide measure of support for the aim of improving the health of mothers and children. No deputy queried making the service free to all who wished to avail of it or suggested that it contravened Catholic social teaching. Deputies were more interested in the financial consequences for the rates of the estimated £550,000 a year the scheme would cost than in its place in a Catholic social order.[24]

The mother and child provisions did arouse the opposition of some doctors, however. The February issue of the *Journal of the Irish Medical Association* reported that the private practitioners group of the Association considered that the Bill was only the beginning of measures 'that might revolutionise the whole of medicine in Eire'.[25] They were alarmed that the provision of free ante-natal and maternity services as well as free attendance on school children 'irrespective of social class' would affect them and obstetricians and paediatricians.[26] They called on the Association to ask that a means test be applied before any free medical attendance was made available. But the private practitioners group was a small group and represented few doctors outside Dublin.

Dr Ward's Downfall

The Bill had reached its final stage when the storm clouds which had been building up around Dr Ward's head burst with a vengence. On 5 June 1946, Mr de Valera read a letter to the Dail from Dr Patrick McCarvill containing serious allegations about the parliamentary secretary's conduct.[27] Dr MacCarvill was a skin specialist in Dublin and a former president of the Irish Medical Association. He and Dr Ward had been close friends as young men, and during the Civil War, they acted as locum to each other when one or the other was in prison for their republican activities. However, their friendship turned into a bitter enmity. The bad feeling between the two was a symptom of the wider antagonism that had developed between Dr Ward and the profession. He was hated because of the high-handed way he dealt with medical issues. He had refused to consult the Medical Association about the Health

Bill, accusing them of being 'rabid politicians', more interested in obstruction than co-operation.[28] Dr MacCarvill certainly had the sympathy of the organised profession when he wrote to the Taoiseach, to the extent that the Association was subsequently to organise a collection to pay for legal expenses incurred in pressing home his allegations. The profession was particularly alarmed about the prospect of Dr Ward's becoming Minister for Health. Dr Ward's reaction was that Dr MacCarvill's allegations were part of a conspiracy against him.[29]

Dr MacCarvill's allegations ranged wide, from the conduct of Dr Ward's bacon business to the manner in which he retained his appointment as a dispensary doctor in Monaghan. Mr de Valera's unusual decision to read the allegations before the House left Dr Ward with little room for manoeuvre. Dr Ward wanted to challenge Dr MacCarvill in the courts as a private person but was told by Mr de Valera that he would have to resign his parliamentary secretaryship, prejudicing his case from the start.[30] The alternative, to which he agreed, was the establishment of a judicial tribunal to investigate Dr MacCarvill's allegations. The tribunal reported in July, clearing Dr Ward of all but one charge, that of failing to return complete tax returns on the profits of his bacon business.[31] Dr Ward had no choice but to resign.

Pending the establishment of a separate department of health, Mr MacEntee resumed responsibility directly for health matters in his Department.[32] Dr Ward's departure, although an embarrassment to the government, does not seem to have weakened Mr MacEntee's commitment to reforming the health services. 'It is small consolation', the Minister reminded the IMA in June 1946, 'for a patient to realise that we have in this country great men in medicine — if that same patient is unable through lack of means or organisation to secure their services'.[33]

A National Health Service

In March 1946 the Minister had circulated a memorandum seeking government approval in principle to the proposals which he intended to announce in the White Paper, to provide 'free medical treatment detached from public assistance administration'.[34] The memorandum proposed that the first phase of the new health service would provide a family doctor service for all members of the family, including special services for mothers and children and enlarged specialist and institutional services, such as the regional sanatoria which were being planned. The family doctor service would initially embrace approximately two million persons or three-quarters of the population, made up of the following: farmers and their dependants with property assessed at a rateable valuation of £25 or less; insured persons and their dependants earning less than £500 and employees exempted from insurance but earning less than that amount; persons eligible for public assistance; and those electing to join the scheme on a contributory basis. The Minister sought agreement to the establishment of a department of health, the constitution of local and regional councils to administer the service and an advisory national health council. The proposed scheme would cost £7.8 million.

The strongest opposition to the proposals again came from the Department of Finance but this time their objections went beyond alarm at the cost of the proposals. The Minister for Finance thought the proposals would 'amount in effect to the socialisation of medicine, and would entail an extension of benefit at the expense of individual liberty'.[35] They would lead to the disappearance of private practitioners; they would limit the right of private citizens to choose their medical attendants; and 'at a time when the public is most vocal in its opinion — however uninformed — of what it terms bureaucracy, the remedies or improvements suggested all lead to the appointment of large numbers of additional officials'.[36] The Department of Finance had raised what would be the main arguments in the approaching battle.

The Minister must have successfully defended himself from the charge of socialism because the proposals were agreed in principle on 10 May and he was given the authority to submit a White Paper to government. He subsequently put forward revised proposals to simplify the financing of local authorities and to increase the number of medical officers.[37] He proposed that the piecemeal grants paid to health authorities towards the cost of different services be replaced by a single health services grant amounting to 50 per cent of the approved expenditure of the authority. He recommended that the number of district medical officers be increased from the 750 proposed to 800 and that ultimately 250 assistant medical officers be appointed to cope with the increased workload on medical officers with 'the establishment of a free service for three-fourths of the population'.[38] The assistants would provide a choice of doctor in the districts to which they were appointed and the posts would furnish a valuable training ground for future district medical officers. The Minister proposed to increase the salary scale of the district officers from £650-£800 to £750-£900 and to pay the assistants £400-£600 a year. He pointed out that the proposed salary for senior general practitioners in Britain under the national health service was £1,300 and the best Irish graduates would be attracted out of the country in increasing numbers if salaries were not raised in Ireland, particularly 'when account is taken of the very limited scope which will be left for private practice'.[39]

The Cabinet at its meeting on 3 September agreed to the proposals for the 50 per cent financing of local authorities but decided to reduce the income limit for eligibility from £500 to £350 a year and postponed a decision on the employment of additional medical officers and assistants.[40] A revised memorandum was submitted in October 1946 but does not seem to have been agreed by early 1947, Mr de Valera considered the proposals very far-reaching.[41] The government did reach agreement later that year on radical proposals for reform of the health services, published as a White Paper in September 1947 and discussed in detail later in this chapter. In the meantime, Mr MacEntee persuaded Mr de Valera of the importance of establishing separate departments of health and social welfare.[42]

In November 1946, Mr MacEntee introduced the Ministers and Secretaries (Amendment) Bill to provide the legal framework for a new health ministry. The new Minister would address himself to the introduction of a comprehensive health service, beginning with co-ordinated schemes for mothers and children, a complete tuberculosis service, and the integration of specialist and regional hospital services 'so that no person who needs it will lack anything that medical skill can do to make him well or to keep him well'.[43] The new Minister would also concern himself with improving the laboratory services, medical education and post-graduate training and research. And in an explicit reference to the Department's intentions said:

> we have now in existence the blueprints of a health structure completely divorced from the old public assistance system, based upon a greatly improved family doctor service, and providing for every scientific agent that may be utilised for the preservation of health and the prolongation of life.[44]

The new comprehensive service would also be divorced from the national insurance system.

The purpose of going into such detail on the health memoranda submitted to the Cabinet and the Minister's view of the priorities of the new Minister for Health is to show how serious were the government's intentions of establishing a health service with free general practitioner and hospital care for the vast majority of the population and, in the process, carrying out a radical overhaul of medical education and organisation. The caution with which the Cabinet approached the details of the scheme indicates ministers' appreciation of just how far-reaching those proposals were. Dr Ward's downfall, while a blow to the reforming spirits in the Custom House, seems to have little impact on Mr MacEntee's commitment to the new health service or the momentum towards reform.

The Opposition Forms

The question arises as to how much those outside departmental and government circles knew of the government's intentions. A judicious reader of Dr Ward's and Mr MacEntee's speeches in the Dail would certainly have concluded that something was afoot. They both made it clear that the Public Health Bill, 1945 and the Ministers and Secretaries Act, 1946 were the first steps on the road to a comprehensive health service for the whole population in which the state would play a much greater part. Dr Ward, in his inspired leaks to journalists, hinted at the shape of the new scheme. Irish society is small enough for information to travel quickly by contacts through marriage and friendship which often transcend political or professional barriers. The medical profession knew that a scheme of 'state medicine' was being planned, even if they were hazy about the details.[45]

The first rumblings of discontent in the medical profession came not from the Dublin headquarters of the Association but from a group of doctors in County Limerick led by Dr James McPolin. Dr McPolin is a difficult personality to assess. He had been a consultant pathologist at the Mater Hospital in Belfast and for a while carried out surgery at his own private hospital. In the late 1920s, he was appointed one of the first county medical officers (CMOs), a position he still held in 1946. Those who knew him describe him as a highly intelligent man with an eccentric character. Dr McPolin was deeply interested in moral philosophy and the application of Catholic social teaching to medical issues and there is little doubt that it was he who initiated medical opposition to the government's health plans and gave the profession ammunition to fight 'state medicine' on a broad front.

There were a number of reasons why Dr McPolin exercised such an influence. Well read in Catholic moral and social teaching, he wrote extensively on the subject and on the dangers of state encroachment in the lay and specialist press.[46] Close family connections with the clergy gave him ready access to ecclesiastical circles. An active member of the executive council of the Irish Medical Association throughout the 1940s and early 1950s, he was in a position to influence his medical colleagues. As medical officer for health he was probably in a better position than most doctors to know the intentions of the Department and as a salaried doctor he had more time to devote to agitation than colleagues dependent on fees for a living. It is ironic that the most vociferous voice against state medicine should himself be a full-time employee of a local authority. Dr McPolin had nothing to gain personally from perpetuating private practice; on the contrary, his status as CMO in any scheme of 'state medicine' would have been increased.

Dr McPolin's stand was largely disinterested. He did, however, have reason to fear the power of central bureaucracy.[47] Following a dispute with the Limerick city manager in the mid-1940s, Dr McPolin was suspended from his position as superintendent medical officer of health for the city, a position he combined with medical officer to County Limerick.[48] Dr Deeny's arrival in the Department in late 1944 greatly increased the pressures on CMOs to take action to improve preventive health services. In the Department's opinion the health services in Limerick were a 'black spot' and serious consideration was given to suspending Dr McPolin from duty. But the Department was reluctant to take any action against him which might be 'regarded as victimisation or could even be misrepresented as persecution, because of the unorthodoxy of his views — since this would have a serious effect on the minds of medical men whom we expect and hope will operate the services'.[49]

In June 1946, the Medical Association *Journal* reported that the Limerick Branch of the IMA had passed a resolution opposing the principle that well-to-do patients be treated free of charge.[50] Over the following months a series of articles appeared in the *Journal* by Dr McPolin arguing that a state medical service contravened the moral law.[51] Because of the importance of similar arguments in subsequent controversies, it is worthwhile examining the thrust of Dr McPolin's case.

The starting point for Dr McPolin, as for the Church, was the family, an institution which he endowed with almost mystical qualities. The parents of each family had certain rights and duties such as the right to privacy in relation to medical records and the duty to provide for the physical and moral well-being of their children. One of a father's duties was to provide medical care for his dependants. The doctor, as the family's medical adviser, was part of the divine role ordained for the family. Any interference by a third party in the doctor/family relationship, by restricting clinical freedom or changing methods of remuneration, was a limitation on the rights of the family. For Dr McPolin, the integrity of the family's relationship with its doctor could only be guaranteed where the doctor was an independent contractor and the family paid for services received. A free medical service undermined the role of the family because it interfered with the duty of parents to provide for the physical welfare of their children. Furthermore, the state was in error in presuming it had a responsibility to educate mothers and children about health; that was the role of the family doctor in conjunction with the Church, the arbiter of when questions of health touched on matters of faith and morals.

Dr McPolin's justification of private medicine and his objection to state medicine were not altogether logical and he relied on a one-sided interpretation of papal encyclicals to reinforce his argument. His defence of the individual and family from state interference owed as much to Benthamite liberalism of the early nineteenth century as it did to pronouncements on social policy from Rome. He applied the natural law to social issues in the way a scientist might use a physical law to explain physical phenomena; the operation of the natural law and the Catholic moral and social code were one and the same thing and obvious to any right-minded observer. In the intellectual climate of the 1940s, few queried Dr McPolin's understanding or application of Catholic social teaching to Irish social problems or suggested that a different interpretation might be given to them in other countries, even to the extent of justifying state medicine.[52]

Dr McPolin's role at this stage was to translate genuine medical objections to a state medical service into moral objections to state medicine which made sense to the more conservative elements of Irish public opinion, most importantly to the leaders of the Catholic Hierarchy and the Fine Gael party. The success of Dr McPolin in raising debate on the issue of a state-controlled medical service was probably responsible for the hesitation shown by the government in late 1946 to commit itself to the details of the proposed national health service. By early 1947, Fine Gael leaders were openly using arguments similar to those of Dr McPolin to warn the government of the dangers of state medicine.[53]

Health Act, 1947

In mid-January 1947, Dr James Ryan was appointed the first Minister for Health. Mr de Valera's choice of a senior and highly

181

respected minister is interesting, reflecting perhaps his apprehensions at the possible troubles which lay in the path of implementing government health policy. Dr Ryan had been medical officer in the General Post Office during the 1916 Rising and was a founder member of Fianna Fail. He had been Minister for Agriculture from 1932 to 1947, during the difficult years of the economic war with Britain and of the Emergency, emerging as a successful and popular minister. A most unprepossessing speaker, his chief political gifts were an ability to win agreement from the most intractable opponents and an astute sense of strategy and tactics. Where Dr Ward antagonised his opponents, Dr Ryan appealed to them for assistance. A medical doctor by training, he had not practised for over twenty years.

The Health Bill, 1947 received its second reading in May of that year. While substantially the same as its predecessor, the Bill had been amended to remove some of the most controversial provisions. Many contentious issues in the earlier Bill were now to be governed by ministerial regulation. The powers given to control infectious diseases and infectious persons were restricted by safeguards on personal freedom. Medical officers were no longer obliged to notify the CMO of verminous persons. No child would be obliged to undergo medical inspection if the family doctor certified that the child was receiving adequate medical attention. The Bill also provided that the state would pay half the cost of maintenance allowances to patients undergoing treatment for tuberculosis promised in the White Paper, *Tuberculosis*.

The most controversial sections of this Bill were those concerning health services for mothers and children. The Bill obliged health authorities to 'make arrangements for safe-guarding the health of women in respect of motherhood and for their education in that respect,' and to provide a comprehensive health (including health education) and treatment service for children before and during their school years.[54] Inspection of children would be compulsory in national schools and every other school unless a family doctor certified that a child was receiving adequate medical attention.[55] The Minister was given wide powers in the Bill to make regulations under this part of the Act. In the context of developing the health services, these sections seemed to do no more than make effective the inadequate provisions of earlier legislation. The real issue was the Department's proposal to reorganise general practice to achieve comprehensive health services for mothers and children, particularly by the recruitment of more dispensary doctors and the free treatment of mothers and children.

While Fine Gael strongly opposed the Bill, there was none of the bitterness of the debate on the earlier Bill. Dr Ryan was conciliatory towards the opposition and accepted many amendments. Two issues dominated the debate: the threat posed by the mother and child sections to the medical profession and the attack on the rights of the family represented by compulsory medical inspection, even with safeguards. Deputy Tom O'Higgins, the CMO for Meath, argued that the Bill was a major threat to the private practice of general practitioners who, he claimed, normally made between 70 and 80 per cent of their income from looking after young children.[56] A free service would have dire financial consequences for private doctors and an increase in the number of salaried medical officers would reduce the size of dispensary districts and the scope for private practice. He thought that the medical profession was being 'walked into a rat-trap in blinkers'.[57]

Deputies Dillon and Mulcahy led the opposition to the Bill from the stance of Catholic teaching on the family. They objected in particular to compulsory medical inspection, free treatment and the danger of breaches of confidentiality between doctor and patient under a salaried medical service. James Dillon thought it an 'astonishing and most undesirable proceeding' that 'every man's child ... whether his parents desire it or not, must become the responsibility of the State in so far as the maintenance of its health is concerned'.[58] The proper responsibility, he argued, lay with the parents and family. General Mulcahy called on those who considered national life from the point of view of Catholic sociology to be alert to the possibility of a serious attack on the integrity and privacy of the family from a free state medical service for mothers and children and warned the doctors to be careful that they were not 'moulded into a state regimented service'.[59] Mr

183

Dillon announced his intention of petitioning the President to consult the Council of State on the Bill, with a view to referring it to the Supreme Court to test its constitutionality.[60]

The Minister professed his pride in the mother and child sections of the Bill. He considered them to be the most important provisions in the Bill and had placed them ahead of other sections to give them greater prominence. He justified compulsory medical inspection on the same grounds as compulsory education: those who were most in need of it were least likely to avail of it if it was left to parents' discretion.[61] He offered to meet the IMA when the Bill was passed to discuss in detail the regulations governing the mother and child service.[62] He suggested that doctors whose practice was reduced by the new scheme would be compensated and many new opportunities offered to young doctors in private practice to seek employment as salaried medical officers.[63] He thought that the exemption of children with medical certificates from their family doctors from compulsory medical inspection would generate a lot of private work.[64] He reminded the House that under the original 1915 legislation many of the existing services provided for mothers and children were free to everyone who applied and that there had been no objection to the free service when the previous Bill was discussed.[65] He took a pragmatic approach to the question of a free service arguing that charges would deter 'those on the border-line' from adopting 'the best treatment for their wives and children'.[66]

He regretted that General Mulcahy should give the impression that he and his Fine Gael colleagues were burdened with the responsibility of maintaining Catholic moral principles or that the medical profession should keep watch on the Department of Health to see that those principles were maintained.[67] He promised amendments that medical inspection would be compulsory only in counties where the Minister made an order to that effect, and that parents would be given the right to be present at the examination. But these two concessions failed to satisfy the opposition.

With the publication of the Bill, Dr McPolin stepped up his campaign against state medicine. In May 1947, the Limerick Branch of the Association convened a meeting of all Limerick doctors to discuss the Health Bill.[68] The doctors passed resolutions condemning the dictatorial powers given to the Minister and refusing to accept the status of state-directed officials. The meeting opposed compulsory medical inspection and free medical attendance for persons other than those in the necessitous classes.[69] In July, Dr McPolin published an article in the influential Catholic journal, *Christus Rex*, outlining his objections to the Bill.[70] Dr McPolin informed Limerick County Council that steps were being taken to seek the protection of the Constitution against the Bill, according to the *Irish Independent* of 1 July. In the same month he sent a document to the Taoiseach and Dr Ryan which claimed that the Bill contravened the natural law and the Constitution on eleven counts.[71] The Taoiseach's Department was sufficiently alarmed to ask the Minister for Health if it was his intention to consult the Attorney General on the constitutionality of the Bill.[72] Testing the constitutionality of legislation was a novelty in Irish law and politics and no one was sure of the consequences.

The Department of Health sought a formal opinion from the Attorney General on the points raised by Dr McPolin. The Attorney General replied that he did not consider that the Bill encroached on the rights of the family nor that any of the mother and child sections were unconstitutional.[73] He did, however, consider that the Minister's powers to control infectious diseases could contravene the Constitution. In August, the President consulted the Council of State on the constitutionality of the mother and child sections of the Bill but they recommended that he sign the Bill.[74]

The opponents of the Act continued their campaign to prevent it taking effect. James Dillon took out a High Court summons challenging the Act and suing the Minister for Health. The Limerick doctors lobbied the Central Council of the IMA to strengthen resistance to operating it.[75] Dr McPolin took his case to the Bishop of Limerick, Dr Patrick O'Neill, seeking his opinion as a churchman on whether the obligation in the Act on doctors to disclose records of their patients constituted a menace to professional secrecy and whether compulsory medical inspection was a threat to parents' rights.[76] The Bishop answered both questions in the affirmative.[77] The full significance of that reply was not publicly known until some years later.

After its 7 October meeting, the Hierarchy sent a private protest to the government about the new Health Act, the text of which has not been analysed in detail before.[78] The Hierarchy's statement opened with a reaffirmation of the principles of Catholic teaching that the state must respect the rights of individuals, the family, the professions and voluntary institutions. The bishops claimed that in the Health Act, the Minister had infringed the rights of individuals by taking the power to detain and isolate a person who was a probable source of infection, to declare what was an infectious disease, and to require an infectious person to submit to medical examination. The rights of the family and Church in education were infringed by the power given to health authorities to educate women in regard to motherhood and children in regard to health. The Hierarchy were most concerned about this issue: 'It is precisely in this sphere of health education, where so many moral questions arise, that conflicts with totalitarian systems have developed elsewhere'.[79] The rights of the medical profession were threatened by the power of the Minister to define 'infectious disease' and by the requirement that medical officers record case histories and notify cases of infectious disease. Finally, they alleged that the rights of voluntary institutions were undermined by the Minister's power to prohibit the treatment of some patients in certain institutions.

There are several points to make about this statement. It was the first time that an Irish government had received a formal protest from the Hierarchy about a specific piece of legislation.[80] The bishops did not argue a case for their opposition to the Act; it was sufficient to state the danger as they saw it and to make their opinions known to the government. There is no mention of compulsory inspection of school children, the main objection raised by Dr McQuaid to Dr Ward's Bill in 1945, the main plank of Fine Gael's opposition to the Bill and the subject of James Dillon's constitutional challenge. Having accepted Dr Ward's amendment to permit those with certificates from their own doctor to opt out of the compulsory inspection, the Hierarchy were not, at this stage, prepared to argue the point of compulsion any further. Instead they objected to the danger posed to the morals of women and children by health education. But if the principle of public authorities advising women and children about health infringed the rights of the family and the Church, these rights had been infringed since the passage of the Notification of Births Act, 1915 and the Public Health (Medical Treatment of Children) Act, 1919. Their condemnation of these sections suggests the extent of their worries in the 1940s about exposing Irish women to information about contraception and abortion and children to sex education. Interestingly, the bishops did not express any opinion at this stage on the universal nature of the proposed service for mothers and children or the absence of charges, issues which were to predominate at a later stage of the controversy and which could be considered to be new principles.

It is difficult to understand the objection to the infectious disease provisions. The isolation of infectious persons, the practice of keeping case histories and the notification of infectious diseases were introduced by the Public Health Act, 1878 and the Minister had emergency powers to detain infectious persons since 1940. Since the nineteenth century it had been widely accepted that the general good took precedence over individual liberty and professional secrecy in out-breaks of infectious diseases. The bishops' stance on these questions is suspiciously close to that of Dr McPolin and the Limerick doctors and suggests an ignorance of the problems posed to public health by infectious persons. The alleged attack on voluntary institutions was intended as no more than an effort to prevent hospitals treating infectious persons, especially tuberculosis patients, when they had no facilities to do so. What the Hierarchy seemed to be saying was that much of the foundation of public health policy laid down in the nineteenth century was contrary to Catholic social teaching and posed a danger to morals. The statement signalled a major breakdown of communication between churchmen and statesmen. What persuaded the Hierarchy to contest an Act of the Oireachtas whose constitutionality had satisfied the President and the Council of

State? In February 1946, Archbishop McQuaid had expressed himself satisfied with almost identical provisions in the Public Health Bill, 1945. What factors were at work in the meantime to bring about this chilling condemnation of a humanitarian measure? The most likely explanation, in the absence of firm evidence from the ecclesiastical records, is that a number of events in 1947 drew their attention to the hitherto-unforeseen dangers in the Act and in health policy and encouraged them to make their views known to the government.

At their meeting in October 1947, the bishops would have been acutely aware of the introduction of a national health service in the United Kingdom. In August 1947, the Stormont government published a Health Services Bill to extend the British National Health Service to Northern Ireland; this included a controversial proposal that all voluntary hospitals be taken over by a government-appointed Hospitals Authority. This would have meant that the largest Catholic hospital in Belfast, the Mater, would be controlled by a state body in which the Hierarchy had little or no confidence. Following protests from the Northern bishops, the Stormont government agreed that, at the cost of losing all public funds, the Mater could opt out of the scheme. While the issues North and South were different, they indicated to the bishops that the state was stepping outside its legitimate sphere.

A further factor may have been the publication of the Department of Health White Paper in late September 1947.[81] A toned-down version of the *Report of the Departmental Committee on Health Services,* it was nonetheless a radical document. It made it clear that the 1947 Act was only the first step in a fuller 'programme of reform'.[82] The simplest solution to the administrative problems of running a health service was to make the service available to all citizens free of charge; but it rejected this option in the short term because some people preferred to exercise the right of choosing their own medical advisers and because it would 'strain unduly the resources of the service in its still undeveloped condition to the detriment of patients in more exigent circumstances'.[83] But in identifying women, children and 'the public assistance classes' as the priority groups to benefit from

188

improved medical services, it promised a 'further widening of their scope' as the long term aim.[84]

The immediate scope of the scheme was less than the Department had originally proposed. Specialist services were to be free of charge to those entitled to public assistance. The mother and child service and treatment of tuberculosis were to be free to the whole population irrespective of income as intended but the upper income limit for eligibility for general practitioner services was to be £250 a year or a rateable valuation of less than £25 for farmers. However, eligibility for hospital services was maintained as originally envisaged. The upper income limit was set at £500 or £50 rateable valuation for farmers. The new services were not to be entirely without charge. Token payments would be expected from all but the public assistance classes.

The administration of the new services required much greater involvement by the state than heretofore. The foundation stone was the district medical officer who would provide general practitioner services for eligible classes and a mother and child service regardless of income, conduct preventive health work and register births, deaths and marriages. The doctor's work would be assessed by local health councils, by medical inspectors of the Department of Health resident in the area and by the regional and county medical officers. Health centres and clinics would replace the dispensaries and specialist hospital services co-ordinated in three regions based on Dublin, Cork and Galway. Special arrangements were suggested for Dublin, including a joint health authority to co-ordinate the activities of the public health authorities, private practitioners and voluntary hospitals. For those who feared state medicine, the danger of its implementation must now have seemed acute.

This writer has no evidence that the Hierarchy had studied the White Paper or were aware of its contents. The wording of their letter suggests that they were only concerned with the provisions of the 1947 Act. But if they were aware of the White Paper proposals it would have reaffirmed what Dr McPolin and the Limerick doctors were saying about the dangers posed by the 1947 Act to the family, the medical profession and the educational authority of the church.

189

For the reasons discussed in the previous chapter, the bishops were also particularly sensitive about the influence of contraception, abortion and certain kinds of sex education on Irish women and youth. Since it was not obvious from the wording of the Act that the public authorities would instruct women in family planning or children in sex education, somebody must have alerted them to the possible misuse of the powers in the Bill. The opposition of Fine Gael deputies may have influenced them, but it is more likely that Dr McPolin's campaign was the deciding factor. And for reasons also discussed in the last chapter, it is likely that the bishops would listen with great attention to the complaints of doctors against the encroaching powers of the state, particularly one as well versed in Catholic thought as Dr McPolin.

Just how controversial an issue contraception was in Ireland at this time can be illustrated by a few examples. The importation, sale and advertising of contraceptives had been prohibited under the Criminal Law (Amendment) Act, 1935. In October 1949, the Censorship of Publications Board banned the report of the British Royal Commission on Population because it advocated 'the un-natural prevention of conception or the procurement of abortion or miscarriage'.[85] It was the first action against an official government publication and caused such an outcry that the ban was revoked the following year. But that decision did not prevent Vogt's *Road to Survival*, where the author pointed out the dangers of uncontrolled growth of the world's population, from being banned shortly afterwards. Even a work by Dr Halliday Sutherland on approved Catholic methods of contraception, with the imprimatur of an English bishop, was banned, although allowed on appeal.

The bishops may also have been alarmed by the enthusiasm of the new Department of Health. Some of them had had personal experience of the heat generated by the missionary zeal of the health reformers. Dr McQuaid had been embarrassed by a report prepared by the Department and the public health section of Dublin County Council on the atrocious conditions in some national schools for which he had overall responsibility, one of which was in Ballybrack, close to the Archbishop's private house. Mr de Valera sent the report, which included photographs, to the Archbishop with a covering note to say that the chief medical officer of the Department, Dr Deeny, would be available to discuss how the situation could be improved. The Archbishop replied that he did not deal with junior civil servants.[86]

A row had also developed with Dr Lucey, the Bishop of Cork over a home for unmarried mothers in Bessborough, on the outskirts of Cork city. The home was closed following a departmental inspection which found an endemic staphylococcal infection, resulting in an extremely high death rate among the babies over a number of years. The Bishop took the matter up with the Papal Nuncio and Mr de Valera but both agreed with the Department's decision.[87]

Faced with the collapse of the tuberculosis service in Limerick, the officials of the Department, going beyond their legal authority, gave the incumbent tuberculosis officer the choice of resigning or a public enquiry. The officer resigned, a fact which would not have escaped the notice of the theological doctors of Limerick, or their bishop, Dr O'Neill.[88] These incidents, while small in themselves, illustrate the clash between the old lackadaisical attitude to public health and the Department's determination to improve health standards. Health reform posed a threat to the status quo and to the authority of some of the most powerful men in the country.

In conclusion, one can say that the Hierarchy's protest to the government was a defensive action. They felt threatened by the establishment of a national health service in Northern Ireland, by the zeal for reform in the Custom House and by the proposals to reorganise the health services in the Republic. They had only to look to Eastern Europe for examples of the state taking over control of society and Church. The 'ferocious chastity' of the Irish was under threat from the growing acceptance of contraception and abortion in Britain.[89] The increasing centralism of Irish government and the refusal to consider seriously the vocational alternative made them suspicious of the motives of the politicians and civil servants and credulous of alarmist views of the dangers of the Act. When it was suggested to them that the state would provide contraceptive advice to women and sex education for children through state-appointed and -directed 'civil servant' doctors, who might not necessarily be Catholics, they let their opposition be known in an unprecedented way. Their action indicates at least two similarities with that of their predecessors in 1911: how out of touch they were with the physical needs of mothers and children for better health care and with the real intentions of those who planned the service and secondly, their liability to take the side of those with the greatest interest in protecting the status quo.

The government reacted slowly to the Hierarchy's letter. Mr de Valera did not reply until 16 February 1948, two days before his government fell.[90] The reason he gave for the delay was that the Act was being challenged, a reference to James Dillon's action before the courts. The Taoiseach included a memorandum on the points raised by the Hierarchy which has not been made available with the state papers of the period.

Meanwhile the medical profession had been mobilising opposition to the White Paper and its proposals for an extended medical service. On becoming Minister, Dr Ryan had made it his business to improve relations with the profession after the stormy days of Dr Ward. He softened the Association's attitude to the Health Bill by retrospectively increasing the salaries of dispensary medical officers.[91] The IMA welcomed the Health Bill as 'a very great improvement on its predecessor'.[92] In his speech at their annual dinner in June 1947, the Minister seemed to calm the fears of the profession when he said:

> I have been asked the question more than once whether we are aiming at State Medicine in this country. As far as I understand what State Medicine means I say 'No'. We have here a splendid foundation to build upon, namely, the family doctor.[93]

Under these circumstances, the White Paper must have come as quite a shock. The Association was particularly critical of the absence of a choice of doctor, state interference in parents' responsibility for the health of their children and the abolition of charges for certain sections of the population. On 13 November

1947, the Central Council passed a resolution opposing 'the taking over or directing of all medical services by the State and ... the degree of State control and direction visualised in the White Paper'.[94]

There is some evidence to suggest that the Association was aware of the Hierarchy's intervention in October. In January 1948 the editorial of the *Journal* said:

> high ecclesiastical authorities are apparently not satisfied that certain sections of the Health Act of 1947 do not mean too great an intrusion of the State into the rights of the individual. We cannot say more than has appeared in the public Press, but obviously the matter is not going to be allowed to rest.[95]

The editor may have been simply referring to Dr O'Neill's letter to Dr McPolin which appeared in the press in December 1947 but he seems to suggest that there is more than is generally known. In February the Association announced that it had set up a committee to deal with the Act and the White Paper. Meanwhile, they watched developments in Britain, supporting the BMA in its opposition to the introduction of the National Health Service, and anxiously awaited the results of the Irish general election of February 1948.

Conclusion

By early 1948, opinion on reform of the Irish health services had polarised. The Minister for Health in the Health Act, 1947 and the White Paper had made clear his government's intention to develop a new and expanded health service available to many more people. It was a modified form of the departmental committee's report, though the prospect of a comprehensive service free of direct charge to all was not ruled out. These proposals were sufficient to alarm the Hierarchy that the state was over-stepping its rightful bounds. Their attention seems to have been drawn to the dangers of the Act by the Fine Gael spokesmen against the Bill and more particularly by the lobbying of Dr McPolin. The organised medical profession, which had accepted the Minister's peace offerings and had been slow to oppose the 1947 Health Act, discovered with the publication of the White Paper that the government planned reforms in the health service which, if not as far-reaching as those proposed in Britain, would radically upset the traditional privileges of the profession. The conditions for a powerful alliance between the profession and the Church against radical changes in the health services had been fulfilled.

9
The Sport of Politics
1948~1951

FIANNA FAIL'S DEFEAT in the general election of 1948 interrupted Dr Ryan's plans to implement the proposals of the White Paper. The party actually increased its number of seats by one but the opposition parties showed an unprecedented desire to exclude Mr de Valera from government. Five parties formed a government under the leadership of John A. Costello of Fine Gael. The most dynamic party in the coalition was Clann na Poblachta, founded in 1946 by republicans disaffected from Fianna Fail and campaigning on a mildly radical economic and social programme.

The conduct of the new government was in sharp contrast to that of its predecessor. The participants stressed that theirs was an 'inter-party' rather than a coalition government. Conducting a Cabinet of five different parties, differing greatly in tradition and outlook, was a difficult task for even the most experienced and skilful Taoiseach. Mr Costello's previous experience in government was confined to the Attorney General's office and he was chosen as Taoiseach because the leader of Fine Gael, General Mulcahy, was unacceptable to the other parties. Although a member of the Dail since 1933, Mr Costello was better known for his skill as a barrister. A compassionate and popular man, he lacked Mr de Valera's leadership qualities. As a result of some members of the new Cabinet having an inordinate suspicion of the civil service, the secretary to the government was excluded from Cabinet meetings and procedure seems to have been extremely lax. The lack of cohesion of the government and its casual attitude to Cabinet government, played an important part in subsequent controversies over health policies. Clann na Poblachta was allocated two ministries in the new government: External Affairs, going to the party leader, Sean MacBride and Health, to Dr Noel Browne.

Dr Browne had campaigned on the single issue of the inadequacy of facilities for treating tuberculosis. Aged 32, he was appointed Minister on his first day in the Dail. Dr Browne's life had been dominated by tuberculosis.[1] His father, mother and two sisters had died from the disease and two other siblings had suffered from tubercular infections. He succumbed to the disease as a medical student at Trinity College and might have died but for wealthy benefactors who sent him to an English sanatorium to receive the best surgical treatment. On qualifying, Dr Browne specialised in the treatment of tuberculosis, working in sanatoria in England and returning as assistant medical superintendent to Newcastle Sanatorium, County Wicklow. He was shocked by the lack of surgical facilities for treating the disease and the wastage of young life, and campaigned for radical improvements. He organised a pressure group of former sanatorium patients and joined Clann na Poblachta with the intention of making tuberculosis a political issue. His campaign led him into conflict with Dr Deeny, the chief medical officer of the Department. Dr Browne disputed Deeny's research findings on the clustering of tuberculosis cases in a northern town in the Irish Medical Association *Journal*; and a Department of Health meeting at which Dr Browne was present, was terminated by Dr Deeny because he found it impossible to have a useful discussion about the implementation of the Department's plan to combat the disease.[2] Dr Browne's election campaign had been emotional and somewhat extravagant. He accused the out-going government of criminal neglect in letting 60,000 people die from the disease in the previous sixteen years.[3] He was not prepared to accept that any progress had been made in fighting the disease. He later admitted that he was unaware until just prior to the election that regulations had been passed to pay maintenance allowances to sufferers from the disease.[4]

Dr Browne had the good fortune to become Minister at the moment when the groundwork had been done and the system was already in motion. The new Department of Health was just a year old and full of enthusiasm for reform. The war-time restrictions on building materials were easing and it was possible to build sanatoria and hospitals at a much faster pace. Sites for the sanatoria had been bought and a high-powered team of architects and engineers, under the direction of Norman White, had been recruited to the Department. The Health Act, 1947 gave the health services a firm statutory basis and wide scope to an active Minister. The Health (Financial Provisions) Act, 1947, also passed when Dr Ryan was Minister, empowered the new Minister to spend money on the health services until the state's share of expenditure rose from 16 to 50 per cent of total expenditure on the health services, an amount equivalent to £3 million in 1948.[5] The Hospitals Sweepstakes was in business again after the war-time interruption and was accumulating funds, though not on the same scale as before. The Department was in the process of taking over beds in existing institutions to meet the immediate need for segregation and treatment of tubercular patients. The first mass x-ray and BCG vaccination programmes were initiated by Dublin Corporation and arrangements to appoint thoracic surgeons to local authority hospitals were underway.

While Dr Browne brought few new ideas to the Department, he brought a drive and momentum to action that were unprecedented in the traditions of the Custom House. As Minister, he would brook no delay in the planning of a hospital or the provision of a service. He kept pressure on his senior officials to achieve what in normal times would be considered impossible. A large planning chart on his wall kept a record of the stage of development of every sanatorium, hospital and clinic under construction. He toured the country visiting the forgotten parts of the most neglected institutions. He drove himself and his officials hard. Not fully recovered from his own tubercular problems, he was frequently ill during his period in office.

Dr Browne also seems to have been the first Minister to use the media extensively to publicise policies. He broadcast regularly on the radio on health topics. He used the opportunity of opening every new facility to inform the public of the progress of the tuberculosis campaign. In April 1949, he recruited a journalist to run a publicity section in the Department which produced stylish pamphlets in the Irish and English languages on health topics and a film on tuberculosis. Dr Browne's high profile was most effective in persuading people to seek treatment for tuberculosis. Because of his youth, obvious compassion, his own history of illness and his commitment to eradicating the disease, Dr Browne overcame the reluctance of people to admit to having the disease and to seeking treatment. He offered hope and people were prepared to trust him. Maintenance allowances and additional beds were necessary elements of the campaign but Dr Browne's mobilisation of the people's will to fight the disease was equally important.

A more dangerous effect of his high profile was the personalising of the job of Minister for Health. The fact that Dr Browne had no previous experience of politics and had never had to compromise his ideals for party or national interest put him outside the ordinary run of politicians and permitted him to cultivate the image of a knight in shining armour. The lack of a sense of collective responsibility around the Cabinet table allowed him to take more of the credit and of the responsibility for his policies than was common in Irish government up to then. His accusation that nothing had been done by his predecessors in office to improve the health of the people, brought the counter charge from the Fianna Fail opposition that he was bringing politics into the health services.[6] By identifying himself so closely with policies which were not exclusively his, Dr Browne raised the political stakes surrounding his ministry and left himself vulnerable to personal attack.

Tuberculosis

Progress with the tuberculosis programme was rapid. By the end of 1949, 1,200 additional beds for tuberculosis patients had been provided in institutions as diverse as the new mental hospital in Castlerea, Mallow district hospital and a former military college in the Phoenix Park, Dublin.[7] There was a net gain of 2,000 beds by 1953 when unsuitable beds were abandoned, an increase of 50 per cent more than the number of beds in 1943.[8] Work continued on the elaborate sanatoria at Dublin (Blanchardstown), Galway (Newcastle), Cork (Sarsfieldscourt) and Waterford (Ardkeen), the first of which opened in 1953.

The ratio of beds to deaths increased from 0.72:1 in 1943 to 4:1 in 1953.[9] In 1948, the first thoracic surgeons were appointed to local authority hospitals through the Local Appointments Commission. For the first time, advanced surgical procedures such as lobectomy and pneumonectomy were made available to low income patients. By 1953, there were six fully equipped chest surgery centres in operation in local authority hospitals.[10] Surgery offered the only form of treatment for chronic sufferers of the disease. Even for those susceptible to chemotherapy, the cost of treating one patient with streptomycin in 1948 at £400 was prohibitive and the drug was not in effective use until 1950.[11] A National Blood Transfusion Association was established by the Minister in August 1948 to ensure an efficient supply of blood for thoracic and other surgery. Blood donation was organised on a voluntary basis and hospitals contributed towards the running expenses of the Association. Laboratory services were improved, with the first regional laboratory service provided in Galway in 1949.

Services for detecting new cases of tuberculosis developed alongside the hospital facilities. In 1949, a national BCG committee was established to extend vaccination throughout the country. At the Dublin mass radiography centre, 27,000 persons were x-rayed between June 1946 and March 1949, giving a result of 9 previously undiagnosed cases per 1,000 x-rayed.[12] By 1953, there were six mobile x-ray units in vans touring the country providing a mass x-ray service under the direction of a specially formed limited company, the National Mass Radiography Association.[13] Advertising in newspapers, on the radio, on buses and in schools encouraged people to come forward for treatment. In 1950 a major survey of the disease was initiated to examine the effectiveness of preventive services and treatment facilities. The results of the survey were published in 1953 in a major report on the disease, *Tuberculosis in Ireland*.

The effect of this concerted campaign was dramatic. There was a significant reduction in deaths from a rate of 1.25 per 1,000 population in 1945 to 0.91 per 1,000 in 1949.[14] By 1952, this ratio had nearly halved, giving a rate of .54.[15] The figure was still high by international standards (the rate for England and Wales was 0.24, for Denmark, 0.13) but it was a remarkable improvement.[16] The effect of BCG vaccination on child deaths from the disease was equally remarkable. Between 1948 and 1953, an 82 per cent decline was recorded in childhood deaths from tuberculosis in Dublin city.[17] The number of new cases of the disease diagnosed in 1952, 6,685 or 2.26 per 1,000 population (a rate twice as high as that for England, Wales and Northern Ireland) indicated the size of the task which still remained, but the corner had been turned.[18] The 'national epidemic', which had defied earlier attempts at eradication, was under control.

Hospital Programme

At the same time as the tuberculosis campaign, Dr Browne pursued a massive hospital-building programme. On arrival in the Department, he found 135 proposals for new hospitals or for the adaptation or repair of existing hospitals, at a total estimated cost of £27 million.[19] These were scaled down to a programme costing £15 million over a seven-year period, of which £13.5 million would come from the Hospitals Sweepstakes.[20] It was the most intensive hospital-building plan since the foundation of the state. At a time when local authority expenditure on health and public assistance services was £4.7 million, this was an enormous investment.[21] Little thought appears to have been given to the revenue implications of the additional beds. The Minister did not require the approval of the government or the Minister for Finance to spend sweepstake funds and had little sympathy for those who objected to paying higher taxes and rates for a first class health service.

The plan included the sanatoria, new hospitals for St Vincent's and St Laurence's in Dublin, new regional hospitals at Cork, Galway and Limerick, six new county hospitals, four district hospitals, and cancer and fever hospitals. The Minister's priority was to develop hospitals outside Dublin and to concentrate on providing facilities before widening the scope of the service.[22] In conjunction with the building programme, specialist medical services outside Dublin were improved. Orthopaedic surgeons were appointed in the west, south-east, Limerick, Cork and the north-east. Radiologists, pathologists, and bacteriologists were to be appointed on a similar basis and posts of obstetrician/gynaecologist and anaesthetist introduced in selected county hospitals. Nurse training was expanded and the social status of nursing as a career for women meant that there was no shortage of applicants. The plan to turn St Kevin's in Dublin into an acute hospital with a post-graduate medical school took shape with the appointment of medical directors of medicine, surgery and pathology.

Mother and Child Scheme

Dr Browne was under pressure from the Fianna Fail opposition to introduce a mother and child health scheme from the day he took up office. The first problem to overcome was Fine Gael's opposition to certain sections of the Health Act, 1947 dealing with mothers and children. Deputies Costello, Dillon, Mulcahy and O'Higgins, who had been the strongest opponents of the compulsory and universal nature of the mother and child sections, were now members of the Cabinet. Shortly after the new government took office, the Attorney General, Mr Cecil Lavery, said that the sections of the Act obliging parents to submit children for medical inspection and managers of schools to make facilities available for inspections were unconstitutional. (His predecessor had taken the opposite view during the 1947 debate.) Mr Lavery also thought that the sections empowering health authorities to provide services for mothers and children would be unconstitutional if the implementing regulations made the services compulsory.[23] On the strength of this opinion, the Minister for Health proposed

201

to repeal the offending provisions for compulsory medical inspection and to impose charges by regulation for the remaining services for mothers and children. The reason given by Dr Browne for the charges was that they would lessen the opposition of the medical profession to the proposed services.[24] The Minister was also convinced at this stage of the need to separate as far as possible the new service from any association with the dispensary system and felt that people would attach more value to a service to which they contributed.[25]

In the Cabinet discussion on 25 June, he won agreement to amend the sections on compulsory health inspection but not to the imposition of charges.[26] The Cabinet would not agree to charges because the Labour members of the coalition opposed any capitulation to the medical profession and without their support, the amending Bill would not pass through the House.[27]

The Minister took his time in bringing forward his amending Bill and a scheme for mothers and children, a delay which is hardly surprising given his commitment to the tuberculosis and hospital programmes. In May 1948 he set up a consultative Child Health Council with thirteen members, including four paediatricians and one obstetrician/gynaecologist – all Dublin based – with a remit to recommend improvements in health services for children. Surprisingly, their terms of reference did not extend to services for mothers. Dr Browne's subsequent proposals were based, at least in part, on the reports of the Council.[28] In July 1949, Dr Browne received the Department of Finance's approval in principle to a mother and child scheme, although detailed agreement was not forthcoming until March 1950.[29] The Department of Finance opposed even the limited choice of doctor offered in the Minister's scheme, arguing, on the grounds of economy, for the service to be provided by full-time, salaried doctors. On 10 June 1950, Dr Browne sent a draft scheme to the IMA and a copy to each member of the government about the same time.[30] Crucially, the details of the scheme were not formally discussed or agreed by the Cabinet; Dr Browne apparently relied on government agreement in 1948 to amend the Health Act for authority to act on the mother and child scheme.[31] This failure to secure the commitment of the government to the details of the scheme greatly weakened Dr Browne's hand in subsequent negotiations. The contrast with the previous government, where all proposals were discussed and agreed in detail by the Cabinet, is striking.

Dr Browne's mother and child proposals must be one of the most complex schemes ever produced by the Department of Health.[32] For the county boroughs, the scheme proposed that district medical officers would provide a medical service for children, remunerated by annual capitation payments of 10s per child aged six weeks to sixteen years. Parents would be given a limited choice of doctor. The dispensary officer's salary would be reduced to take account of capitation income because it was estimated that under the new scheme, his or her income from public funds would increase from about £900 to £1,500 at the top of the scale. In Dublin, the maternity hospitals would provide care for expectant and post-partum mothers and for infants up to six weeks. In the other county boroughs, a maternity and infant service would be provided by local authority hospitals.

Outside the cities, the scheme distinguished between interim and final proposals. In the interim period, maternity care by general practitioners would be provided by district medical officers and by private practitioners willing to participate in the scheme. District medical officers would provide a health care service for children at health centres but the introduction of a domiciliary health service for all children would be deferred to the final period. In the long term, a comprehensive service for mothers and children would be provided by district medical officers only; the doctors would be paid a mixture of reduced dispensary salary, capitation fees and lump sums. The income of district medical officers in the final period would rise by the same proportion as their colleagues in the county boroughs. Specialist obstetrical and gynaecological services would be provided by consultants in local clinics and county hospitals.

The scheme emphasised three things: there would be no compulsion to use the services, there would be no means test and there would be no charges. The chief medical officer of each health authority would be responsible for the direction and supervision of the scheme, and doctors participating in the service would keep records of their patients' illnesses under arrangements made by health authorities.

Relations between the Minister and the medical profession, which had been deteriorating for some time, were badly strained by the proposals for a mother and child scheme. The profession had admired the early achievements of the Minister in combating tuberculosis and quickening the tempo of health administration. Relations between the Department and the Association had been described as 'most cordial' by the IMA's president in summer 1949.[33] But thereafter, things began to go wrong. The Association would not agree to a proposal from the Minister that medical cards, entitling the holder and dependants to free medical care for an indefinite period, be substituted for the once-off dispensary tickets.[34] Nor would the dispensary doctors agree to see poor patients with paying patients in their private surgeries, or to a proposal that they, rather than assistance officers, would admit poor patients to district and county hospitals.[35] The dispensary doctors were infuriated by an advertisement in the public press in which Dr Browne announced that local authorities had been instructed to inform him within 24 hours of any complaints made by a patient against a dispensary doctor. For the Association this was tantamount to an invitation to patients to make 'frivolous and perhaps malicious complaints'.[36] Private medical practitioners were angered by the Minister's decision to restrict the use of streptomycin to approved hospitals, because they would be unable to treat their private patients with the drug.[37]

Perhaps most serious of all was the Minister's proposed use of the sweepstakes funds. The Minister had initiated an enormous hospital-building programme which would consume all sweepstake moneys for the foreseeable future, most of which would be spent on local authority hospitals. The Dublin consultant establishment were incensed by what they considered to be an act of piracy by the Minister. Dr Browne compounded the insult by announcing in July 1950 that the amount of sweepstake funds which would be paid towards the deficits of the voluntary hospitals in 1950, 1951 and 1952 would be no more than was paid in 1948.[38] Local authorities would instead increase the payment per public patient treated in the hospitals by one-third, making it clear to the hospitals that if they wished to increase income they would have to treat more of the poor.[39]

These were perhaps no more than the usual storms which cloud the relationship between any Minister for Health and the medical profession but in Dr Browne's case there was something more. The Minister seems to have set out deliberately to provoke the profession, in particular the Dublin consultants, by criticising in public their manner of practice and preoccupation with money. As a house officer in Newcastle sanatorium, Dr Browne had been at the receiving end of consultant arrogance and as a salaried doctor had little sympathy with the fee-for-service ethic of the medical establishment.[40] But a junior doctor who takes on the leading members of his profession is on weak grounds in any circumstances; when he is also Minister for Health, it is most unwise, unless he has strong forces on his side. The Minister's refusal to maintain good relations with the profession was the cause of the final break between him and his medical adviser, Dr Deeny.[41] In early 1950, Dr Deeny left the Department on special assignment as director of the National Tuberculosis Survey.

The IMA had been disappointed when the government in 1948 had decided against imposing charges for mother and child services and wrote to the Minister stating its opposition to 'the provision of Free Medical Treatment to non-necessitous persons'.[42] The profession remained on the alert for signs of increased state medicine. Their concern was not so much the over-night transformation of the health services into a state medical service but a gradual 'Fabian' extension of state control to all medical services. This 'Fabian technique', according to the IMA *Journal*, took the form of 'starvation of voluntary services and boosting of State services; of control of more and more of the profession by whole-time appointments and salaries'.[43] The *Journal* admitted that this approach was politically popular because the cost of the expanded health services was met from taxation, not personal contributions but warned that it would bring in its train an unacceptable degree of control by lay bureaucrats.[44] Medical morale was lowered by the surrender, as the doctors saw it, of the British Medical Association to Aneurin Bevan on the issue of a national health service.

The proposed mother and child scheme had major financial implications for many doctors, presenting them with a crisis of more extensive proportions than in 1911. The group of doctors most obviously affected by the proposals were private general practitioners, for whom no role was envisaged in the long term. Since much of such doctors' incomes came from treating childhood disorders and attending women in confinement, and since the doctor who treated the mother and children usually treated the remainder of the family, private practitioners were threatened with the abolition of private practice and with enrolment as full-time, salaried medical officers.[45]

Less obviously, specialists and consultants were affected by the proposals. At that time, most consultants were not paid for treating poor and national insurance patients in hospital. Their income came from treating those not entitled to free treatment. The Minister was proposing a free specialist service for all mothers and children without any reference to whether or not the consultants would be paid. Paediatricians, gynaecologists and surgeons were most directly affected. County physicians feared that the appointment of obstetrician/gynaecologists in the provinces would reduce their private maternity work. Even the dispensary doctors were less than happy with the proposals. They believed that there would be intolerable demands on the dispensary doctor if the service was extended to the whole population and that the dispensaries would repel the better off if they found themselves 'sitting alongside tinkers' wives and others of a similar type'.[46] The Association believed that if the scheme went through, it would lead to a full-time state medical service in which doctors would become civil servants. They demanded an income limit for the service, a demand which coincided with their financial interests and their interpretation of Catholic social teaching on the role of the state.

Dr McPolin was particularly alarmed by the threat to Catholic teaching, as he understood it, of the policies pursued by Dr Browne. He intensified his campaign against the extension of free health services, arguing that the medical profession had a duty to discourage all schemes that undermined the rights of the family and the Church.[47] He denounced the availability of the tuberculosis service to all patients irrespective of income; and said that the proposal to develop a post-graduate medical school at St Kevin's Hospital in Dublin interfered with the rights of the existing medical schools and of the profession.[48] At least one doctor consulted a 'moralist' about the ethical aspects of the mother and child scheme who gave his view that it was based 'on the false philosophy of the Supreme State, and that there was the danger from the gynaecological point of view that (it) might lead to false teaching in regard to contraceptives and other matters'.[49] Whether by conviction, conscious design or osmosis, it was on the moral ground prepared by Dr McPolin that the Association chose to fight Dr Browne's proposed mother and child scheme.[50]

The Association mobilised its strength to oppose the mother and child scheme in late June 1950.[51] In early October, the Executive Council appointed a press relations officer and held a referendum of its members to test reaction to the scheme.[52] The results of the questionnaire were announced at an extraordinary annual general meeting on 23 November at which 330 doctors were present.[53] To the first question – 'Do you agree to work a Mother and Child Health Scheme which includes free treatment for people who are able to pay for their own medical care?' – 78 per cent of the 994 replies were negative and 22 per cent positive.[54] On the question of working a scheme providing free treatment if private practitioners were included, 24 per cent of the total said that they would.[55] While the results showed a clear majority opposed to the scheme, they also brought some comfort to the Minister, particularly the fact that only 53 per cent of the balloted membership had answered the questionnaire. They also suggested that a sizeable proportion were prepared to work a scheme without charge if private practitioners were included. In November 1950, the Association formally conveyed its objections to the proposed scheme to the Hierarchy and the heads of the other churches.[56]

The IMA was vulnerable on a number of points. There were

up to 500 doctors who were not in the Association, most of whom were young and struggling to make a living. Irish medicine had become much more competitive since war-time restrictions in Britain had reduced the opportunities for Irish graduates to emigrate. These doctors might be tempted by a well structured state scheme which offered a good salary and conditions of employment. There was also the possibility that such a scheme would attract Irish doctors back from Britain.[57] At the only meeting held with the profession to discuss the scheme, the Minister made the acceptance of a free service the condition for detailed negotiation and threatened that he would force through a scheme without the co-operation of the doctors if necessary.

The climate for negotiation was not improved by the Minister's forthrightness. On at least two occasions, he announced his personal preference for an eventual salaried medical service.[58] He disapproved of the money transaction between doctor and patient, announcing that doctors should not need 'the constant carrot of a fee for services dangled in front of them in order to flog their flagging morality and high principles'.[59] Towards the end of 1950, the Minister seems to have developed what one of his ministerial colleagues described as a 'pathological hatred' of doctors.[60] In November or December, Association members came by copies of a document, entitled *The Mother and Child Scheme — Is it Needed?* which was circulated among branches of Dr Browne's party, Clann na Poblachta. The document was unsigned but there were enough clues to suggest that the Minister was the author.[61] It was a hard-hitting attack on the arguments put forward by the medical profession against the mother and child service but the language was inflammatory, to say the least. The profession was accused of making fortunes out of the misfortunes of sick children, of accepting a free tuberculosis service because it was 'largely a poor man's disease' with little money in it, and of objecting to the proposed scheme because they would have to pay income tax for the first time.[62] The document queried the credentials of doctors in 'the Medical Squares or Crescents of our big cities and towns' to pronounce on ethical and moral principles.[63] When called upon to deny he wrote the document,

Dr Browne was equivocal, suggesting that the Association had circulated it for its own ends.[64]

The Medical Association took the document seriously enough to employ a private detective who found sufficient evidence in the Custom House to satisfy the Association that the document had originated there. Dr Browne's Cabinet colleagues also took the document seriously. Dr O'Higgins, the Minister of Defence, termed it 'as foul a piece of muddy-minded scurrility as ever poured out on a clean-minded people'.[65] Dr O'Higgins, a regular attender at council meetings of the Association at this time, was present at the meeting when any doubts about the authorship of the document were removed.[66]

The incident brought a sharp deterioration in relations between the Minister and the Association and weakened any remaining support which Dr Browne might have enjoyed from his Cabinet colleagues. It also seems to have undermined his position in his own party, with newspapers linking his resignation from the standing committee of Clann na Poblachta to a committee discussion of the intemperate language of the document.[67] Dr Browne seems to have neglected to keep any lines open to the leadership of the profession and was in no position to play conflicting medical interests against each other, as his counterpart in Britain, Aneurin Bevan, had done so successfully. Nor does he seem to have paid sufficient attention to securing his flank by maintaining the support of fellow ministers and party colleagues. This omission was all the more serious given the instinctive sympathy of the Fine Gael ministers for the arguments of the doctors and their close links with the profession.[68] Mr Costello had declared his determination not to take part in any government which favoured or tried in any way to socialise medicine and Dr Browne was aware of his views.[69] The leadership of the Association was in no doubt that Dr Browne's scheme was far from enjoying the whole-hearted support of the Cabinet and that he was increasingly isolated from his colleagues. Dr Browne was also having difficulties with his party leader, Sean MacBride, who was soon to make it clear that he was not prepared to support Dr Browne's stance on the mother and child scheme.[70]

Dr Browne took an equally uncompromising stand in hi.
dealings with the Hierarchy and the religious orders which playec
so prominent a part in the organisation of health services. He
refused a request from Dr McQuaid to exempt religious nursing
sisters at St Kevin's Hospital from night duty.[71] He attemptec
without success, to transfer control of the new Children's Hospita
in Crumlin from Dr McQuaid (on whose initiative it had beer
built) and his nominees to the Dublin Health Authority.[72] He
refused a proposal from the Sisters of Charity that they turn a
vacated building into a private hospital.[73] As with the medica
profession, these events were not significant in themselves, but
assumed significance in the growing climate of opposition to the
Minister's mother and child proposals.

While Dr Browne expected conflict with the medical profession
over his proposals, he did not, by his own account, have any reason
to believe that there would be any opposition from the
Hierarchy.[74] In this he had seriously misjudged the opposition to
the scheme. The Hierarchy had received a copy of the mother and
child scheme and following discussion at their October meeting,
the Archbishop of Dublin was deputed to make their objections
to the scheme known to the government. On 12 October at Dr
McQuaid's request, Dr Browne visited the Archbishop's House
and was informed by the Archbishop, the Bishop of Galway, Dr
Michael Browne and the Bishop of Ferns, Dr James Staunton,
of the contents of a letter from the Hierarchy to the Taoiseach
objecting to the scheme.[75] In the Hierarchy's opinion, the
scheme, while 'motivated by a sincere desire to improve public
health', was 'in direct opposition to the rights of the family and
of the individual' and constituted 'a ready made instrument for
future totalitarian aggression'.[76] The physical education of
children raised important moral questions on which the Church
had definite teaching. They expressed particular concern about the
education of women for motherhood, which they assumed would
include instruction in 'sex relations, chastity and marriage' where
the state had no competence to act.[77] Gynaecological care could,
they argued, include instruction on contraception and abortion
and, in a veiled reference to Trinity College, expressed alarm that

210

district medical officers employed to provide the service might have 'trained in institutions in which we have no confidence'.[78]

So far the Hierarchy was consistent with its objections to the Health Act, 1947. But now an additional reason for objecting to the scheme was raised. The bishops queried the right of the state to provide a free service to all. In their view, the state was not entitled to relieve the '10 per cent necessitous or negligent parents' by a state medical service which infringed the rights of the other 90 per cent of parents to provide for the health of their children.[79] They repeated their warning of October 1947 that the confidential relationship between doctor and patient would be destroyed by the requirement to keep records and added that:

> elimination of private medical practitioners by a State-paid service has not been shown to be necessary or even advantageous to the patient, the public in general or the medical profession.[80]

They advised that the government develop more maternity hospitals, provide adequate maternity benefits and greater tax relief for large families.

The bishops' objections to the proposed scheme display the same defensiveness as those of 1947, as well as a certain naivety about the percentage of necessitous parents in the population. Although statistics on poverty were few, it was generally believed that about one-third of the population received free medical care from dispensary doctors, a figure which roughly coincided with those in poverty.[81] Furthermore, the bishops did not refer to the main argument against a means test (used by Dr Ryan and Dr Noel Browne), namely, that it would deter those on the borderline from seeking the medical assistance which they needed but could not afford. Nor did they raise any objection to the free tuberculosis service already available. Caught up in principles more suited to the nineteenth century than the twentieth, sheltered from the harsher side of Irish life, fearful of hidden dangers to faith and morals, and susceptible to the arguments of the medical profession against the pretensions of the state, the bishops' objections to the scheme seem wide of the mark. The similarity of the Hierarchy's and medical profession's objections to the scheme illustrate how

211

well the doctors chose their weapons to fight Dr Browne.

Dr Browne and the bishops disagreed about the outcome of the meeting, Dr Browne maintaining that he thought he had satisfied them on the points raised, especially their fears about the education of mothers, and the bishops claiming that the Minister had refused to discuss their objections and had walked out.[82] The following day, the Taoiseach visited Archbishop McQuaid and was informed of the Hierarchy's objections to the scheme and of what Dr McQuaid considered to be Dr Browne's unreasonable behaviour the day before. Mr Costello undertook to try to reconcile the Hierarchy's views with the Minister's policy.[83] He maintained constant contact with Dr McQuaid up to the crisis of April 1951.[84] In what became a point of controversy, the Hierarchy's letter of 10 October was never answered by the government, although the Department of Health prepared an able defence of the scheme for transmission to the bishops. The Taoiseach hoped to settle the problems between the bishops and Dr Browne without taking issue with the bishops on their objections.[85]

Mr Costello was now under pressure from the Hierarchy and the medical profession to reach agreement on the mother and child scheme. He proposed to Dr Browne that the Bill to amend the Health Act, 1947, agreed in 1948 but not yet introduced, should amend the section which referred to the education of women for motherhood.[86] Assisted by James Dillon, Dr O'Higgins and Mr Norton, he attempted to mediate between Dr Browne and the medical profession. Since Dr O'Higgins was very close to Mr Costello and in direct contact with the Association, it is unlikely that the profession's negotiators were unaware of the Hierarchy's intervention. Dr O'Higgins advised the Association to meet the Taoiseach. On 29 November 1950, Mr Costello, accompanied by Mr Norton, reassured the doctors that he was firmly opposed to the socialisation of the medical profession but that he would be compelled to implement the mother and child scheme which would be available without charge. If this point were accepted, he felt that there could be concessions on the inclusion of all general practitioners in the scheme and safeguards for professional secrecy.[87] Until then the Taoiseach had been under the impression that any scheme would have to be free under the enabling section of the Act. On re-reading the section, he came to the conclusion that there was no binding obligation on the government to have a free scheme and that a means test or payment on a contributory basis would be legal. According to his own account, he did not inform the doctors at the 29 November meeting of his re-interpretation.[88]

Nevertheless, Dr Browne felt betrayed by this meeting and accused the Taoiseach of acting treacherously.[89] On 16 December, Dr Browne wrote to the Taoiseach complaining that the Medical Association had been given the impression that negotiations in future were to be conducted with the Taoiseach and not with him.[90] He repeated his position that 'there can be no compromise on the principles of a free service and no means test'.[91] It seems that there was no further open negotiation by the Taoiseach with the profession at this stage.

The medical profession played for time. In December, the Minister pressed the IMA for a decision and was told it was preparing a scheme of its own.[92] By the end of January 1951, the Association had still not informed the Minister of its views or of its alternative. On 3 February, the Association responded by repeating its general objections to the scheme, namely, that it was the first step towards the introduction of a full-time salaried medical service under central bureaucracy and that it heralded the destruction of the private practitioner.[93] The Association maintained its opposition to the principle of free treatment for the well-to-do. Detailed objections were confined to the question of a service for Dublin. As an alternative to the Minister's scheme, the Association proposed a mother and infant scheme in which each mother below a certain income would be given a cash grant to spend on maternity care.[94]

Dr Browne at first seemed to take a conciliatory line, informing the Association on 19 February that he was prepared to continue negotiations on the possibility of reconciling his proposals with those of the profession.[95] He asked the Association on 25 February for a date to open negotiations but the medical negotiators asked for deferment until 8 March.[96] This was too much for Dr

213

Browne and on 5 March he abruptly broke off relations with the Association, informing the Taoiseach that it was because the Association had made telephone threats to the Secretary of the Department and did not wish to reach agreement.[97] Dr Browne then set about introducing his scheme, despite the opposition of the profession and the unresolved objections of the Hierarchy, and without the support of his ministerial colleagues. He released details of the scheme to the press on 6 March promising an end to 'doctors' bills'.[98] Copies of pamphlets announcing the scheme were sent to the Hierarchy and to leaders of the other churches but apparently not to government members.[99] He wrote to every doctor in the country inviting them to participate in the scheme, announcing his intention to employ additional district medical officers if enough general practitioners did not come forward.[100] On 8 March, Dr Browne gave a radio broadcast in which he explained the purpose of the scheme. He said that private general practitioners would be welcome into the scheme provided they let the Minister know their intentions within the next month. He assured his listeners:

> there will be no interference whatsoever with what is called the 'doctor-patient relationship'; the only change that you will notice and the doctor will notice is that in future in relation to the birth of your child and the growth of that child up to the age of 16 years, you will have no more doctors' bills to pay.[101]

As Dr Browne made that broadcast he had a letter in his pocket received earlier that day from Dr McQuaid, the Archbishop of Dublin, repeating, in strong terms, his opposition to the scheme.[102]

Perhaps Dr Browne did not fully appreciate the impact of Dr McQuaid's letter on the Taoiseach or his Cabinet colleagues or perhaps he thought that his only chance of success was to appeal over the heads of the doctors, the bishops and the politicians to the people of Ireland. Whatever his motives, he did not contact the Taoiseach or acknowledge the Archbishop's letter.[103] He continued to publicise the scheme and agreed to reopen discussion with the IMA if they agreed in advance to the absence of a means test for all mothers and children under sixteen.[104] He put pressure on the Department of Finance to make extra funds available to pay private general practitioners whom he had now proposed to include more fully in the scheme, particularly to provide domiciliary treatment of children in areas outside the county boroughs. The Minister for Finance, Mr McGilligan, refused to agree to the increased expenditure without a government decision on the revised scheme.[105] On receipt of that letter, Dr Browne asked the Taoiseach to hold an emergency Cabinet meeting to approve an additional £30,000 with which to 'kill' the doctors.[106] The Taoiseach refused to call such a meeting, telling Dr Browne that:

> *Whatever about fighting the doctors, I am not going to fight the Bishops and whatever about fighting the Bishops, I am not going to fight the doctors and the Bishops.*[107]

He withheld permission to proceed further with the scheme until the bishops' objections had been met.

On 15 March, the Taoiseach wrote to Dr Browne emphasising how serious he considered the Archbishop's objections to be and announced that the government would:

> *not be party to any proposals affecting moral questions which would or might come into conflict with the definite teaching of the Catholic Church.*[108]

He suggested that Dr Browne consult the Hierarchy to remove their objections to the scheme.[109] Dr Browne replied that as far as he was concerned he had completely satisfied the bishops when he met their representatives in October and suggested that Dr McQuaid's views did not represent those of the Hierarchy.[110]

On 21 March, the issue came to a head. The IMA inserted advertisements in the national newspapers condemning the Minister's scheme on the grounds of politically controlled medicine, cost to the taxpayer, invasion of patients' privacy and administration by state-appointed doctors.[111] In response to this attack, the Minister proposed to publish a letter from the Secretary of his Department to the Secretary of the IMA referring to the introduction of a scheme without a means test as 'Government policy' and condemning the Association's advertisements.[112] The Taoiseach stopped publication of the letter because he did not accept that a scheme without a means test was government policy.[113] The ground on which Dr Browne had chosen to fight the profession was being taken from under his feet. In an increasingly weak position, he came to the conclusion that he would have to satisfy the Hierarchy on the question of the means test and on their other objections and sought an interview with Dr McQuaid the next day, Holy Thursday.

At that meeting, Dr Browne was persuaded that far from satisfying the objections of the Hierarchy to his scheme, their objections remained as strong as ever.[114] He requested that the scheme be referred to the whole Hierarchy for adjudication as to whether it conflicted with Catholic faith and morals. He agreed to abide by the Hierarchy's ruling and raised the question of his resignation from the Cabinet.[115]

Dr Browne prepared a memorandum on his scheme for the Hierarchy, similar to that prepared by the Department of Health in October 1950 but which had not been sent by Mr Costello. There were, however, three new points. The Minister now proposed to include private practitioners; he emphasised that the scheme would not interfere with the confidential relationship between the doctor and his patient; and it would not reduce the amount of private practice.[116] The memorandum ended with a request for a decision from the Hierarchy as to whether the scheme was contrary to Catholic moral teaching.

A special meeting of the Hierarchy was arranged for 4 April. In the days before the meeting, Dr Browne toured the country visiting bishops and lobbying their support. He felt confident that the Hierarchy would not find his scheme contrary to Catholic *moral* teaching, whatever their understanding of Catholic *social* teaching. He had been advised by a moral theologian since the dispute with the bishops had arisen who had assured him that nothing in the scheme contravened Catholic faith and morals.[117]

But Dr Browne's confidence was misplaced. The bishops did not answer his query about whether the scheme contravened Catholic moral teaching but pronounced it contrary to Catholic social teaching. In a letter dated 5 April 1951, Dr McQuaid informed the Taoiseach of the reasons why the scheme was unacceptable to the Hierarchy and where they considered it conflicted with Catholic social teaching.[118] The bishops did not refute the arguments put forward in Dr Browne's memorandum nor argue the case for their opposition. They were content to state their objections and leave it at that. The Hierarchy expressed its approval for 'a sane and legitimate Health Service, which will properly safeguard the health of Mothers and Children'. It withheld approval from any scheme which permitted 'undue control by the State in a sphere so delicate and so intimately concerned with morals as that which deals with gynaecology or obstetrics and with the relations between doctor and patient' and which 'lessened the proper initiative of individuals and associations and the undermining of self reliance'.[119]

The bishops accepted the Minister's good intentions to build safeguards into the scheme to prevent abuse of Catholic teaching on sexuality, but they objected to the principle of the state taking on the function of educating mothers and children, an objection which could only be removed by amendment of the enabling section of the Health Act, 1947. They considered that the purpose of the scheme could be achieved for the vast majority of citizens by individual initiative and that the scheme interfered unduly with the activities of parents, children and doctors. So far the bishops were repeating objections which they had made in 1947 and 1950. But now they went further and objected to the burden of taxation which the scheme would entail, taxation which would morally compel citizens to avail of the service and the extent to which the scheme would be determined by ministerial regulation as distinct from legislation passed by the Oireachtas. These objections were hardly within the sphere of the bishops' moral authority and echoed the arguments of the medical profession in resisting Dr Browne's scheme.[120] The letter finished with a reference to the bishop's pleasure that there was no evidence that the government supported the scheme advocated by the Minister.

If there were sound arguments in Catholic social teaching against the mother and child scheme, this letter from the Hierarchy did

217

them no justice. On the contrary, the bishops appear to have overstepped what might reasonably be considered their legitimate concern and to have taken sides in a political dispute between the Minister for Health, the medical profession and the other members of the Cabinet. They seem to have placed less emphasis on the moral dangers and more on the social consequences of the scheme. But as far as Dr Browne's Cabinet colleagues were concerned, it did not matter on what grounds the Hierarchy condemned the scheme, the fact of their condemnation was enough. At a Cabinet meeting on 6 April, Dr Browne tried to convince his colleagues that the bishops' condemnation of the scheme was not the final word because they had not opposed it on moral grounds.[121] Catholic social teaching, he argued, varied from country to country, and even from city to city and pointed out that the introduction of a state health service to Northern Ireland had not been condemned by the Irish bishops as contrary to Catholic social teaching. But his fellow ministers were not prepared to go ahead with the scheme in the teeth of the Hierarchy's opposition. They decided instead to introduce a scheme with a means test and one which conformed to Catholic social teaching.[122] Dr Browne's isolation was complete. The Minister, having promised to accede to the Hierarchy's views and having sworn to introduce a scheme without a means test, was in an impossible situation. He could only resign but postponed this final step until 11 April when his party leader requested him to do so.[123] The IMA could hardly restrain its satisfaction at this outcome.[124]

The whole affair took on a new political dimension with Dr Browne's decision to release to the press copies of the correspondence between the Hierarchy, the Taoiseach and himself. His resignation and the publication of what had been intended as a private communication between Church and government created a political controversy of a scale unprecedented since independence and scarcely equalled since. Opinion polarised on the issues of whether the Church had been justified in the way it intervened. The evidence that real power in the country lay not with elected representatives but with the Catholic Hierarchy generated a crisis of confidence in the democratic institutions of the state and the ideals of republicanism. The anger of a sizeable section of the population with the Hierarchy's intervention took Church authorities aback and if they acted more cautiously in future, it may have been as a result of lessons learned during this affair.

Conclusion

There are a number of reasons why Dr Browne failed to put his mother and child scheme into effect. Foremost among these was his neglect to secure the government's support for the details. The medical profession and the Hierarchy knew from early in the dispute that the Minister did not enjoy even limited support in the Cabinet when he opened negotiations. Dr Browne's inexperience and the difficulty of gaining agreement among ministers from five political parties with divergent views perhaps led him to underestimate the importance of securing this flank. The doctors and the bishops were able to exploit these differences to their advantage. Dr Browne approached the implementation of the mother and child scheme with the same attitude as he dealt with tuberculosis and hospital building; he would brook no opposition until the job was done. But unlike the tuberculosis and hospital programme, little of the spade work had been done on the mother and child service when Dr Browne became Minister. In implementing a service for mothers and children, Dr Browne was taking on much more formidable opponents than civil servants and local authority officials. His scheme affected a much broader section of the medical profession than anything he had attempted hitherto and the determination of the doctors to resist the scheme was strengthened by the knowledge that the scheme was the first step in a much wider national health service. Dr Browne's indiscretions did not assuage fears that they would soon be salaried medical officers in a service run from the Custom House and he did little to persuade any branch of the profession that they had anything to gain from a nationalised health service. Nor did his erratic behaviour and refusal to negotiate on the question of the means test encourage his ministerial colleagues to rally round him.

Another serious tactical error by Dr Browne was the failure to see that, given the constraints of Irish life, he would have to satisfy the Hierarchy before coming to terms with the doctors. If Dr Browne suspected that the profession was lobbying the Hierarchy against his scheme, his strategy should have been to remove the bishops' fears, not increase them by ignoring or belittling them. More skilful handling of the Hierarchy's objections in October 1950 might have satisfied them that they had nothing to fear from the scheme and that they had much to lose by opposing a scheme for which there was a great deal of support throughout the country. But right to the end, the Minister seems to have treated their objections in a somewhat cavalier manner, and considered that the doctors were the chief opponents to be beaten. The Hierarchy's letter of 5 April shows the weakness of the bishops' case.

The Hierarchy was stung at what must have seemed like a snub from Dr Browne when he went ahead with his scheme and, influenced by the medical profession's opposition, they widened their grounds for opposing the scheme. It was a serious misjudgement by Dr Browne to underestimate the strength of the Hierarchy's position. In retrospect it seems strange that Dr Browne should have handed a hostage to fortune by asking the bishops to adjudicate on his scheme and promising his unequivocal agreement in advance to that decision. It would have taken a Hierarchy with a very different character and outlook to have come to any other conclusion than they did.

The acceptance by Mr Costello's government of the Hierarchy's decision, no matter how weak the case, gave rise to the conclusion that the Catholic Church was the effective government of the country, at least during this administration. Comparing the situation created in 1911 when the bishops intervened to prevent the application of the National Health Insurance Bill with that created by the Hierarchy's intervention on the mother and child service, the political skill of the leaders of the Irish Party contrasts strongly with the ineptness of their political successors.

The question for the health services was whether this crisis marked the end of the initiatives begun in the mid-1940s to provide a first class health service for the whole population or whether it was just another battle in the war between the profession and the administration over how the services should be organised.

10
Compromise
1951~1957

IN 1951, THE VICTORY of the medical profession and the Hierarchy over the agents of 'State controlled medicine' seemed to be confirmed.[1] In line with a Cabinet decision of 6 April, Mr Costello began to lay the basis for a new mother and child scheme which would 'fully respect Catholic social teaching in regard to the individual and society' and which would have the support of the medical profession.[2] Mr Costello himself took over the portfolio of Minister for Health. He set up a committee with Dr J.D. McCormack, the acting chief medical officer of the Department, as chairman; the other members were IMA representatives and departmental medical officers. The omission of lay departmental officials from the committee reflected Mr Costello's lack of confidence in, and the IMA's suspicion of, administrative civil servants.[3] The committee's brief was to draft a scheme for an improved health service for the whole community, beginning with mothers and children.[4] The committee's drafting ability was not put to the test, however, as a few weeks after its appointment the government, badly shaken by the mother and child controversy, fell from office.

In the general election, the health services became an issue as in no other. The medical profession was particularly criticised for its part in the affair and Mr Costello accused of handing the fate of mothers and children to doctors because of family connections with the profession.[5] The coalition parties lost the election and the victorious Fianna Fail party pledged 'to extend health services, including a mother and child health service in accordance with the general intentions of the Health Act, 1947, and with the provisions of the Constitution and its social directive'.[6] Dr Browne, standing as an independent, did exceptionally well in the election, increasing his first preference vote by more than 70 per cent.

The absence of any direct reference to Catholic social and moral teaching and the invocation of the intentions of the Health Act, 1947 in this election promise, at a time when politicians feared a 'belt of a crozier' more than anything else, expressed the independent spirit associated with Fianna Fail since its foundation.[7] Fianna Fail interpreted their election victory as a mandate to reform the health services. However, the party needed the support of independent deputies (including Dr Noel Browne) to form a government.

The sense of continuity with the previous Fianna Fail administration was confirmed by the reappointment of Dr James Ryan as Minister for Health. His actions did nothing to reassure the medical profession or the Hierarchy. He disbanded the joint Department of Health and IMA committee, commenting later that he had found the IMA 'in possession' of the Custom House and had told them 'to get out' – in a polite way.[8] He repeated his determination to ensure that 'no person would be denied the best medical treatment through lack of means' and to provide a comprehensive health service when he met an IMA deputation on 27 July 1951.[9] As usual, Dr Ryan was careful to qualify his intentions by declaring that he did not favour a 'complete scheme of state medicine' or 'of going further than is necessary to provide the specialised services necessary to give our people the best possible service'.[10] As a conciliatory gesture, he invited the profession to make proposals for improving the health services by mid-October.

In an important tactical move, the Minister decided not to proceed with the mother and child service on its own but to include it, as originally intended, as part of a wider extension of health services. It was now possible to consider extending services as envisaged in the 1947 White Paper because of progress in building and equipping hospitals, and in appointing specialists to hospitals outside Dublin and Cork. In July 1951, the Minister informed the Dail that the number of hospitals to be reconstructed or extended under the hospital building programme was 128, and that work had started or been completed on 62.[11] The programme included 37 new hospitals, of which 20 had been started or completed, and it was hoped to reconstruct 16 other hospitals by the end of 1951.[12] There were still shortages of beds. There was accommodation for less than half of the 63,000 births in 1953, but the hospital building programme, to be completed by 1956, would meet expected demand.[13]

Extending entitlements to free hospital services was a politically popular move since the burden of hospital and consultant bills was a growing worry for a sizeable section of the population. It would be difficult for those opposed to such an extension to show that it posed a threat to the moral well-being of the population. Furthermore, since the details of the extended health service had not been worked out, it also gave the Minister breathing time in which to allow the passions of spring 1951 to cool.

The decision to move on a broad front also carried risks. One of the chief reasons for medical opposition to the mother and child scheme was the knowledge that it was a major step towards a free health service for the whole population. A move to provide hospital care at reduced cost or without charge to all was what the most powerful group of doctors in the profession, the voluntary hospital consultants, most feared.[14] While relatively few consultants were directly affected by the proposed mother and child scheme, an extension of free hospital services was a direct threat to all of them. It is significant that in April 1952 the IMA *Journal* referred to the 'recent much increased activity of Dublin consultants in the affairs of the Association'.[15] And since many voluntary hospitals were managed by religious orders, the Church had a direct interest in any changes in their status.

On 17 October 1951, the Association presented the Minister with a voluntary, state-subsidised insurance scheme for financing the health services.[16] The scheme was strong on principle but weak on construction. It amounted to little more than the introduction of an insurance scheme for those who wished to contribute covering hospital, and eventually, general practitioner care. The Association called for an end to public assistance but in the event of a person having no insurance or exhausting his benefit, the proposal envisaged that 'his position would be the same as at present'.[17] No attempt was made to cost the proposals.

The Minister's response to the proposed scheme was less than warm. His Department pointed out that in no country did voluntary insurance cover more than a small proportion of the population; and the scheme would do nothing to provide additional specialist and nursing services or reduce the high level of infant mortality.[18] In more colourful language, the Minister regretted that 'any responsible body should have issued a document which would probably have landed a "bucket" share pusher in gaol.'[19] The profession had, unintentionally, strengthened the Minister's hand by showing they had little to offer the majority of the population as protection against medical expenses.

The Minister began to draft a White Paper outlining his proposal for extending eligibility. In the meantime, he quietly resolved issues around which medical and clerical opposition might have grown. In a sharp change of tack from the days of Dr Browne, he proposed that the Exchequer would meet the actual deficits of voluntary hospitals by way of a grant to the Hospitals Trust Fund since the sweepstakes income was no longer large enough to meet the deficits and the capital required by the hospital building plan.[20] He won government agreement to delete the reference to the 'education of women in respect of motherhood' from the Health Act, 1947 on the grounds that 'the wording could be interpreted as including education in matters affecting ethics and religion', and to the removal of the provisions for health education and compulsory medical inspection of children in the same Act.[21]

He was adept at compromise. The IMA had 'banned' the filling of new university and local authority posts of consultant obstetrician/gynaecologist in Galway and Cork by the Local Appointments Commission. It argued that the appointments could 'conceal an attempt to bring clinical teaching under the control of the State' and 'mark the initial step in the ultimate establishment of a State monopoly of Maternity and Child Welfare Services'. The Minister suggested a representative interview board acceptable to the profession.[22] His Department also moved to improve the fabric of dispensaries, condemned by the IMA as 'unsanitary and wretchedly appointed', by drawing up a standard plan for new buildings and making generous building grants available to local authorities.[23]

The medical profession's worst fears were, however, realised with the publication of Dr Ryan's White Paper in July 1952.[24] The document repeated much of the thinking behind the 1947 Health Act and White Paper, although in presenting it to Cabinet the Minister described it as 'a considerable scaling down of the proposals' contained in the earlier White Paper.[25] The new White Paper proposed a major extension of entitlement to hospital services, 'provided without charge to the recipients'.[26] It was emphasised that there would be no compulsion on persons to avail themselves of any service.

Three categories of eligibility for health services were proposed – the lower, middle and upper income groups. The lower income group, those already entitled to all services without charge, would benefit from the expansion and development of the health services. A means test would determine entitlement to free health services as before. Under the new proposals, entitled persons would receive a card giving the holder and dependants access to free health services for the duration of the card's validity. The middle income group was defined as those currently ineligible for public assistance but earning less than £600 per annum and farmers on farms with a rateable valuation of £50 or less. They were to be entitled to hospital and specialist treatment, and to the new mother, infant and child services, without charge, and to the free tuberculosis service as before. This group would continue to pay their general practitioners for services not provided free to all. The upper income group – persons earning above £600 a year and farmers with a rateable valuation of more than £50 – would be entitled to free tuberculosis, mother, infant and child services and, in cases of hardship, to hospital and specialist treatment at reduced cost. They too would continue to pay their family doctors for other services.

The most significant departure from the 1947 proposals was the abandonment of a comprehensive and free health service for all children under sixteen years of age and of plans to extend the general practitioner service to more people. The Minister conceded that the latter restriction was 'a retreat from the intentions of the 1947 Health Act' but justified it on the grounds that it was a 'substantial concession' to the medical profession and because 'the withdrawal of this part of the service is less likely to cause hardship and ... have an adverse effect on the health of the classes concerned' than any other change in the proposals.[27] Despite these concessions, the White Paper presented radical proposals for extending eligibility for health services. Since about 90 per cent of non-agricultural family incomes were less than £600 a year and the vast majority of farms had rateable valuations of less than £50, the proposed extension of hospital services would cover well over 80 per cent of the population.[28]

The proposals posed the biggest threat yet to the position of voluntary hospitals and to the private practice and income of hospital consultants. The White Paper announced that local authorities would pay voluntary hospitals for providing services for eligible patients, but no rate of payment was mentioned. Nor was there reference to whether specialists in voluntary hospitals would be paid for treating eligible patients or be compensated for loss of private practice. The abolition of charges for most of their fee-paying patients, without reference to alternative remuneration, was a major threat. The White Paper made it clear that patients who opted for private or semi-private accommodation and care by a specialist would do so at their own cost and was firm that no payment in respect of them would be made. The Minister had considered imposing charges on eligible patients for hospital and specialist services but felt that they could only be justified in order to prevent abuse, a contingency which he felt was unlikely to arise.[29]

The White Paper reaffirmed the government's intention to introduce a free service for all expectant mothers and newborn infants, including general practitioner, hospital and specialist care.

The main change on previous proposals was the restriction of free general practitioner care to infants under six weeks and of free hospital and specialist care to children under six years. For the first time mothers were promised a choice of doctor for maternity care from a panel of participating private and dispensary doctors. A free and expanded child welfare service in public health clinics (with referral to hospital and specialist services where necessary) would be provided for children between six weeks and six years. School medical examinations would be extended to secondary schools; and all children in national schools would continue to be entitled to free hospital and specialist treatment for defects discovered at school medical examinations.

It might be asked why Dr Ryan did not confine eligibility for the mother, infant and child services to the lower and middle income groups on the pattern of the proposed extension of hospital and specialist services. The Minister justified the wider access to these services partly on the grounds of history: treatment for defects discovered at medical examination in national schools and certain maternity services could legally be provided without regard to means since the relevant Acts of 1919 and 1915.[30] Secondly, he felt that the income limit of £600 for the middle income group was too low as far as maternity care was concerned. Hospital services were seldom required by a family but maternity care could arise frequently, usually when parents were young and had numerous other financial commitments.[31] He had considered an income limit of £1,000 but since no more than five per cent of couples of childbearing age had incomes above that level, he did not think a special means-testing organisation could be justified.[32] Finally, a means test might discourage women from availing themselves of the service, the main purpose of which was to encourage ante-natal care.[33]

In an attempt to meet criticisms of the encroaching power of the state, the White Paper announced that health authorities would be empowered to make financial and other arrangements to assist voluntary agencies to provide services. The district nursing service would be extended to supplement the voluntary efforts of the Jubilee and Lady Dudley nursing organisations to provide a nursing service to the sick poor at home and to ensure the success of the preventive services for mothers, infants and school children.

The IMA condemned the White Paper proposals. They represented a 'further intrusion of a civil service regime' and state control of medicine and medical teaching.[34] It condemned the 'dangerous growth' of state control implied in the free mother, infant and child services and free treatment to all children in secondary and vocational schools.[35] It claimed that the autonomy of voluntary hospitals was under attack and that the 'health authority … will be the County Manager'.[36] It criticised the expense of an extended health service and repeated its proposals for an insurance-based health service. The Minister's refusal to establish a health council with power to administer any new health schemes was a major omission as far as the profession was concerned.[37]

The Minister was conciliatory on the detail but firm on the principles of his proposals. He was prepared to reappoint an advisory health council to which he would submit all draft regulations for discussion but one without the wide powers demanded by the profession.[38] At a meeting with the IMA on 3 October, he suggested that a joint committee of officials and IMA representatives be established to discuss the White Paper. The doctors refused because they disagreed with the principles underlying the Minister's proposals.[39] On the mother and infant service, he reminded the Association that 'the proposals in question were issued after the fullest consideration and with the authority of the Government and he sees no reason to alter them'.[40] In press statements countering the claims of the IMA, the Minister denied any intention of taking over the medical profession or voluntary hospitals, suggesting that those claims were either dishonest or arose from confusion about the role of the medical profession, which was to practise medicine, not administration.[41]

The Association's published objections to the proposals were spiced with quotations from Catholic social and moral teaching.[42] The profession was careful, no doubt for tactical reasons, not to focus its public opposition on the extension of hospital and specialist services to the middle income group. Although this posed the greatest threat to the status and income of the profession, there was an obvious case for such an extension and it was politically popular. The IMA published a statement openly rejecting the Minister's proposals on 6 November. This precipitated a fierce battle of words with the Minister in the national newspapers.[43]

In defending its interests on this occasion, the medical profession was facing a very different constellation of forces from that under the previous government. It now had to deal with the formidable combination of an able and experienced Minister backed by a united government. Fianna Fail, unlike Fine Gael, had little time for the profession's fears about the encroaching state. On the contrary, it was committed to a much greater public involvement in the health services. The doctors' room for exploiting differences in the Cabinet was limited, if it existed at all, and there was a strong likelihood that the Minister would carry the Health Bill implementing the proposals of the White Paper. The profession still had a formidable ally, however: the Catholic Hierarchy.

The Minister had circulated copies of his White Paper to the bishops in July 1952. Dr McQuaid subsequently asked Dr Ryan to call on him as he thought a few points needed to be changed.[44] At that meeting on 16 September, the Archbishop expressed most concern about the absence of an income limit for the mother and infant scheme.[45] The Minister explained his reasoning for omitting an income limit and while the Archbishop accepted his arguments, he warned Dr Ryan that he would 'run into trouble' with the scheme.[46] Dr McQuaid also informed the Minister that he was a member of a committee of bishops appointed by the Hierarchy to examine health proposals.[47]

A significant factor in the subsequent controversy was the departure of Mr de Valera in early autumn 1952 to Utrecht for treatment of a serious eye complaint and his absence from the country until shortly before Christmas. In his absence, Sean Lemass, Minister for Industry and Commerce and Tanaiste, deputised for the Taoiseach, but neither he nor Dr Ryan inspired the confidence of Dr McQuaid to the same extent as Mr de Valera.[48] Conscious of the dangers of alarming the Hierarchy on the health proposals, Mr de Valera asked for frequent briefings on discussions with the

bishops while he was in Holland.[49] On 6 October, the Minister
again met Dr McQuaid, who on this occasion was accompanied
by Dr Browne, Bishop of Galway and Dr Lucey, Bishop of Cork.
Most discussion centred around the mother and infant scheme with
the bishops promising their approval for the scheme if it contained
a means test.[50] Dr Ryan undertook to put their views to the
government. Other issues which concerned the bishops included
the protection of individuals from any compulsion to use the
services, especially the power of county medical officers to detain
persons suffering from infectious diseases in hospital. The Bishop
of Galway was apparently concerned that 'an unscrupulous and
vindictive medical officer of health ... had power to kidnap his
enemy and then detain him against his will in hospital'.[51]

Dr Ryan appears to have been in no hurry to convey the bishops'
views to the government or to get their agreement to a means
test in the mother and infant scheme. On 6 November, Dr
McQuaid, prompted by the IMA statement rejecting the mother
and infant scheme, which had appeared in that morning's press,
wrote an impatient letter to Mr Lemass seeking a government
response to the Hierarchy's objections to the scheme which he
described as 'unacceptable from the moral viewpoint'.[52] Mr
Lemass and Dr Ryan met the episcopal committee on 10 December.
The bishops again insisted that an income limit apply if the mother
and infant scheme were to comply with Catholic principles.[53]
They were content, however, to leave the actual level of income
to the government to decide.[54] Dr Ryan outlined some proposed
amendments to the 1947 Health Act and discussed the position
of the voluntary and teaching hospitals, without the bishops
expressing any definite views.

As a result of these meetings, Dr Ryan made only one significant
change in his proposals. Women in the upper income group who
wished to use the new mother and infant scheme would have to
pay an annual contribution of £1.[55] This was a concession in
principle, but the Minister gave little away in practice. And the
safeguard written into the Bill at the bishops' behest – specifying
that no one was under an obligation to avail of any examination
or treatment under the Act – did not tie the Minister's hands

231

either.[56] No doubt the power in the Bill to charge middle income patients nominal amounts for hospital maintenance also met with the Hierarchy's approval, although the Minister claimed that the pressure for such charges had come from the local authorities.[57]

In late January 1953, the Minister sent drafts of some of the most important sections of the Bill to the Archbishop of Dublin, including those dealing with the mother and infant scheme, the extension of hospital and specialist services and school health examinations.[58] There were further interchanges between the Minister and Dr McQuaid after the Bill had been circulated, with the Minister undertaking to make certain other amendments at committee stage.[59] When the Minister moved the second reading of his Bill on 26 February, he was under the impression that he had met the bishops' objections to his proposals.[60]

Meanwhile, Dr Ryan continued his propaganda war with the medical profession. In a strongly worded speech in February 1953 he denied that the health services had a policy of starving voluntary hospitals of funds through the building of local authority hospitals and the appointment of publicly employed consultants.[61] He suggested that the striking success of these consultants was because they had been appointed by the Local Appointments Commission solely on merit.[62] He dismissed accusations that his proposals would breach medical secrecy as 'humbug' arguing that no one ever raised the issue of secrecy in the dispensary service or the 'free for all' infectious disease services.[63] 'One can only conclude', he said, 'that the importance of medical secrecy increases with the means of the patient or with the critics' hostility to a particular scheme'.[64] In a speech in Wexford in January, 1953, he condemned the 'mischief makers' in the profession who were trying to mislead family doctors about the implications of the proposed changes in the health services. Those doctors, he claimed, belonged either to 'a branch of the profession who fear the Scheme may be detrimental to their interests, and those with political antipathy to the Government. The few who have both the selfish and the political bias are deadly in their opposition and unscrupulous in their methods'.[65]

Despite the frigid relations with the profession, Dr Ryan went ahead and re-appointed the National Health Council in early 1953, with a membership dominated by medical representatives. As he had promised, the Minister widened the Council's terms of reference to allow it to comment on all Bills and regulations sponsored by the Minister. Some of the IMA's principal spokesmen were appointed to the Council, notably T.C.J. (Bob) O'Connell, and the Association used the Council as a forum to negotiate with the Minister. At meetings on 4 and 11 March, the medical spokesmen argued strongly for amendments to the Bill and the Minister, who chaired meetings, accepted some while rejecting others. The most important concession he made was to enable local authorities to pay consultants in voluntary hospitals for treating lower and middle income patients.[66] This was a major and expensive step and Dr Ryan must have thought that it would remove the chief reason for the Association's opposition to the Bill. It would also mean a major change for the voluntary hospitals, as money paid by public authorities had been paid to the hospital up to then, with few exceptions and not to the doctors. The Minister was also prepared to limit local authority involvement in medical education to the power to provide post-graduate instruction for medical officers but this was not acceptable to the profession.[67]

The medical spokesmen fought hard for the introduction of higher contributions or charges for those who could afford them for the mother and infant scheme but the Minister would not make any further concession on this issue.[68] Nor would the Minister grant more powers to the National Health Council, or agree to the establishment of local health councils.

The Association took their case to the public, playing on what can only be described as class prejudice. 'This Bill represented a further and serious stage in the attack upon the middle classes', T.C.J. O'Connell declared in early April, and its proposals threatened to bring down the standard of medical care and 'the pauperisation of large sections of the community'.[69] An IMA document entitled *The White Paper on Health Services* warned that the proposal meant 'the birth of your children in public maternity wards'.[70]

On 18 March, a general meeting of the Association rejected the Bill unanimously.[71] The editor of the IMA *Journal* declared that 'the fight was on', that the Bill 'conceals ... a fuller measure of State control of medical practice than ever a British Minister sought' and that it was 'an undemocratic instrument under the control of a Doctor Tito and his apparatschniks (sic) in the Custom House'.[72] The Minister described the Association's decision to reject the Bill as a 'bombshell' but reaffirmed his intention of going ahead with the legislation without the profession's co-operation.[73]

The Association decided to lobby their former allies, the Catholic Hierarchy. A deputation from the Association visited the Archbishop of Dublin to inform him of their objections to the Bill.[74] A resolution, sent to the heads of all the churches, defended rejection of the Bill on the grounds of state control of the profession, undue interference by the state with the doctor/patient relationship, the impact on taxation, and the scope for ministerial regulation.[75] In early April, a series of articles by leading doctors appeared in the *Irish Independent* which emphasised the threat in the Health Bill to voluntary hospitals, the independence of their consultants and the professional control of medical teaching; and criticised the absence of a choice for patients of hospital or specialist.[76]

The strategy of the medical spokesmen seems to have been effective. To the government's surprise, the Hierarchy's opposition to the Bill unexpectedly stiffened. At a meeting with the Minister on 23 March, the committee of the Hierarchy, which had been negotiating with the government, felt that an impasse had been reached. A formal letter to the government said that the committee was referring the matter to the general body of bishops.[77] Dr Ryan believed that he had satisfied the bishops' objections and did not interpret this letter as a warning.[78] As John Whyte comments, Dr Noel Browne was not the only Minister to experience difficulties in communicating with the Hierarchy.[79]

The Hierarchy discussed the Bill at a special meeting on 13 April 1953 and decided to issue a public statement setting out their objections. By letting their views be publicly known, the bishops were clearly trying to avoid any repetition of the accusation that

234

they secretly dictated to government. On 17 April, a statement signed by Cardinal D'Alton of Armagh, the head of the Hierarchy, was sent to most of the national papers and Catholic press, and a copy was sent to the Taoiseach some twelve hours before publication.[80] The stage was set for a confrontation between Church and state of even greater proportions than that which occurred in 1951. This time there was no question of the government disowning Dr Ryan's policies and sacrificing the Minister for Health to the critics. The Hierarchy was attacking government policy itself and seemed determined on a public trial of strength. The resolution of this crisis would test Mr de Valera's political skill to the utmost.

The bishops' letter was the most detailed contribution yet made by the Hierarchy to the debate on the expansion of the health services. They welcomed the parts of the Health Bill which amended the mother and child provisions of the 1947 Health Act but went on to point out that parts of the Bill conflicted with Catholic teaching. Significantly, the letter did not specify whether this was Catholic social or moral teaching. The letter argued that the Bill infringed the rights of individuals and fathers to provide for their own health and that of their families by giving the state responsibility for the treatment of all mothers in childbirth and extending hospital and specialist services to seven-eighths of the population. It was claimed that this infringement would lower the 'sense of personal responsibility and seriously weaken the moral fibre of the people'.

Secondly, the letter claimed that the Bill infringed the principle of the state's subsidiary role in social activity by greatly expanding the control of the state over medical services. As examples, the bishops listed the:

absence of a choice by patients of which hospital to be treated in;

powers given to the public health authority, described oddly as 'an official entirely subordinate to the Minister' to direct medical services;

excessive power given to the Minister to modify the services by regulation;

absence in the Bill of a guaranteed choice of doctor for women in the proposed maternity service;

tendency towards 'the elimination of the voluntary hospitals and the establishment of a monopoly of State hospitals';

increasing number of state appointed consultants 'forbidden to practise outside state hospitals';

power given to the Minister to establish medical schools.

Finally, it was claimed that the Bill exposed patients to moral dangers because it contained no safeguards to ensure that patients would not be obliged to accept treatment from 'men who are imbued with materialistic principles or advocate practices contrary to the Natural Law'.

It is even more difficult to account for the Hierarchy's opposition to the Health Bill, 1952 on the grounds of Catholic moral and social teaching than their earlier interventions. Dr Ryan had thought that he had already met their objection to a universal service for mothers and children by introducing a nominal contribution for women in the upper income group. The proposal to extend hospital and specialist treatment to the middle income group was done on the basis that these services had become so expensive that fathers could not afford by their own initiative to provide for the treatment of their dependants. The government had refrained from extending the service to the upper income group and under the Minister's latest proposals, local authorities could levy nominal charges on the middle income group for hospital maintenance. A free general practitioner service was restricted to those who were too poor to pay their doctor. The Minister had promised in his White Paper and announced in the Dail that women would have a choice of doctor in the mother and infant scheme; a woman in the lower income group who previously had no alternative to the dispensary doctor could now choose her doctor for maternity and infant care.[81] Participating dispensary doctors would be subject to less control by the local authority in caring for maternity cases than under the old public assistance code. Local authorities were being given the power to assist voluntary bodies to provide services on their behalf.

It could be argued that the Minister had bent over backwards to reconcile Catholic social teaching with the need to improve and extend the health services. It was not obvious how, in Catholic social thinking, a post-graduate medical school at St. Kevin's Hospital, ministerial power to make regulations governing the operation of services, or the role of local authorities in administering health services could conflict in principle with the legitimate role of the state. The Bill as introduced had already provided that no one was compelled to accept treatment under the Act. One can only marvel at the paternalism, indeed lack of confidence in their flock, which led the bishops to demand legal safeguards to protect patients against treatment or advice from persons with 'pernicious Freudian and materialistic principles'.[82]

The objections of the Hierarchy to the Bill were perhaps rooted in more practical considerations than the bishops would care to admit. Their case makes more sense if it is seen as a defence of the powerful Catholic voluntary hospitals, their consultant staff and associated medical schools, from further state encroachment. The Catholic voluntary hospitals had made a major contribution to medical development in Ireland and had been providing services for the sick poor long before the existence of an Irish government.

The bishops were justified to some extent in their accusation that the role of the voluntary hospitals was being undermined. The expansion of the public hospitals system, using the sweepstakes money which the voluntary hospitals viewed as their own, the refusal of Dr Browne when Minister to meet the cost of their deficits, the growth of a corps of highly competent local authority consultants throughout the country, all threatened the primacy of the Dublin and Cork voluntary hospitals. The extension of hospital services to the majority of the population at nominal or no charge with local authorities paying voluntary hospitals and consultants for their treatment, meant that the hospitals would be even more dependent on public funding than previously.

The extension of the health services had inevitably caused a shift in the balance of medical services, away from the voluntary and private towards the publicly organised and funded. The threat of direct state involvement in medical education, with the possible weakening of the influence of Catholic teaching in the main medical schools, could easily be represented to the bishops as further evidence of the state's malevolent intentions. They may also have been convinced that the absence of a choice of hospital for patients, in an extended and publicly financed hospital service, was a weapon which public authorities could use to slowly starve the business of voluntary hospitals.

Since many of the provisions in the Bill to which the Hierarchy objected in their letter had been put forward originally in the White Paper of the previous July and their implications discussed with the episcopal committee, since the committee of the Hierarchy was aware of the contents of the Bill before it was published in February 1953, and since the Minister, no novice in the business of negotiation, was satisfied that he had met the objections of the bishops, the question arises as to why the bishops came out so decisively and openly against the Bill in March and April 1953? It may be that the bishops were slow to see the implications of the Bill for voluntary hospitals and medical education, but it is more likely that the medical profession, alarmed at the compromise which seemed to have been reached between the Hierarchy and the Minister by February 1953 and by its own failure to win more concessions by March 1953, succeeded in persuading the bishops to broaden their grounds of opposition to the Bill. A notable feature of the bishops' letter of 4 April 1953 is the convergence of the medical and ecclesiastical objections to the Bill. As the editor of the *Journal* of the Irish Medical Association commented, there was 'a striking conformity' between the views of the Hierarchy and the profession on the Bill.[83]

The letter came 'as a complete and unpleasant surprise' to Mr de Valera and his government.[84] When Dr Ryan saw a copy, his immediate reaction was that publication of the letter must be stopped, since if it were published, he would have to prove the bishops wrong in public.[85] He had a cogently argued statement prepared the same day in his Department countering the bishops' objections on the government's behalf.[86] Mr de Valera agreed with the Minister but wanted at all costs to avoid a public confrontation with the Hierarchy and considered that 'there was no reason why objections to a health scheme could not be met without resort to a controversy in the papers'.[87]

With the controversy of 1951 still simmering in the public mind, Mr de Valera knew that neither Church nor state had anything to gain in the long run from another unseemly row over the details of the health services. Mr de Valera and Dr Ryan must have had their suspicions about the source of much of the Hierarchy's ill-informed objections to the health proposals and the speed with which they subsequently acted may also have been prompted by a desire to ensure that the bishops would not act this time as storm troopers for the medical profession.[88] Meanwhile the country was full of rumours about an impending showdown between the government and the Hierarchy over the Health Bill.[89]

Mr de Valera acted without delay. Archbishop McQuaid, to whom the Taoiseach might have turned first to avert a confrontation, had recently left for a prolonged visit to Australia.[90] Mr de Valera decided that he must speak to Cardinal D'Alton immediately and, accompanied by Dr Ryan, he drove the same day to Drogheda where the Cardinal was administering confirmation. When they met the Cardinal, Mr de Valera expressed his astonishment at the contents of the letter and requested him to withdraw the letter for two reasons: because it contained incorrect statements, and, less plausibly, because the Taoiseach's absence from the country before Christmas meant that he was not sufficiently up to date with the details of the health proposals.[91] If the letter were withdrawn, the Taoiseach would agree to resume negotiations on the Bill with the episcopal committee and suggested that the venue might be the relatively neutral setting of the President's home.[92] The Cardinal agreed to use his influence with the Hierarchy to have the letter withheld from publication.[93] In this the Cardinal was successful and, on 19 April, copies of the letter which had been sent to the newspapers were returned, but not before several people had read and made copies of its contents. Mr de Valera's primary aim of preventing a public clash of Church and state on the Bill had been achieved, for the moment at least.

Agreement was quickly reached between the Taoiseach, Dr Ryan and the episcopal committee, chaired in Dr McQuaid's absence by Archbishop Kinnane of Cashel, on the outstanding difficulties with the Health Bill. The government representatives agreed to introduce amendments at the committee stage guaranteeing patients a choice of doctor and of hospital, establishing local health advisory councils and further restricting eligibility for the mother and infant scheme.[94] A public debate soon began about whether these amendments represented a capitulation by the government to the Hierarchy or whether they were no more than drafting changes which allowed the Hierarchy to climb down gracefully from the awkward position on which they chose to make their stand. The question has never been fully resolved and it is worth examining these amendments to see, as far as the health services are concerned, whether they implied a defeat for the government.[95]

The amended Bill now included a specific guarantee that no one would be obliged to accept treatment contrary to the teaching of his religion, and that there would be a choice of doctor in the mother and infant scheme.[96] Since there was never any question of obliging patients to accept treatment contrary to their religious principles and since the Minister had committed himself much earlier to a choice of doctor, these amendments were little more than drafting changes, involving no concession of substance. More substantial were amendments to give patients a choice of hospital, with health authorities paying a reduced rate of subvention for those patients who exercised the choice, and providing for the establishment of local health committees.[97]

The Minister, in complicated amendments, also changed the conditions upon which upper income women could participate in the maternity and infant scheme.[98] Such women would not immediately be eligible to participate in the scheme but would have to contribute £1 in each of the first three years of its operation. Thereafter, all new higher income participants in the scheme would pay half the estimated cost of the maternity services for the upper income group or £2, whichever was the less. There were two further significant amendments which appeared to have been inserted with an eye to the Hierarchy's wishes. The proposal to give health authorities the power to run post-graduate medical schools was removed; their role was limited to providing intermittent 'courses of instruction for medical officers'.[99] Secondly, medical inspection of school children would not take place in secondary or vocational schools, thus returning the school health service to the pre-1947 situation.[100]

Despite these concessions, the amendments appear to be more of a victory than a defeat for the government.[101] The Minister retained what he considered to be the chief provision of his Bill: the extension of eligibility for hospital services.[102] If the medical inspection and treatment of children had been curtailed, Dr Ryan had saved the mother and child scheme at the price of no more than a slight increase in the token contributions from the upper income group. The government conceded nothing on the principle that the state had a responsibility for the medical care of the majority of the population and for the welfare of all mothers and infants, a principle contested by the bishops, most recently in their letter of April 1953. Nor had the Minister accepted any real curtailment of his or the health authorities' powers to administer the health services. No brake was placed on the further expansion of public hospitals and finally, no screening mechanism was introduced to protect unsuspecting patients from obstetricians, gynaecologists and psychiatrists with materialistic tendencies. Once the Minister had protected the substance of his Bill, it was easy to compromise on the details, such as the right of patients to choose to be treated in a voluntary hospital even when a perfectly good public hospital was closer. It is unlikely that the conscience clause or concession on local advisory health councils would have given him much cause for concern.

The most significant amendment from the point of view of services was the decision to limit medical inspection to national schools. The original idea of the Department, that every child would be screened and treated for health defects from birth to sixteen years of age, was abandoned and the benefits of a comprehensive school health service limited to those children who went to public primary schools. However, if the bishops' principles had been accepted, the service would have been means-tested. Perhaps most important of all, the government had made it clear

241

that it would not passively accept criticism from the Hierarchy of legislation, regardless of whether or not the criticism was accurate. Mr Costello had accepted the authority of the bishops to determine what was acceptable health policy but Mr de Valera and Dr Ryan accepted only that the bishops had a right to make their views known. It was a crucially important distinction of the respective spheres of Church and state in Irish public life. The government was careful, however, not to give the impression that it had won any victory over the Hierarchy. It is a sign of the skilful handling of the affair by Mr de Valera and Dr Ryan that so many believed, and still believe, that the government made substantial concessions to the bishops on the Health Bill following their intervention in April 1953. That the bishops had to accept much less than they wished is borne out by the manner in which they grudgingly accepted these latest amendments to the Bill. Acceptance of the amendments, they reminded the government in May 1953, 'is not to be construed as positive approval to the Bill. Since the Bill is not in accordance with the Catholic ideal, positive approval of it would be impossible'.[103] Ronan Fanning's conclusion that 'the bishops got virtually everything they asked for and, in effect, rewrote as much of the Bill as they wanted to' seems, on this analysis, unjustified.[104]

The Medical Association did not hide its disappointment at the amendments agreed with the Hierarchy. The amendments, the editor of the Association's *Journal* wrote, 'have served effectively to intensify our objections to the Health Bill, 1952, as an instrument for the further extension and improvement of State control of medical practice and teaching'.[105] By late June, the Medical Association was undecided whether or not to refuse to operate the legislation now that events seemed to have swung against them. Some days before the Association's annual general meeting to be held in Waterford on 1 July, Archbishop McQuaid, who had returned to the country on 6 June, asked to see some of the leading medical representatives.[106] Dr McQuaid asked them if the Association was going to continue to fight the Bill. The doctors replied that it would be difficult to oppose the amended Bill and that there were advantages in it for sections of the profession. The Archbishop expressed his disappointment and asked the doctors to encourage the Association to continue its opposition.

Dr McQuaid's motivation is not clear. He had been out of the country when the amendments to the Bill had been agreed with the government but had returned for the Hierarchy's meeting on 25 June at which the bishops' letter of 14 April was finally withdrawn. However, Dr McQuaid was anxious to secure a further amendment to the Bill which would open public hospitals to the university medical schools for clinical teaching, while at the same time ensuring that the medical schools would control medical appointments with a clinical dimension in those hospitals.[107] The Taoiseach and Dr Ryan met Dr McQuaid at the President's house on 7 July and agreement was reached on a suitable amendment which Dr Ryan included at the report stage of the Bill.[108] Encouraging the IMA to continue its defiance of the Minister may have suited the Archbishop's purpose of maintaining pressure on the government for this last concession. Dr McQuaid was clearly acting on this occasion as a spokesman for the three medical schools of the overwhelmingly Catholic National University.

The annual general meeting of the IMA in Waterford demonstrated the close alliance between the profession and the Catholic Church. The profession, like most in Ireland, contained its share of Protestants and a sprinkling of Jews. It was normal practice for the annual conference of the Association to begin with various denominational services without any political overtones. But in Waterford in 1953 the Catholic Bishop of Waterford and Lismore presided over the opening ceremony and the annual general meeting was preceded by a votive mass at which the faithful were addressed by a senior priest of the diocese, who compared the Association with 'those vocational bodies, which, as the great Pope Pius XI has declared, are not only desirable but necessary in the social order'.[109] He called on doctors to defend the notion of a person's individual responsibility for health, 'just as for his own soul'.[110] The annual general meeting of the Association went on to pass a resolution expressing their continued opposition to the Bill.[111]

It came as somewhat of a surprise to the two medical negotiators when Archbishop McQuaid recalled them some days after the Waterford meeting and informed them that he had changed his mind about the profession's continued opposition to the Bill.[112] Without giving his reasons, he advised the Association to operate the Bill as best they could. One can only surmise that having won the concession on medical education from the Taoiseach and Dr Ryan on 7 July, Dr McQuaid no longer needed the profession's moral support. The doctors, without too much difficulty, persuaded their colleagues to follow the Archbishop's advice.[113] Faced with the withdrawal of their best cavalry, the doctors had little choice but to look for peace terms. A petition to the President by some of Dublin's leading consultants not to sign the Bill, on the grounds that it infringed the rights of patients, doctors and families, fell on deaf ears and the Health Bill became law at the end of October 1953.[114]

The comparison between the inter-party and Fianna Fail governments' handling of the different stages of the crisis over the extension of health services highlights the difference in political skill and judgement between the two administrations and between Dr Browne and Dr Ryan. Dr Browne, inexperienced, isolated in the Cabinet and making many errors of judgement, stood no chance of overcoming the combined resistance of the medical profession, the Hierarchy and his government colleagues. Dr Ryan, on the other hand, made sure of the support of the government, and of Mr de Valera in particular, and was well aware that the key to removing medical opposition to the Bill was to contain the objections of the Hierarchy. With the support of a united Cabinet, he was able to come to terms with the bishops and, indirectly, with the medical profession.

Dr Ryan was not, however, destined to preside over the implementation of the Health Act, 1953. Mr de Valera's minority government found it increasingly difficult to hold onto power and in the spring of 1954 a general election was announced. The Minister moved quickly to set 1 August 1954 as the date for the implementation of the Health Act. Regulations filling in the details of the Act were rushed through the National Health Council and signed on 15 May 1954, just three days before the general election.

Dr Ryan's haste was justified as Fianna Fail was unable to form a government after the election and a second inter-party government, with Mr Costello as Taoiseach, took office in June.

The new Minister for Health was Mr T.F. O'Higgins, son of Dr T. O'Higgins, the former Minister for Defence and member of the IMA Central Council. Mr O'Higgins' brief from the Taoiseach was 'to take health out of politics'. The sympathies of the new Minister and of Fine Gael, the largest party in the government, lay with the medical profession but their room for manoeuvre was circumscribed by the need to retain the support of their partners, especially the Labour Party which supported the Act. The Minister, working on the assumption that he could repeal his predecessor's regulations by a further regulation, began negotiation with the different medical interests affected by the Act, beginning with the general practitioners.[115] At these meetings the Minister was accompanied only by a notetaker from the Department, so intense was the doctors' distrust of the administrative civil servants in the Custom House. The negotiations with the other medical interests proved more difficult and it was clear that no agreement would be reached by 1 August. The Minister decided to alter the implementation date by regulation but discovered to his consternation that the date could be changed only by a new Act. He had difficulty persuading his Labour colleagues that legislation was necessary.[116] About this time, the Minister sought a private meeting with T.C.J. O'Connell, the leading medical negotiator and explained his difficulties with the implementation date.[117] He could only postpone the implementation of the Bill if public opinion, and particularly the Labour Party, could be persuaded that genuine grounds for delay existed. It was agreed that a recommendation for postponement from the National Health Council would help the Minister's case. The Minister promised to set up a commission to inquire into the feasibility of a voluntary scheme of insurance against medical expenses, a proposal close to the profession's heart.

Mr O'Connell fulfilled his part of the bargain by persuading the National Health Council to recommend to the Minister that the sections providing for hospital and specialist services for the middle income group be postponed on the grounds that the existing accommodation was inadequate to cope with the demand which this extension of eligibility was expected to bring about.[118] On 7 July, the Minister introduced a Health Bill which allowed him to stagger the extension of services under the Act.[119] The net effect of this legislation was that the extension of hospital and specialist services to the middle and upper income groups envisaged in the Health Act, 1953 was postponed until 31 March 1956 and the maternity and infant scheme for the upper income group, a major source of controversy since 1947, was never implemented.

There were other changes which signalled a new rapport between the profession and the Minister for Health. The Medical Practitioner Acts were amended, reducing ministerial control over the activities of the Medical Registration Council, and the conditions of appointment of county surgeons were revised to permit them to engage in private practice outside local authority hospitals.[120] The Minister also kept his promise to establish a body to advise on a voluntary health insurance scheme. A committee, chaired by H.B. O'Hanlon with prominent representatives of the medical profession including Oliver Fitzgerald, T.C.J. O'Connell and Patrick Meenan, was appointed in January 1955. The committee was charged with the task of advising the Minister on the feasibility of introducing a scheme 'which would enable citizens to insure themselves and their dependants voluntarily' against the cost of hospital, specialist, maternity and dental services and medicines and appliances, and on the organisation of such a scheme.[121] In a well argued report, the committee found that a voluntary health insurance scheme for the upper income group and for those in the middle income group who wished to choose private care, was feasible.[122] A scheme was suggested to meet the cost of hospital maintenance, surgical and medical services in hospital and of a cash grant for maternity. The possibility of including general practitioner services within a scheme was ruled out early in the committee's deliberation. Routine dental services and long term care for the chronically and mentally ill were excluded and an age limit of seventy years for contributors suggested. It recommended that the scheme be organised by a non-profit public company established

246

by the Minister for Health, with a government subsidy to guarantee its initial solvency.

Mr O'Higgins accepted the committee's report and introduced legislation to establish a company called the Voluntary Health Insurance Board (VHI), on lines similar to those recommended by the committee.[123] The Minister advanced £13,000 to the fledgling Board to get it off the ground. The Board had hardly begun its operations when the second inter-party government fell and Fianna Fail was returned to office. The new Minister, the veteran Mr MacEntee, threatened that if the VHI was not financially independent within a year he would close it down.[124] The new scheme proved as popular with the upper income group as its promoters had predicted and the VHI was able without any difficulty to repay the Minister his £13,000 by the appointed day. Mr MacEntee soon became one of the VHI's staunchest defenders.

Conclusion

The dramatic events of the late 1940s and early 1950s have been ably analysed in terms of the clash of Church and state by J.H. Whyte and most recently by Ronan Fanning.[125] Less attention has been paid to the health issues at stake or to the role of the medical profession in bringing conflict to a head. This analysis highlights the extent to which radical proposals to improve the health services in the mid-1940s drew fierce opposition from the medical profession and alarmed the bishops. The opposition of the medical profession was to be expected since their status, traditions and income were threatened. The intervention of the Hierarchy was less predictable, but it can be explained in terms of a dislike of bureaucracy, fear that abortion and contraception would be imported to Ireland, concern about the abuse of state power, and the belief in the medical profession as one of the ideal vocational groups advocated by Catholic social teaching. These factors predisposed them to accept the doctors' opinion that the government's proposals contained serious infringements of Catholic teaching. Secondly, church control of voluntary hospitals and influence in medical education made the Hierarchy suspicious of government proposals which seemed to undermine their prestige and power. The authority exercised by the Hierarchy, especially in this aspect of Irish life, meant that their intervention would be a critical factor in disputes between ministers and the medical profession.

Who gained and who lost as a result of these battles? The answer, as to many such questions, is that each group had its victories and defeats. The original departmental goal of a gradual move towards a universal and first class health service without charge for the whole population, in which most doctors would be employed by salary, was severely modified. The organisation of general practice was left unchanged by the Health Act, 1953, except that all general practitioners could apply to provide a mother and infant service for lower and middle income patients in their area. Far from extending the scope of the dispensary service to include an ever widening group of the population, private medical practitioners were allowed to provide a service for patients who previously could only go to the dispensary doctor. The proposal to provide a comprehensive health service for children from birth to sixteen years of age through district medical officers was reduced to one scheme for infants up to six weeks, another providing advice and treatment in health clinics for all children aged six weeks to six years, and a third providing inspection and treatment for children in national schools. The legislative provision for a contributory maternity and infant service for mothers and infants in the upper income group was never implemented. Hospital and specialist services, which the Department had proposed extending to the whole population without charge (on the model of the tuberculosis service), were restricted to the lower and middle income groups, and many middle income patients could be charged nominal charges for hospital maintenance. The notion of access to all services on the basis of medical need alone gave way to complex eligibility criteria, largely based on income, varying from service to service.

On the other hand, the health services in the 1950s were a vast improvement on those which existed in the early 1940s. Tuberculosis and other infectious diseases had been brought under control. Services for mothers and babies were greatly improved, and maternal and infant mortality reduced significantly in a short time. Modern hospital and specialist treatment was made available at nominal or no charge to the majority of the population, on the principle that the state had a responsibility for those who could not afford to pay for hospital treatment. The VHI protected those not covered by public schemes. The expansion of eligibility was given practical effect by the vast hospital-building programme which between 1949 and 1956 provided 4,000 tuberculosis beds, 2,400 general medical and surgical, 176 maternity, 200 orthopaedic, and 450 children's beds, and by the appointment of highly qualified specialists to hospitals throughout the country.[126] Pathology, radiology, and blood transfusion services, vital to the success of physicians and surgeons, were greatly improved. In the space of a dozen years, Ireland had developed a modern health service which compared favourably with those of more prosperous countries.

The Hierarchy's successive interventions on health issues clearly put a brake on the Department's drive towards a publicly controlled health service, and ensured greater legal protection for the individual and voluntary groups in the health service. But the Catholic Church paid much in terms of credibility and good will as a result of the vehement reaction from many people to their opposition to Dr Browne's mother and child scheme and because of their dignified retreat before the firm stance of Mr de Valera and Dr Ryan on the Health Bill, 1953.

The medical profession could be satisfied that it had, at least for the moment, stopped the momentum towards a nationalised health service in which there would be little or no private practice and in which they would be remunerated mainly by salary or capitation. Their case for health insurance for those not covered by public provision was recognised by the establishment of the VHI. But they had to accept the growing strength of publicly organised and funded health services and the extension of maternity, infant, hospital and specialist services at no or a nominal charge to the majority of the population.

By 1957, the passions which had raged over the extension of the health services seem to have spent themselves and a spirit of compromise had emerged. It would be hardly surprising if all parties had lost the stomach for further conflict. The administration modified its original ambitions, the Hierarchy accepted much greater involvement by public authorities in providing health services and the medical profession found that the extension of services, which they had so bitterly opposed, held considerable advantages for them. The establishment and success of the Voluntary Health Insurance Board indicated a new kind of partnership between government, the medical profession and the idealised 'voluntary' spirit of Irish Catholic moralists.

Perhaps those who gained most from the controversies of these years were the ordinary Irish people, whose chances of dying from an infectious disease in infancy, of tuberculosis in adulthood, of complications in childbirth or of suffering throughout life from disabling but treatable diseases, were greatly reduced. They now benefited from a health service of an incomparably higher standard than in the 1940s; and the extension of eligibility and provision of publicly guaranteed insurance had removed the fear of crippling medical costs. It was an achievement about which politicians, health administrators, doctors, and even bishops, could be proud.

11
Taking Health out of Politics
1957~1970

THE GENERAL ELECTION of 1957 was a turning point in the recent history of Ireland, according to F.S.L. Lyons.[1] The faces which made up the victorious Fianna Fail Cabinet did not portend any new departure. Many were the same as those which had formed the first Fianna Fail government in 1932. But change stirred beneath the apparent continuity. This was exemplified in a new approach to the economic problems of the country. A White Paper, the result of a fortuitous partnership between Dr James Ryan, now Minister for Finance and Kenneth Whitaker, the young Secretary of the Department, was published in 1958 as *Programme for Economic Expansion,* setting out priorities for public investment to expand the economy over a five-year period.[2] This economic initiative was remarkably successful because it gave a sense of purpose to public and private activity and enabled Ireland to take advantage of the economic growth in other Western countries. The Programme's target was a modest 2 per cent growth of GNP a year. In the event, average growth over the period of the Programme was twice this amount. Economic growth was sustained throughout the 1960s, at close to an annual average of 4 per cent, bringing an unprecedented level of prosperity to the country.

The White Paper also emphasised that Ireland's economic future lay through the development of an export-oriented industry and agriculture and the attraction of foreign investment. This outward-looking economic policy coincided with and encouraged a decline in the introspection and isolation which had characterised Irish life for decades. The prospect of joining the European Economic Community and the liberalising impact of the Second Vatican Council on Irish Catholicism helped widen national horizons. The intellectual climate of the 1960s was remarkably liberal and adventurous by comparison with that of the 1940s and 1950s. Tensions between bureaucratic and corporatist views of the state, and between civil servants and vocational groups, gave way to conflicts more familiar to Western democracies as workers strove for a larger share of the new prosperity, farmers resented the gains made by city dwellers, and women and young people questioned social values. A pre-occupation with the principles of organising society yielded to a concern with technology, business techniques and more efficient administration. A sign of the times was that bishops asked for increased state intervention in the affairs of the community, not less.[3] Debate on social issues was dominated by the belief that social progress must follow, rather than accompany, economic growth and by the assumption that 'a rising tide lifts all boats'.[4] Few doubted that the key to economic development had been found, and that continued growth and prosperity were inevitable. A further sign of the loosening of old attitudes was the attempted reconciliation with Northern Ireland in the mid-1960s, an attempt which seems only to have fuelled the flames of the approaching conflict. By 1970, when this study ends, policy towards Northern Ireland had divided the Cabinet and created a major crisis for the government.

The approaching prosperity was hardly apparent in 1957 as the country struggled with economic depression and psychological despondency. An attempt in 1955 to stimulate the economy by heavy investment in social infrastructure failed, creating a budget deficit crisis which the incoming Fianna Fail government only resolved in 1957 by stringent economies. It soon became clear that the new Minister for Health, Sean MacEntee, while he had lost none of his pugnacity or zeal, was opposed to the kind of radical changes in the health services which he had supported in the 1940s.

He believed that the changes which had occurred since his days in the Custom House had given the country a health service which, if not ideal, was as good as any in the world.[5] He could not justify additional expenditure on improving the services, given the other demands on public resources. When he took up his new job, he let it be known that he was not interested in any major overhaul but simply in 'oiling the machine'.[6]

Perhaps the Minister was forced to make a virtue of necessity. The momentum towards increased revenue expenditure on health services had been initiated by the generous financial provisions of the Health (Financial Provisions) Act, 1947. In the late 1950s, the cost of running the additional 7,000 beds provided by the hospital-building programme and the extension of hospital and specialist services to 85 per cent of the population greatly increased the pressure on spending. Expenditure by local authorities on general hospital services in the financial year 1956/7 was £4.6 million, £1 million more than in 1955/6 and double the increase in the previous year.[7] Grants from the Hospitals Trust Fund in 1956 to cover the voluntary hospitals' deficits, at £1.2 million, were twice those paid in 1955.[8] In response to the fiscal crisis, one of Mr MacEntee's first actions as Minister was to raise hospital charges, and introduce charges for specialist consultations and x-rays for the middle income group at out-patient clinics.[9] Charges on the middle income group, which Dr Ryan had reluctantly included in the Health Act 1953, were defended by Mr MacEntee as a matter of principle on the basis that it was 'only right, just, fair and equitable' that those who could afford to contribute something should do so.[10]

Given the Minister's elevation of pragmatism to principle, it is hardly surprising that he showed no interest in extending the mother and infant scheme to the upper income group as provided in the Health Act, 1953, but postponed indefinitely by the previous Minister, nor in extending eligibility for other services, apart from keeping pace with changes in the social insurance code. It explains too his warm support for the voluntary health insurance scheme once his initial fears of insolvency had been allayed.

A Choice of Doctor

Mr MacEntee's period as Minister for Health was not devoid of innovation, however. One important initiative which he was prepared to contemplate was the introduction of a choice of doctor in the dispensary service. Mr MacEntee was no doubt influenced by the success of the mother and infant scheme under which eligible women could choose their doctor and which was popular with doctors and patients alike. Extending a choice of doctor could not be faulted in principle by the authorities of the Catholic Church or the medical profession, on previous form. Granting this choice, however, posed major questions for the future of the dispensary service. It was unclear if a choice of doctor was compatible with the notion of one doctor providing services for eligible patients within a defined geographical area.

The task of examining the practicability of providing a choice was assigned to a small group of officials, chaired by Brendan Hensey (who was later to become Secretary of the Department). Their report, which was not published, proposed the most radical overhaul of the dispensary service since its inauguration more than a hundred years previously.[11] The group found that a choice of doctor would be practicable. It favoured a panel system, on the model of the mother and infant scheme, with private practitioners competing for business with former dispensary doctors.

Salary was rejected as a method of paying doctors participating in the scheme. The-fee-for-service method was also ruled out, because it would be 'administratively difficult and inconvenient and would probably work out much more expensive'.[12] The committee supported a capitation system, because of its success in the mother and infant scheme and its use in the UK. It recommended an average capitation rate of £1 5s a year for each eligible person, with special payments to doctors in remote areas and a rural travelling allowance.

A choice of doctor would improve the service to eligible patients although the report did not discuss this in detail. The dependence of public patients on one doctor under the dispensary system, irrespective of the doctor's willingness to give them a good service, was a constant irritant. Choosing a doctor from a panel of general practitioners in the area would give a public patient the same kind of hold over the doctor as a private patient. If a patient were being treated badly, he or she could change doctor. At the same time, it would encourage competition between doctors for public patients and provide incentives to the more energetic and able practitioners. It also offered a way of bridging the divide between public and private general practice in a way which suited the ethos of Irish general practice.

Relations with the Medical Profession

It might have been expected that Mr MacEntee's vigorous defence of the principles on which the health services were organised would lead to improved relations with doctors. But, on the contrary, relations between the medical profession and the Custom House were seldom worse than while he was Minister. Suspicious of the close links between the leaders of the profession and Fine Gael and wary of their tactics, the Minister conducted a campaign to keep the profession in its place, as he saw it, a campaign which was punctuated with moments of heated passion and high comedy.

Hostilities began over the issue of whether the Minister had the right, in cases where a complaint was brought against a dispensary doctor, to inspect the patient's medical records. IMA dissatisfaction with salaries and conditions of doctors employed by health authorities was met with a refusal by the Ministers to recognise the IMA's mandate to negotiate on behalf of the profession under the Trades Union Act, 1941.[13] The Association responded with its time-honoured tactic of blacking posts by inserting 'important notices' in its *Journal* instructing doctors not to apply for public medical posts. The Minister countered by accusing the IMA of resorting to the tactics of the boycott.[14] The row deepened with the Minister's refusal to consult the profession on the Health and Mental Treatment (Amendment) Act, 1958 which increased the income limit for entitlement to hospital and specialist services from £600 to £800 a year.

An attempt by both sides to mend fences after the general

election of June 1959 backfired. The Association, against the wishes of a substantial number of members, invited the Minister, Mrs MacEntee and senior officials of the Department, to their annual dinner in Killarney. The Minister, with some reluctance, agreed to go. At the dinner the Minister confirmed his willingness to meet a delegation of the Association in the near future, provided, he later claimed, that the 'important notices' were removed.[15] When the notices continued to appear in the *Journal,* the Minister withdrew his offer of a meeting and sent the Association £5 for the cost of his and Mrs MacEntee's dinner in Killarney. The editor of the *Journal,* William Doolin, published a blistering attack on Mr MacEntee in which he castigated the Minister for being so undignified as to send a cheque 'to cover the expense of the entertainment of himself and his formidable escort' in Killarney.[16] The reference to the Minister's 'formidable escort' could have referred to Padraig O Cinneide, the Secretary and Patrick O Muireadhaigh, Assistant Secretary of the Department, who had accompanied the Minister, both of whom were big men. It was, however, intended to be, and understood by the Minister as, an insult to Mrs MacEntee, a lady of generous proportions.[17] The incident was followed by a complete breakdown in communication between the Custom House and the profession.

Compromise was eventually reached in 1963 between the profession and the Minister on the question of seeing the medical records of patients who complained about their doctors and the profession agreed to set up the Irish Medical Union to negotiate salaries and conditions with the Department. From then on relations between the Department and the profession improved steadily. By the end of the decade a virtual alliance of interests had developed between the Minister, the Department and the profession, an alliance cemented in the Health Act, 1970.

Select Committee on the Health Services

By the early 1960s an unusual situation had developed whereby the main impetus for change in the health services was coming, not from Fianna Fail, but from the Labour Party and Fine Gael.

In 1959, the Labour Party published its proposals for a free health service for all financed from central taxation and insurance contributions.[18] Fine Gael favoured a comprehensive health service funded largely by insurance contributions for 85 per cent of the population, providing a free choice of doctor, free hospital and specialist services and the abolition of medical cards.[19] In the 1961 general election, the extension and financing of the health services were major issues. Fianna Fail was able to form a government after the election, but only with the support of independents.

Vulnerable on health issues, the new government was forced to respond to a Dail motion from Deputy T.F. O'Higgins demanding the introduction of a health scheme on the lines proposed by Fine Gael.[20] Mr MacEntee's response was uncharacteristically and superficially accommodating. He proposed the establishment of a select committee of the Dail to examine 'to what extent the existing system of health services did not reasonably meet the essential medical needs of the population'.[21] Since such committees were unusual in Irish parliamentary life, the Minister's motives were immediately suspect. Deputy O'Higgins condemned the committee as a ploy 'to put (health) into the political limbo of forgotten things'.[22]

The extent to which the Minister and the Department had curtailed their ambitions for the health service became apparent early on in the committee's deliberations. Referring to the 'general principles' of the health services, a submission from the Department to the committee announced that:

> *In developing the services ... the Government did not accept the proposition that the State had a duty to provide unconditionally all medical, dental and ancillary services free of cost for everyone, no matter what their individual need or circumstances might be. On the other hand, the services are not designed so that a person must show dire need before he can avail himself of them.*[23]

Interestingly, this statement did not say what principles the government had pursued in developing services, referring only to those which it had eschewed. It claimed that 'the pursuit of this broad principle' had resulted in more effective use of resources than if 'an effort had been made to develop ... a comprehensive free-for-all national health service or ... a general practitioner service for a much wider group of the population'.[24]

These official sentiments should be understood less as a statement of historical accuracy than as an expression of repentance and a promise not to offend again. The Minister and the Department were reassuring those with a stake in the health services that they no longer contemplated any radical change in eligibility or in the role of the state. Their formulation, while hardly a statement of principle, made sense of what had been achieved, was immediately acceptable to the mores of Irish society and, over the next decade, provided a rationale for public activity in medical services.

A number of themes emerged from the evidence submitted to the committee. There was support for an extension of the general medical service to a wider group of the population and for a choice of doctor in an existing or extended medical service.[25] While some submissions favoured small increases in the income limit for hospital and specialist services and the removal of charges on the middle income group, the system of eligibility set out in the Health Act, 1953 seems to have been widely accepted. Indeed, the Department noted with some satisfaction that in only one submission was a demand made for an extension of hospital and specialist services to those earning over £1,100 a year.[26]

Less satisfaction was expressed with the quality of the hospital services. The Irish Medical Association, influenced by the British White Paper, *A Hospital Plan for England and Wales,* argued that hospitals providing services at consultant level should cater not only for medicine and surgery but also for maternity, psychiatry, geriatrics and infectious diseases.[27] It recommended that a hospital with 350 beds should be the minimum acceptable size. It conceded that it would be impracticable to abolish the county hospitals in order to replace them with hospitals of the desired size but suggested that some county hospitals might be amalgamated in groups or associations. It considered that the existing arrangements, whereby consultants based in regional hospitals visited county hospitals, was a poor substitute for a specialist who was a member of the hospital staff. The need to develop specialist medical facilities throughout the country was a major theme of other submissions from medical bodies.[28]

The Department was defensive. Thanks to the work of the departmental committee on a choice of doctor, it conceded that it was feasible to provide a choice in all but a few areas of the country.[29] The Department was also prepared to accept the case made in medical submissions for the concentration of specialist services in larger hospitals. It agreed that for technological and staffing reasons, and 'to avoid making a shuttlecock of the patient', the team of specialists should be available under one roof.[30]

The Department's memoranda to the committee also indicated a growing concern with the problem of financing the health services. The generous terms of the Health Services (Financial Provisions) Act, 1947, whereby the state had expanded its contribution from 16 to 50 per cent of the total cost of health services, had been fully exploited by the financial year 1953/4.[31] Further increases in health expenditure had to be met equally by the Exchequer and local rates. At a time of low inflation, the cost of health services showed a disturbing rate of increase, rising from £13 million in the financial year ending 31 March 1955 to £21.2 million in the year to 31 March 1963.[32] This rate of increase was slightly higher than growth in gross national product – public health expenditure grew from 2.5 to 2.7 per cent of GNP in the period.[33] More significant was the impact on local taxation. Between 1954 and 1965, the rate in the pound in Dublin increased from 32s to 45s and in Galway from 43s to 74s, increases due largely to higher spending on health services.[34] In response to demands that health charges should no longer fall on the rates, the Department warned that if the state bore all or most of the costs of the health services, there would no longer be a case for leaving the administration of the services in the hands of local authorities, with only direction and supervision from the Department.[35] The Department's attitude illustrated three things – a distrust of the capacity of local authorities to spend money wisely, a belief that additional funds would be made available to improve health services and an assumption that it was the most responsible body to decide how this money should be spent.[36]

259

Suspicions about the Minister's motives in establishing the select committee were confirmed by the manner of its demise. Despite the weight of evidence presented to it and of analysis by the Department, the committee issued only two interim reports, neither of any importance.[37] The committee finally fell apart in March 1965, a month before a general election, when the Labour and Fine Gael members formally withdrew.

Mr MacEntee's reluctance to contemplate change in the health services may have contributed to his undignified departure from the Custom House. A few days before the election, the Taoiseach, Mr Lemass announced that Mr MacEntee would not be taking up ministerial office if Fianna Fail won the election and he pledged his party to the introduction of a choice of doctor in the general medical service. The enforced retirement of Mr MacEntee was fully in line with Mr Lemass's views on the need to retire older ministers to make way for new blood, but it was an ignominious end to Mr MacEntee's long association with the health services.

The 1966 White Paper

The quality and organisation of the health services were important issues in the general election of 1965. Fine Gael, in their policy document *Winning through to a Just Society*, reiterated their criticisms of the existing services and the principles behind them. If elected, Fine Gael promised to introduce a comprehensive health service based on insurance.[38] General medical services would be extended to all but the wealthiest 15 per cent of the population. Significantly, their proposals included a promise to remove the cost of financing personal health services from the rates. The Labour Party in its policy statement repeated its objections to the existing services and called for the establishment of 'a free medical health service for all citizens' under the direction of a 'national health authority' which would 'take over voluntary hospitals'.[39]

As if to prove that elections are won and lost on issues other than the health services, Fianna Fail was again returned to power. The new Minister for Health, Mr Donogh O'Malley, could hardly have differed more in temperament from the elderly Mr MacEntee.

Mr O'Malley, young and energetic, and in his first Cabinet post, was a politician in search of issues. He had a lively, flamboyant style, not conducive to detailed administrative work but an asset in persuading fellow politicans and the electorate of the merits of his policies. On arrival in the Department, Mr O'Malley lent his support to those officials with ideas for action and more specifically, he agreed to publish a White Paper outlining the changes considered necessary in the health services.

The White Paper, *The Health Services and their Further Development*, was published in January 1966.[40] While all White Papers are composite documents, the hand of Dr Brendan Hensey is generally considered to have played the main part in drafting this document. Acknowledging the importance of the submissions made to the Dail Select Committee in forming the government's proposals, the White Paper condensed and integrated strands of thought which, to officials at least, had become familiar. It disarmed potential critics by repeating the disclaimer, first made in 1962 to the select committee, that the government did not accept the proposition that the state had a duty to provide unconditionally for all medical services free of cost for everyone.[41] In fact, the White Paper proposed only one significant extension of service. It announced that persons in the middle income group would be formally entitled to assistance towards the cost of obtaining drugs where undue expense arose. Such assistance could be justified by the White Paper's pragmatic philosophy of helping those in genuine need, while weakening the case for extending general practitioner care to the same group. The White Paper argued that since 'hardship is seldom caused in the middle income group through family doctor's bills', an extension of state-organised general medical services was unnecessary.[42] The bulk of the White Paper was devoted to detailing improvements in services and, most importantly, proposing administrative changes in the hospital service and ways of paying for the increasing cost of the health services.

The White Paper reaffirmed the government's decision to introduce a choice of doctor in the general medical service; it went further than before in specifying that participating doctors would have to provide the same facilities for public and private patients and make no distinction in treating them.[43] While the method of payment to doctors would have to be negotiated, the government expressed its preference for capitation.[44] The government accepted the logic that if eligible patients were to be given a choice of doctor and not treated differently from private patients, they should also be entitled to have their prescriptions filled in the retail chemist of their choice. Eligibility for the new scheme would be specified in legislation and widely publicised.

The White Paper drew firm conclusions on what needed to be done in the hospital services but did not present strong arguments to support them. The increase in the proportion of patients treated in voluntary teaching and regional hospitals between 1951 and 1964 was evidence 'for considering the future planning of our hospital services in geographical units larger than the county'.[45] Similarly, the White Paper claimed that the increasing complexity of medical care and the sub-division of medical specialities 'must lead to a recognition that a county hospital is not entirely suited to be a self-contained unit'.[46] The solution proposed was that county hospitals should become closely associated with each other and with teaching and regional hospitals in some form of regional administration.

A new form of administration for the health services was justified for financial reasons. Harassed local representatives were offered financial relief on the rates in return for surrendering their control of health services. The rates, the White Paper announced, 'are not a form of taxation suitable for collecting additional money'.[47] It promised that the cost of improving the health services would not be met from the rates. The government had not, however, decided on who was going to pay for the improvements. In the meantime, the White Paper promised that the share of the total cost of health services falling on the rates in 1966/7 would not exceed the cost in the previous year. In return, health authorities would have to surrender their autonomy.[48]

What the government had in mind was to transfer the administration of the health services from the existing health authorities to regional boards. It was envisaged that the new health boards would be composed of representatives of the medical and related professions and others appointed by the Minister for Health and local authority members, representing 'a partnership between local government, central government and the vocational organisations'.[49] It was made clear that the voluntary hospitals would remain in their present ownership. The principles of the county management system, with a manager carrying out executive functions under the general direction of the body of members, would apply in the new boards and the Department of Health would exercise a more general control. It would 'become oriented towards broad forward planning for the health services'.[50]

Although the regional health boards were later proclaimed to be an exercise in decentralisation, the word was not mentioned in the White Paper. On the contrary, the distrust of local authorities, the bureaucratic traditions of the Department and the desire to trade more Exchequer funding for local control of services point towards centralisation. Introducing the debate on the White Paper in the Dail, Mr O'Malley expressed the view that the county was too small a unit for the organisation of many health services and described the development of regional boards as 'the logical outcome, not only of the other proposals in the White Paper, but of the long-term trend in the administration of the health services'.[51]

Mr O'Malley's promise of legislation to implement the White Paper by autumn 1966 proved optimistic.[52] Had he remained Minister for Health, the process of negotiation and preparation before the Bill appeared might have been quicker but in August 1966, Mr O'Malley became Minister for Education. It is no coincidence that education policy became the main focus of public attention.

Mr Sean Flanagan, who succeeded Mr O'Malley as Minister for Health, was less enthusiastic about the choice of doctor scheme than his predecessor, fearing that rural patients would lose out under the scheme. His fears were shared by many of the local authorities he visited in autumn 1966 to explain the White Paper proposals. As a result of this tour, he asked for a detailed and time-consuming examination of the implications of a choice of doctor in each dispensary district.[53]

263

Perhaps as a way of disarming potential critics of the Bill, the Minister was at pains to stress his view of the minimalist role of the state in the provision of health services. Mr Flanagan announced his opposition to large extensions of the health services 'not because we are afraid to raise the money, but because we see no justification for such an extension'.[54] He saw no reason why it should be accepted that it was the duty of the state to provide health services for all the people any more than it had a duty to reorganise free transport or free bread for all. 'Our health policy', he argued, 'has been, is and will be based on a different philosophy and one I think which is more in accord with our national traditions'.[55] As John Whyte comments, 'one might question the antiquity of the national tradition to which Mr Flanagan referred'.[56] The Minister's espousal of an approach to health services which would have been shared by bishops and the medical profession meant that the preparation and passage of the Health Bill, 1969 was remarkably free of the ideological conflict which marked debate on earlier health legislation. While there was much to bargain about, negotiations were conducted on the same plane as is normal between government and powerful interest groups. The main issues facing Mr Flanagan in implementing the White Paper were how the health services should be financed, how the administration of the health and hospital services were to be regionalised, and, most intractable of all, how doctors would be paid in the proposed choice of doctor scheme.

Financing the Health Services

The link made in the White Paper between reducing the burden of health costs on the rates and the establishment of the regional health boards was a tactical success.[57] In response to the wishes of local councillors, the Minister promised that the number of public representatives on the new regional authorities would equal the number of professional nominees.[58] That concession helped sweeten the pill of losing local control. Criticism increased, however, when, in the financial year 1967/8, the Minister was unable to honour the White Paper promise that the cost of any further extension of the services would not be met from the rates. The Minister was clearly unable to get Cabinet approval to an open-ended commitment from the Exchequer. The question of financing the health services continued to be handled on a 'hand to mouth' basis over the next few years, without evidence of the fundamental rethinking promised in the White Paper. While the 'freeze' on local contributions which operated in 1966/7 was not continued in subsequent years, annual discretionary grants from the Exchequer helped alleviate the burden on rates.

Meanwhile public expenditure on health services was rising at an alarming rate, reaching £47 million in the financial year 1968/9 or 3.5 per cent of GNP.[59] In real terms, this represented an increase of 1.7 times the expenditure in the financial year 1962/3.[60] Most of the increase was due to expenditure on the general hospital service, which rose from £7.2 million to £15.3 million in the same period, an increase of 1.8 in real terms.[61] Some of this increase can be explained by more admissions which grew from 229,000 in 1957 to 372,000 in 1971.[62] Although there was little overall change in the number of hospital beds, most of the sanatoria beds had been reclassified as general hospital beds as the number of persons undergoing treatment for tuberculosis declined. The change meant these beds were used more intensively and more expensively. Staff numbers in the health services also grew. While it is difficult to be precise, there appears to have been a rise of more than 4,000 general nurses between 1951 and 1971.[63] A fourth factor was the effect of pay settlements on the labour-intensive hospital service. Wage rates in the 1960s rose faster than national output.[64]

The role of the Hospital Sweepstakes as a source of funding for hospital deficits and building had become increasingly marginal. After 1961, the annual income of the Hospital Trust Fund from sweepstakes never exceeded £3 million. In 1969, an Exchequer grant in aid of £4 million was by far the Fund's largest source of income.[65] By the end of the 1960s, the state paid for most of the voluntary hospitals' annual deficits of £5 million. The Fund had become little more than an accounting mechanism.

The political opposition to financing health services from the rates continued to grow. By 1969, the rate in the pound in Dublin had reached 63s and in Galway 101s. Health expenditure as a proportion of total local authority expenditure had grown from 37 per cent in 1962 to 51 per cent in 1969.[66] The political issue was not how to control health expenditure but how to remove health charges from the rates. The Department, by offering to trade relief on the rates for the loss of local autonomy, encouraged the idea that rates were no longer a suitable source of financing health services. No one appears to have questioned the general taxpayer's ability to pay the full cost of the expanding services.

The issue became acute in April 1969 when, shortly before a general election, the Dublin city council refused to strike a rate because of the burden of the health charge required by the Dublin Health Authority. The city council was unceremoniously removed en bloc from office by the Minister for Local Government and a commissioner appointed to run the affairs of the city. A more acceptable way of financing the health services, however, remained to be found.

Regionalisation

If the White Paper had underlined the need to regionalise hospital services, it gave little idea how the new administrative structure would work. The question was which hospitals should develop as regional centres and what ought to be the relationship of the voluntary hospitals and their consultant staff to any new regional structure. Early in 1967, the medical organisations had a series of discussions with Department of Health officials.[67] While there was a substantial measure of agreement about the changes necessary in the public hospital sector, there was less consensus about the role of the voluntary hospitals. To resolve the problem, the Minister appointed a Consultative Council on the General Hospitals Services in November 1967 to make recommendations on reorganisation.

It is clear from the composition of the council what it was supposed to do. Every member was a consultant of either a local authority or a voluntary hospital. The Department intended that it should come to a purely 'technical' decision as to the best structure for hospital administration. The Department hoped that once the leading consultants had agreed to a solution, the authority of an unanimous report would enable changes to be made. It was asked to report in an exceptionally short time of seven months. Its chairman was Professor Patrick Fitzgerald, a former joint editor of the IMA *Journal,* a leading voluntary hospital consultant and professor of surgery at University College Dublin, with strong views on the need to rationalise the Irish hospital system. The council's report, better known as the Fitzgerald Report, proved to be one of the most controversial reports on any issue in Irish public life.[68]

The most politically explosive recommendation of the report concerned the number of hospital centres to be developed. In a manner reminiscent of the Hospitals Commission thirty years before, the report recommended that the hospitals be developed at twelve locations in the country, involving four regional and twelve general hospitals. Each general hospital would have 300 beds, servicing a population of at least 120,000, and provide services such as general medicine, surgery, obstetrics, gynaecology, pathology and radiology. A minimum of two consultants would be employed in each speciality. The case for fewer but larger hospitals was based on arguments of patient safety, economics and medical and nurse training. County hospitals not chosen to be general hospitals were to become 'community health centres'.[69] The regional hospitals would be based in Dublin (two), Cork and Galway. Each would have at least 600 beds and provide both a general service for the immediate catchment area and a highly specialised service for the region.

The council calculated that, even with the reduced number of hospitals recommended, few areas of the Republic would be more than sixty miles from a hospital or more than one hour's driving in excess of existing driving time to hospital. In Dublin, the Report recommended the development of two regional hospitals based, significantly, at the Catholic St Vincent's and Mater hospitals, and two general hospitals, at St Kevin's and at the former sanatorium in Blanchardstown. All the other Dublin hospitals were to be regrouped around these centres.

With apparent disregard for the decisions of the White Paper that all health services should be administered by the same authority, the report recommended a separate administrative system for hospitals. It recommended that three regional hospital boards be set up based on the medical teaching centres of Dublin, Cork and Galway, with responsibility for the general policy and supervision of the public and voluntary hospitals in their regions. Below the hospital board, special management committees would administer individual hospitals or groups of hospitals. The proposal was radical since it envisaged a single administrative system for public and voluntary hospitals. Recognising that the control of the number and type of consultants was as important in shaping the structure of the future hospital system as control of bricks and mortar, the council recommended the establishment of a central body to decide on the distribution of specialities and the appointment of consultants.

It would be hard to fault the logic or presentation of the Fitzgerald Report. Part of the explanation for the controversy it caused must lie in the sheer clarity of its argument and presentation, its major flaw stemming from its very strength. It assumed that the hospital system could be administered separately from the rest of the health services. It viewed hospital development with 'a cold medical eye', and hospitals as purely medical institutions whose development should be guided by the principles of the best medical practice.[70]

The Department and the profession were surprised by the vehement opposition to the report. What they had considered a purely 'technical' question — how to organise hospitals so as to provide the best medical care — was far from being a technical issue for local communities and their public representatives. The 'downgrading' (the word became synonymous with discussion of the report) of a local hospital to a community health centre would mean a loss of prestige, revenue and employment and could mean that patients and their relatives would have to travel relatively long distances to hospitals. The report was criticised in the Dail as 'purely a consultants' scheme which is totally unacceptable to rural Ireland'.[71] Other deputies were quick to point to the correspondence between the hospitals marked out for development and those to which the consultants on the council belonged.[72]

In the months following the report's publication, consultation took place between the Department and representatives of voluntary hospitals. The voluntary hospitals agreed to the proposals for regional hospital boards and for a central body to control specialist appointments. However, the plans for developing regional and general hospitals in Dublin were not so well received. Predictably, St. Vincent's was not enthusiastic about co-operating with the Protestant Dublin voluntary hospitals to establish a regional hospital on its campus.[73] Nor, one can surmise, were the Protestant hospitals too enthusiastic about the proposals either.

Doctors' Remuneration

The issue which gave rise to most difficulty in implementing the White Paper was the payment of doctors in the proposed choice of doctor scheme. Given the strength of doctors' traditional opposition to capitation as a method of payment, difficult negotiations could have been predicted. While the profession had given a positive welcome to the proposals of the White Paper, Dr Bryan Alton, a leading medical spokesman and senator, warned that 'the point on which there will be the most likely disagreement will be on the mode of remuneration'.[74] He claimed that the medical profession 'by a very great majority in this country, are anxious for fee-per-service'.[75] The profession lobbied public representatives on its case for a fee-for-service method of payment and a number of deputies who were also doctors spoke in favour of the profession's stand.[76]

Mr O'Malley's open-minded approach to the proposals of the White Paper soon turned to impatience with the tactics used by the medical profession. In the Senate he criticised Dr Alton for rousing doctors on the issue of payment and blamed 'hot-heads' and 'wild-catters' in the IMA for stirring up trouble.[77] In an intemperate television interview, Mr O'Malley claimed that some five per cent of dispensary doctors treated some of their patients like 'pigs'. He warned the profession that he did not want 'to use the big stick', and that he would not be 'blackmailed into coming down on any particular side'.[78] The expected show-down between the Minister and the profession was averted in August 1966 when Mr O'Malley was appointed Minister for Education. The urgency evident in Mr O'Malley's attempt to introduce the choice of doctor scheme died following his departure from Health.

When serious negotiations began under the new Minister, Mr Flanagan, it was clear that there was a wide gulf between what the Department was prepared to offer and what the profession would accept. The Department proposed a sophisticated version of the capitation system then being introduced in the United Kingdom. This involved extra payment for special services over and above a flat rate payment for each patient. The Department maintained its dislike of fee for service because of the anticipated expense and possibility of abuse by unscrupulous doctors. The profession, on the other hand, argued that the most appropriate way to ensure the main objective of the choice of doctor scheme – the abolition of the distinction between public and private patients – was through the fee-for-service method of payment. Capitation, since it presented no incentive to give the best service to a public patient, encouraged a minimal standard of care. A further disadvantage of capitation identified by the doctors was that only a certain number of doctors would be able to participate because of the need to get and keep worthwhile panels of patients. Since fee-for-service payment would make it worthwhile for a large number of doctors to participate in the scheme, a more realistic choice of doctor would be available to patients. Despite protracted negotiations, and agreement on most other aspects of the new service, no agreement had been reached between the doctors and the Department on payment by the time the Health Bill was introduced to the House in 1969.

Health Act, 1970

The government was under considerable pressure to produce its long-promised Health Bill. It only received its second reading in April 1969, when the shadow of a general election hung over the debate. The Minister, Sean Flanagan, emphasised that the philosophy behind the Bill, first announced to the Select Committee in 1962, repeated in the 1966 White Paper and by him subsequently, remained unchanged in the Bill. He made no apology 'for its not being something else, such as a Bill for the introduction of a comprehensive national health service'.[79] He offered it as 'the most rational solution to a number of problems'.[80] The cost of the health services, which had risen from £33 million in 1965/6 to £51 million in 1969/70 (mainly due to increased wages and salaries) was evidence in the Minister's view of the wisdom of continuing the existing policy towards eligibility, and of concentrating any additional resources on those with real need.[81] Any sizeable extension of eligibility, such as providing a general medical service to the middle income group, would cost an extra £20 million, he warned. This figure was designed to dampen the enthusiasm of deputies ever sensitive to the interests of the ratepaying electorate.[82]

The Minister emphasised the improvements in services contained in the Bill, particularly the replacement of the dispensary service with a choice of doctor scheme. Vulnerable because he had not agreed a method of payment with the medical profession, he announced that a working party had been set up to examine ways of preventing abuse under fee-for-service payment.[83] Without admitting it, the Minister had conceded the principle of fee for service under the new scheme.

The Bill changed the terminology of eligibility for health services. The population was no longer classified into lower, middle and upper income groups. Instead the Bill referred to those with 'full eligibility' and 'limited eligibility' and persons with entitlements to certain services.[84] The Bill actually reduced the entitlements of one group. Children of higher income parents would no longer be entitled to free hospital and specialist services for problems discovered at national school examinations, an entitlement first granted in 1919. The Minister sugared the pill by making all handicapped or disabled children eligible for permanent or long-term care, regardless of income.

The Bill extended eligibility in one significant way. It provided

271

for a scheme to compensate persons with limited eligibility for expenditure above a specified amount each month on drugs and to meet the full cost of drugs for persons with certain diseases, regardless of income. It provided for the abolition of out-patient charges on the middle income group and for the future abolition of in-patient charges if replaced by a scheme of contributions deducted from earnings. One important change seems to have passed unnoticed, one which in former times might have sounded alarm bells with the profession and the Hierarchy. This was a provision to change the definition of eligibility for health services by ministerial regulation. As a safeguard against abuse, such regulations would require the positive approval of the Dail. The Minister explained that this change was being introduced to take account of changes in the value of money, and possibly to 'change the general formula for eligibility'.[85]

The other important changes concerned the administration of the health services. The Minister indicated that about eight health boards would be created, following county boundaries and taking into account the parallel development of regions for planning and other purposes. Local representatives would have at least half the seats on the new boards; and advisory committees in each county would be established to advise the health board. Faced with the administrative dilemma posed by the desire to have a unified administration for all health services and the Fitzgerald recommendations for a separate regional structure for hospitals, the Bill attempted a compromise. The management of public hospitals would transfer to the new health boards. A central co-ordinating body would be established to advise the Minister on the appointment of specialists in health boards and voluntary hospitals, and three regional hospital boards would co-ordinate the activities of public and voluntary hospitals at regional level.[86] The hospital boards would have power to employ consultants. At least half the members of the central body, to be known as Comhairle na n-Ospideal, would be hospital consultants and half the members of the regional hospital boards would be local representatives. The Minister reassured the voluntary hospitals that he had no intention of ending their traditional independence but appealed to them to accept some restrictions in the interests of the hospital system as a whole. He thought that these arrangements were 'a compromise' between the interests of hospital consultants and the aspirations of public representatives.[87] He pointed out that doctors were 'being brought into health administration' and that the Custom House was 'delegating power to outside bodies with professional representation'.[88]

The proposals for financing the new health boards showed little advance on the promises of the 1966 White Paper. The boards would be funded, as were their predecessors, by a mixture of fixed and variable state grants and contributions from the local rates. The Minister was given power to set the level of health board expenditure each year and, provided the Minister for Local Government agreed, county and borough councils would have to strike a rate to meet their obligations to the health boards or risk abolition.

Fine Gael opposed the Bill on the grounds that it did not provide a comprehensive, insurance-based health service, it retained 'the injustice' of financing half of health costs from rates, and it gave central government excessive powers at the expense of local authorities and hospital administrators.[89] The Labour Party welcomed the improvements provided by the Bill but expressed concern at the establishment of the new boards on which local representatives would not have a majority vote.[90] The debate, while conducted in the knowledge of an imminent general election, exhibited none of the bitterness of debates on earlier health Bills.

The general election of June 1969 left government and policy unchanged. There was, however, a change of Minister. Mr Erskine Childers was appointed Tanaiste (deputy prime minister) and Minister for Health. Mr Childers, a senior member of the Party, brought to the office an interest in health administration and an ability to compromise that stood him in good stead in negotiations on the Bill. The advanced stage of the legislation meant that broad policy had been set down and he saw it as his task to implement it with as little fuss as possible. The government was riven by the crisis which followed the sacking of two Cabinet ministers by the Taoiseach on suspicion of illegally importing arms for use

273

in Northern Ireland. Mr Childers, however, managed to give the impression of 'business as usual' as he sat long hours in the Dail guiding his Bill through the remaining stages. Thanks to his willingness to entertain amendments, the committee stage of the Bill was remarkably even-tempered.

Mr Childers made several important concessions during the passage of the Bill. To relieve the fears of local councillors, he agreed to give public representatives a majority on the new health boards, to the appointment of chairpersons of the health boards by the board members and to hold a public inquiry before closing a hospital.[91] The reluctance of the voluntary hospitals to abide by national rules for the development of specialities and the appointment of consultants was overcome by an amendment giving the new central body, Comhairle na n-Ospideal, power to regulate these matters, instead of merely advising the Minister on them, the Minister emphasising that the Bill was 'an exercise in decentralisation and co-ordination'.[92] Amendments were also introduced to protect the rights of consultants in voluntary hospitals and to restrict the appointment of consultants by the Local Appointments Commission to health board hospitals only. In an attempt to standardise conditions for consultants in public and voluntary hospitals, the Minister introduced an amendment giving health boards explicit power to provide private and semi-private accommodation in their hospitals for those without eligibility and for those with limited eligibility but who preferred to be treated privately.[93]

The Bill became law in February 1970. Eight health boards were established in October of that year, assuming responsibility for services in April 1971. Three regional hospital boards were established but their lack of power over the management of either the voluntary or health board hospitals deprived them of an effective role. The members of the first Comhairle na n-Ospideal were appointed in 1972 and quickly began to make an impact on the organisation of specialist hospital services through their power to regulate consultant appointments. The Comhairle also turned its attention to regionalising hospital services by revising the criteria laid down by the Fitzgerald Report. The reorganised general medical service with a choice of doctor for patients and payment of doctors by fee for service was implemented in 1972, following agreement between the Department and the profession on the method of payment.

The financing of health services became increasingly controversial. In 1971, legislation was passed imposing flat rate health contributions on persons with limited eligibility and at the same time, hospital charges on this group were abolished.[94] While contributions were welcomed by Fine Gael as a step towards an insurance-funded health service, the Minister attributed the existence of the Bill to Department of Finance pressure to find another source of income besides rates and taxes to finance 'the heavy and growing burden of health costs'.[95] Paying contributions did not of itself entitle a person to limited eligibility status. It was in effect a special health levy on some income earners.

The burden of financing the health services from the rates was a central issue in the 1973 general election. Fianna Fail lost office and a coalition government of Fine Gael and the Labour Party assumed power. True to their election pledge, the new government announced that the share of health costs paid for by the rates would be phased out by 1977. While this decision might have been expected to increase central control over health expenditure and the development of services, in practice its effect, by removing the 'brake' of local taxation, may have helped to stimulate a dramatic increase in expenditure on health services, rising from 3.73 per cent of GNP in 1971 to 7.01 in 1979.[96] One consequence was to jeopardise plans for regionalisation of hospital services. With no financial consequences falling locally, every community had an incentive to fight for the development of its hospital to the standard envisaged for a few by Fitzgerald and by Comhairle na n-Ospideal.

Conclusion

Brendan Hensey has described the 1961-72 period as 'a decade of scrutiny of the existing services ... and of a change in emphasis in the aims of health services'.[97] Between 1957 and 1972, there was a remarkable defusing of ideological conflict over the purpose and nature of state involvement in the health services. On assuming office, Mr MacEntee signalled an end to ambitions his party might have once entertained to provide a free health service to the majority of the population. The removal of the glaring deficiencies in coverage for health services by the Health Acts, 1947 and 1953 had also removed the pragmatic case for universal coverage. The opposition of the medical profession and the Catholic Church to an extension of payment by salary or increased public control of medical services reduced the capacity of ministers and administrators to plan a health service which would provide services for the whole population and be economical at the same time. The rapid increase in the cost of health services was another reason for caution in removing all price barriers to the use of services. Under such circumstances it made sense to argue that the state should only provide services free of charge to those who could not afford to pay for them, and to assist others towards the cost of those services which otherwise would be beyond their means. It was easier to claim the mantle of tradition for this approach and defend the means test than to justify and face further conflict and expense in extending eligibility significantly. The Minister could, with some justification, claim that there was little demand for such an extension – people were more concerned by the mid-1960s with the level of their rates bill than with an extension of eligibility or the removal of charges for health services.

It was also necessary to disclaim any intention of increasing state interference in medical services if the Department was to achieve the radical administrative changes it regarded as necessary to modernise the health services. The fervent wish of politicians, doctors and administrators during these years that 'health be taken out of politics' expressed their desire to see an end to the bitter debates of earlier years on health policy and the relegation of health issues to the realm of experts and technocrats.[98] The Health Act, 1970 was largely an attempt to do just that. That this approach was successful, not only in defusing potential conflict in the 1960s and 1970s but also in obscuring the reasons for previous controversies, is clear from at least one informed commentator who has written that 'in Ireland it has never been government policy to provide or to endeavour to provide a fully free health service'.[99]

The replacement of the dispensary service by the choice of doctor scheme was one important innovation. The dispensary service, virtually unchanged in 120 years, was dismantled and the option of treating public patients offered to all general practitioners fulfilling certain conditions. The participation of private practitioners and the concession of fee-for-service payment for doctors in the new service meant that the Department and health boards surrendered their considerable powers over the organisation of general practice through control of dispensary medical officers. They retained only minimal controls over excessive visiting and abuse of the new system. The chief power remaining with local health officials was the authority to decide on eligibility. In addition, the agreed method of payment reinforced many of the defects of Irish general practice: the reluctance to form group practices, poor practice premises, minimal record keeping, excessive competition for patients, and a preoccupation with treatment rather than prevention.

The radical changes in the administrative structure of the health services implemented during this period had their origin in the mid-1940s when doubts were first raised about the adequacy of the county as a unit of administration for health, or more precisely, hospital services. For the Custom House, regionalisation was the key to modernising the hospital system by developing some hospitals rather than others and breaking what was seen as the stranglehold of rate-conscious councillors over the development of health services. There are hints during these years that the Department would have been perfectly happy to see the state take on the entire funding of health services, with rates playing little or no part in health financing, on the assumption that 'he who pays the piper calls the tune'. The offer to exchange local authority control of health services for relief on the rates was an important card in gaining political acceptance of the health boards.

A final aspect of health policy in these years is the extent to which Ministers and the Department were prepared to involve the doctors and the voluntary hospitals in administration. This was part of the process of de-politicising health conflicts and a recognition that alliance with the medical profession was one way of carrying out the administrative changes necessary to provide a modern and co-ordinated health service. The composition of the Fitzgerald council, of the health boards and regional hospital boards, the role of Comhairle na n-Ospideal, the concession of fee-for-service remuneration in the choice of doctor scheme and the safeguards built into the Health Act, 1970 to protect the position of the profession and the voluntary hospitals, reflected a new approach based on partnership rather than confrontation. The alliance of interests between the Department and hospital consultants in the interest of hospital reorganisation is particularly marked. Without such an alliance, it would not be possible to regionalise the county hospital system or to co-ordinate the activities of the voluntary and public hospitals. The Health Act, 1970 was intended to provide a framework for the harmonious development of public and professional interests in health services: the mutual suspicion of the past was to be replaced by teamwork. The price of 'taking health out of politics' was to increase the role of those interest groups which had most at stake in the system and most power. It also meant the formation of an alliance in the treatment of disease rather than in the protection of health.

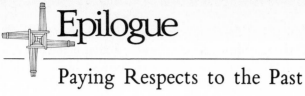

Epilogue

Paying Respects to the Past

ON THE TRANSFORMATION of government in Western societies in the last hundred years, Hugh Heclo has commented that 'one of the things most astonishing to posterity about our own times will be not how much we understood but how much we took for granted'.[1] This study has attempted to lift the veil on one small aspect of this transformation, namely, the growth of public responsibility for health and medical services in Ireland between 1900 and 1970. The extent of change in seventy years – one modern lifespan – was immense, both in terms of reduced mortality and control of disease and in the relationship of patients, doctors and public authorities.

In 1900, government responsibility for the health of the population was limited to controlling outbreaks of the most serious epidemic diseases and ensuring access by the poor to general practitioner services and poor law infirmaries. By 1970, government had accepted responsibility for providing a high standard of medical care for all sections of the population at no or at a heavily subsidised cost to the recipient. The benefit to the poor was not so much the extension of entitlement to services – the nineteenth century poor law and dispensary codes entitled them to all services without charge – but the improvement in the quality of services available to them and the control of diseases which affected them primarily. The poor now had access to the same services as other people.

The extension of eligibility for services primarily benefited the better-off working and middle classes who found it increasingly difficult to pay the price of more sophisticated and expensive medical treatment.

The benefits of this transformation to the medical profession are less obvious and more contentious. There is little doubt, however, that in Ireland, private and voluntary effort alone would have been insufficient to finance the modernisation of medical facilities or to maintain the standard of medical services achieved by the 1970s. As the cost of medical treatment grew, the predominantly private arrangements between doctors, patients and hospitals which existed in the early part of the period were replaced by publicly funded or publicly assisted ones. By 1970, the hospital and specialist charges of even the wealthiest people were heavily subsidised by public funds. While the medical profession bitterly resisted this trend in the 1940s and 1950s, by 1970 they seemed reconciled to working in a publicly financed and planned health service. Their co-operation was secured in return for commitments on the perpetuation of private practice and the maintenance of high incomes, the independence of voluntary hospitals and professional involvement at all levels in the administration of the health services.

The change from a locally controlled and locally financed system to an increasingly centralised and centrally financed one is another striking feature of this period. Change was already under way by 1900 as the new county system of local government offered opportunities for improving services which the boards of guardians or smaller sanitary authorities were unable or unwilling to entertain. The county was enshrined as the main unit of health administration in the 1920s but by the mid-1940s was considered too small to meet the requirements of a modern hospital system. At the same time, central government, through the Health (Financial Provisions) Act, 1947, took the radical step of guaranteeing to meet the full cost of health authorities' spending until local rates and Exchequer contributions were equal. The promise of further relief on rates proved an irresistible attraction to local representatives in the late 1960s in return for surrendering direct control over the administration of health services and for agreeing to the establishment of the regional health boards. By 1977, almost the entire cost of the health services was met from central funds.

If these are the most significant changes which occurred in public arrangements for the medical care of the physically ill between 1900 and 1970, why did they occur and what factors were at work in shaping policy and services? It was suggested in chapter 1 that twentieth-century advances in medicine raised questions about equity of access and quality of service which had not arisen as sharply before. The reports of the Viceregal Commission in 1905, of the Carnegie Trust in 1917 and of the departmental committee on health services in 1945 are evidence of the strong desire of health officials to translate the potential of medicine into services which would benefit people. The increased potential of medicine to cure and prevent illness would not, however, have been so significant had it not occurred at the same time as the consolidation of democracy in Ireland and as popularly elected governments became more responsive to the social and economic demands of the electorate. The health policies of the Fianna Fail governments of 1932 and 1952 and of the inter-party government of 1948-51 are examples of a wider trend in Western democracies to ensure equity in access to medical treatment.

Advances in medicine, the widening of democracy and rising living standards are, in retrospect, the necessary conditions for change but they are not sufficient to explain the specific development of the health services. The answer to this question lies in the particular historical, social and cultural experience of the country, before and during the period under discussion. It would be difficult, for example, to over-emphasise the importance of the historical legacy of the poor law, the dispensary service and the voluntary hospitals in shaping medical services in the twentieth century.

The dispensary service, to judge from its longevity, was particularly well suited to the conditions of the country and helped ensure the survival of individual general practice into the era of hospital medicine. It was the attempt by the Department of Health to develop a salaried medical service for the whole community based on the dispensary service that sparked off the dramatic conflicts between governments, the medical profession and the Catholic Hierarchy in the late 1940s. The dispensary service also shaped policy indirectly: its existence was a major argument against the extension of medical benefit to Ireland in 1911. The dissatisfaction of dispensary doctors with salary as a method of remuneration, the profession's traditional dislike of capitation and their perception of what had happened to their British colleagues account for the determination of medical negotiators to secure fee-for-service payments in the 1960s.

The institutional legacy had an enormous influence on health policy in this century. The poor law infirmaries and voluntary hospitals had been provided for a population in the eighteenth and nineteenth centuries which, at its peak, was twice that of 1900. The proliferation of buildings encouraged a bias towards institutional care and fostered an intense local loyalty to hospitals. Only the determination of the Sinn Fein provisional government, against the backdrop of the abnormal conditions of the war of independence, was strong enough to overcome, at least temporarily, this institutional bias and local loyalty.

The absence of certain factors could also be said to have had an important influence on the development of Irish medical services. The relative weakness of the labour movement, the absence of a socialist tradition or of a strong friendly society or 'help to self help' movement, so characteristic of the Danish experience, underlined the state's role in Ireland as the mediating party between doctor and patient.[2] The large number of doctors in Ireland in 1900 whose salaries came from taxation represented an unusual level of public responsibility for the medical treatment of the poor for the time. The rejection of insurance as a way of organising access to medical services in 1911 ruled out the use of a mechanism by which an increasing proportion of the population might have gradually been covered for medical expenses as in Germany and Scandinavia, with the insurance funds acting as third parties between doctors and patients.[3]

By the outbreak of the Second World War, coverage in Ireland for medical services was relatively restricted by the standards of other Western countries. The National Health Insurance Society was that only in name and Bishop Dignan had few supporters in arguing that it should provide comprehensive coverage against illness for the whole population. The state had little alternative but to step in to improve the quality and widen access to medical services. This role of the state as the sole mediator in Ireland between doctor and patient may have contributed to the particular vehemence of the struggle between successive governments and the profession over extending entitlement to free medical treatment. The state's determination to take on this role in the interest of improving the health of the population alarmed a defensive Catholic Hierarchy and made them susceptible to the arguments of the medical profession in support of the status quo. The extreme distrust of the state which the profession began to exhibit in the early 1940s is understandable from this point of view. Given the ferocity of the subsequent battles, the extent of the rapprochement between government and the profession by 1970 is all the more remarkable.

Comparisons with developments in Britain help to throw some light on the organisation of medical services in Ireland, but the relationship is by no means simple. British policy had a direct influence on public health and the administration of services. But even when Ireland was part of the United Kingdom it did not necessarily follow, as the medical benefit debate of 1911-13 illustrates, that British policy would apply in Ireland. The independence of twenty-six counties in 1921 broke the power of British governments to shape developments in Ireland directly but the indirect effect of events in Britain remained immense. The Beveridge Report and the formation of the National Health Service were particularly important in this respect. The proximity of the two islands, the ease with which Irish people moved to Britain and the close links between professional groups such as the IMA and the BMA, encouraged constant comparisons between services and wage levels on both sides of the Irish sea and stimulated demands for a health service of a standard arguably beyond the means of a country at Ireland's level of economic development.

Developments in Britain, more than any other country, have acted as catalysts for change in Ireland, without determining the precise nature of that change.

Economic growth alone does not explain the high level of gross national product spent on the health services in the 1970s and 1980s.[4] Economic considerations were dominant in the 1920s, when the drive for economy in public services restricted spending on medical services, and in the 1960s, when rising living standards created expectations for improved services. But the expansion and modernisation of the hospital system which took place between 1930 and the early 1950s occurred while living standards hardly rose at all. The cost was met, not from taxation or economic development, but from the funds which the Irish Hospitals Sweepstakes attracted from abroad. The availability of sweepstakes money enabled a level of investment in hospitals which, arguably, could not or would not have been provided otherwise. Of equal significance was the enormous revenue costs generated by such an extensive hospital system, which had to be met from taxation or fees. The relatively high usage of hospital beds in Ireland reflects the level of past and current investment.[5] It is hardly a coincidence that the cost of health services falling on local rates became a major political issue in the 1960s and 1970s and that demand increased for the full cost of current expenditure on health services to be met from the Exchequer. In the 1980s, attention has turned to controlling the rate of increase of spending on health services as pressure from taxpayers and foreign debt commitments increased.

Ireland is perhaps unique in the extent to which the Catholic Church has influenced the development of health policy. The involvement of religious orders in voluntary hospitals and clerical influence over some medical schools gave the Church an important place in the organisation of health services. In 1911, the Catholic Hierarchy played a prominent part in ensuring that medical benefit was not applied to Ireland, basing their opposition on largely economic and capitalist grounds. By the 1940s, their opposition to increasing state involvement in medical services was based on quasi-moral grounds as Church leaders became increasingly nervous of developments in reproductive medicine, and the undermining of individual, family and church autonomy in totalitarian societies. Their influence with a native and overwhelmingly Catholic government was immense. Their power and defensiveness left them vulnerable to the arguments of the medical profession who, for baser motives, opposed increasing state involvement in medicine. Their repeated interventions had a significant but not an overwhelming impact on the development of Irish medical services.

The synthesis of the triangular conflict between the Church, the medical profession and the state left its mark in four distinct ways on Irish medical services. First, it helped to enshrine means tests or income limits as determinants for many services. The means test, the Hierarchy insisted in 1950 and 1953, was the method of deciding where public responsibility for health ended and where individual and family responsibility began. It also coincided with the medical profession's desire to maintain the distinction between those who paid their doctor and those who did not. Dr. Ryan's concession that women in the upper income group would contribute half the cost of a mother and infant service was a symbolic way out of the impasse, saving face on all sides. Of more significance was that means tests or income limits continued to be an important part of public arrangements for medical care. The result was a highly complex set of eligibility requirements for services. When in 1979 eligibility for treatment in public hospitals without charge was extended to the entire population, an income limit was retained excluding those above a certain income from free consultant services.

Second, the conflict encouraged an extraordinary symbiosis of public and private medicine. If, in the late 1940s, the medical profession feared the end or at least the very severe curtailment of private medicine, by 1970 their right to private practice was accepted and facilitated in a number of ways. Means testing ensured that roughly seventy per cent of the population had to pay their general practitioner and fifteen per cent, their hospital specialist. Hospital consultants had the use of the staff and facilities of the expanded hospital service to treat their private patients at little or no cost to the doctor and at subsidised cost to the patient. Private patients in public hospitals or in private accommodation associated with public hospitals were charged only the marginal cost of their accommodation on the principle that they had already contributed through taxation towards the greater part of the cost. The relatively low cost of private medical and hospital bills and significant tax relief on Voluntary Health Insurance premiums provided an attractive package to the public and many more people insured for private care than the fifteen per cent ineligible for public services. By 1984, roughly one-third of the population was insured with the Board for private medical care.[6] One of the consequences of the continued subsidies to private care has been to jeopardise the principle, established first in the 1930s, that all patients, whether rich or poor, should be treated in the same hospital by the same medical and nursing staff. The boom in private medicine has encouraged the appearance of separate private hospitals and clinics, independent of any public hospital or having little connection with a public hospital. What is not generally understood is the extent to which this trend has been encouraged by public subsidies and policies. Third, the conflict cemented an alliance between the Church and the medical profession in the interests of maintaining Catholic ethical standards in medical practice. This alliance continues to influence the development of health services in certain ways, particularly on sensitive issues such as abortion, sterilisation and family planning.[7] The Catholic voluntary hospitals and their medical staff maintain a wariness of public control over their activities and retain a considerable degree of independence despite their almost complete reliance on public funding.

These appear to be the main factors which give Irish medical services their unique character – the legacy of the nineteenth century, the role of the state as the chief mediating force between the medical profession and the patient, the impact of the Hospitals Sweepstakes, the aspiration for a health service comparable to Britain's and the limits set by the formidable alliance of the Catholic Church and the medical profession. These factors have shaped and continue to shape the development of medical services but they are not generally understood and have, to some extent, been taken for granted.

Referring to the need for a more informed approach to the formulation of social policies, R.M. Titmuss commented that 'to plan and guide wisely, we have also to pay our respects to the past. We have to ask questions about past trends; about where we have come from; about what we have tried to achieve, and with what success'.[8] This study has tried to pay respects to the past, to show where Irish health services have come from, what was attempted and with what results. There is room for debate on how past events have shaped the intricate relationships between government, doctor and patient. What cannot be disputed is that a debt exists and that to recognise this debt is a crucial key to understanding the present organisation of the Irish health services.

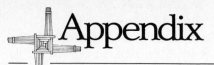

Appendix

Notes for Readers Unfamiliar with Irish History

CHRONOLOGY OF IMPORTANT POLITICAL AND ECONOMIC EVENTS REFERRED TO IN THE TEXT

1800	Act of Union; political and administrative union of Great Britain and Ireland.
1829	Catholic Emancipation Act passed.
1845-50	The Great Famine.
1880	Charles Stewart Parnell becomes leader of the Irish Parliamentary Party (popularly known as the Irish Party).
1886	First Home Rule Bill defeated.
1891	Death of Parnell.
1893	Second Home Rule Bill defeated.
1900	John Redmond becomes leader of the Irish Party.
1906	Liberal Party comes to power.
1909	Lloyd George's budget defeated by House of Lords.
1910	General elections result in the Irish Party holding the balance of power.
1911	National Insurance Act, 1911 passed.
1912	Third Home Rule Bill introduced.
1914-18	First World War.
1914	Irish Party no longer holds balance of power. Home Rule postponed.
1916	Easter Rising in Dublin.
1918	Sinn Fein victory in general election and withdrawal from Westminster.
1919	First Dail (parliament) of the Irish Republic established.
1919-21	Guerilla war against British rule.
1920	Government of Ireland Act passed providing for Home Rule parliaments in Dublin and Belfast. State of Northern Ireland established in six northern counties.
1921	Treaty signed establishing the Irish Free State in 26 of the 32 counties. Cumann na nGaedheal government takes office.
1921-2	Civil war between the pro-Treaty and anti-Treaty forces.
1922	World economic recession deepens.
1927	Fianna Fail, a party formed from those defeated in the civil war, takes its seats in the Dail.

1932	Fianna Fail, under the leadership of Eamon de Valera, forms first government. Remains in office until 1948.
1937	New Constitution passed by referendum.
1939-45	Second World War.
1948	First inter-party government takes office.
1949	Ireland declared a Republic. Formal links to Commonwealth ended.
1951	Inter-party government falls following Mother and Child crisis. Fianna Fail takes office.
1954	Second inter-party government formed.
1957	Second inter-party government falls. Fianna Fail returns to office and retains power until 1973. First Programme for Economic Development published.
1963	Second Vatican Council opens.
1969-	Present cycle of violence begins in Northern Ireland.

GLOSSARY

Clann na Poblachta	Political party. Member of the first inter-party government, 1948-51.
Comhairle na n-Ospideal	Hospitals Council established under Health Act, 1970.
Cumann na nGaedheal	Political party. In government from 1922 to 1932.
Dail Eireann	Lower house of parliament.
Eire	Official title of Ireland in the Irish language.
Fianna Fail	Political party. In government for much of the period, 1932-70.
Fine Gael	Political party, successor to Cumann na nGaedheal. Largest party in the Inter Party Governments of 1948-51 and 1954-57.
Ireland	In this book, refers to the whole island from 1900-1922 and to the twenty-six independent counties from 1921 to 1970.
Irish Free State	Official title of the independent state of Ireland from 1921 to 1937.
Northern Ireland	Title of the six Irish counties which remained part of the United Kingdom in 1921.
Oireachtas	Parliament.
Seanad	Senate.
Sinn Fein	Political movement for the achievement of an independent Ireland. Founded in 1905 and particularly influential between 1918 and 1921.
Tanaiste	Deputy Prime Minister.
Taoiseach	Prime Minister.

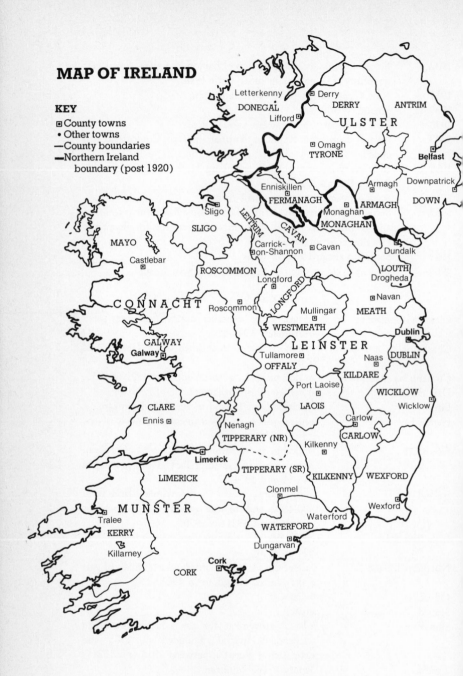

MAP OF IRELAND

KEY
- ⊡ County towns
- • Other towns
- — County boundaries
- ▬ Northern Ireland boundary (post 1920)

Letterkenny
DONEGAL
Lifford

⊡ Derry
DERRY
ANTRIM
U L S T E R

⊡ Omagh
TYRONE

Belfast

Enniskillen
FERMANAGH
Armagh
Downpatrick
⊡ ARMAGH
DOWN

Sligo
SLIGO

LEITRIM
CAVAN
Monaghan
MONAGHAN

MAYO
Castlebar

Carrick-on-Shannon
⊡ Cavan
Dundalk

ROSCOMMON
Longford
LONGFORD
LOUTH
Drogheda

C O N N A C H T
Roscommon
⊡ Navan
MEATH

Mullingar
WESTMEATH

GALWAY
Galway

L E I N S T E R
Tullamore
OFFALY
Naas
KILDARE
Dublin
DUBLIN

Port Laoise
LAOIS
WICKLOW
Wicklow

CLARE
Ennis ⊡

Nenagh
TIPPERARY (NR)
Carlow
CARLOW

Kilkenny

Limerick

TIPPERARY (SR)
KILKENNY
WEXFORD

LIMERICK

Clonmel

Wexford

M U N S T E R
Tralee
KERRY

Waterford
WATERFORD
Dungarvan

Killarney

Cork

CORK

290

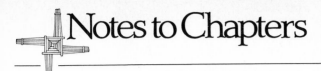# Notes to Chapters

ABBREVIATIONS USED IN NOTES TO CHAPTERS

BMJ	British Medical Journal
DD	Dail Debates
DLG	Department of Local Government, 1919-22
DLGPH	Department of Local Government and Public Health, 1922-47
DOH	Department of Health, 1947 –
HC	House of Commons
HL	House of Lords
IMA	Irish Medical Association
JIMA	Journal of the Free State Medical Association/the Medical Association of Eire/the Irish Medical Association (title varies)
LGB	Local Government Board for Ireland, 1872-1921
RCSI	Royal College of Surgeons in Ireland
SPO	State Paper Office, Dublin

NOTES TO CHAPTER 1
HEALTH, MEDICINE AND IRISH SOCIETY IN 1900

1. Hugh Heclo, *Modern Social Politics in Britain and Sweden — From Relief to Income Maintenance* (London, 1974) p. 13.
2. J.J. Lee, *The Modernisation of Irish Society*, 1814-1918 (Dublin 1973), p. 3.
3. Ibid. p. 6.
4. F.S.L. Lyons, *Ireland Since the Famine* (London, 1971), p. 42.

5. J.J. Lee, op.cit., p. 3.

6. Ibid. p. 35.

7. F.S.L. Lyons, op.cit., p. 57.

8. New Ireland Forum, *The Economic Consequences of the Division of Ireland* (Dublin, 1984), p. 11.

9. Ibid. p. 12.

10. F.S.L. Lyons, op.cit. p. 57.

11. For a profile of admissions to Dublin hospitals at the turn of the century, see Association of Charities, *Dublin Charities* (Dublin, 1902), pp. 68-91.

12. *The Medical Press and Circular*, June 14, 1911, pp. 631-2 and *Committee appointed to consider the Extension of Medical Benefit under the National Insurance Act to Ireland, Report*, Cd. 6963, 1913, xxxvii, 1. p.7.

13. *Standard Time Rates of Wages in the United Kingdom at 1st January 1912*, 1912-13, Cd. 6054, XCII, 573, p. 30.

14. 5th and 6th of George 3.

15. Poor Law Commissioners, *Ireland: Report on Medical Charities*, 1841 (324) XI 1.

16. *Viceregal Commission on Poor Law Reform in Ireland, Report Vol. 1*, 1906 Cd. 3202 Li 349 p. 20.

17. *Commissioners for Inquiring into the Condition of the Poorer Classes in Ireland, Third Report*, 1836 (43) XXX. 1.

18. Helen Burke, 'The Poor Law in Ireland in the 19th Century with particular Reference to the Social Services provided by the South Dublin Union,' Unpublished Ph.D. thesis, University College Dublin, 1976, p. 136.

19. *Commissioners for Inquiring into the Condition of the Poorer Classes in Ireland, First Report*, 1835 (369) XXXII 1.

20. *Act for the more effectual relief of the Destitute Poor in Ireland*, C. 56 1 and 2 Victoria, 1838, Section XLI.

21. Ibid. Section XLVI.

22. *Relief of the Destitute Poor in Ireland (Amendment) Act*, 1862.

23. Ibid.

24. *5th Annual Report of the Irish Poor Law Commissioners*, 1852, (1530) XXIII, 155, p. 2. and *Viceregal Commission, Report, Vol. 1*, op.cit., p. 14.

25. *Viceregal Commission, Report, Vol. 1*, op.cit., p. 33.

26. Phelan, as Assistant Poor Law Commissioner, compiled the *Report on Medical Charities, 1841*, op.cit., on which much of the Medical Charities Act, 1851 was based.

27. Ibid.

28. *Medical Charities Act, 1851*. Helen Burke, op.cit., p. 401.

29. By the *Medical (Amendment) Act, 1886*.

30. *Royal Commission on the Poor Laws and Relief of Distress, Report on Ireland*, 1909 Cd 4630 XXXVIII, 1. p. 63.

31. *Royal Commission on the Poor Laws and Relief of Distress, Appendix Vol.*

X Evidence (with Appendices) relating to Ireland, 1910 Cd. 5070 L. 195, p. 114.

32. Transactions of the Sanitary Institute of Great Britain, VI (1884-5). Quoted in Anthony S. Wohl, *Endangered Lives — Public Health in Victorian Britain* (London, 1983) p. 201. See also the remarks in the *LGB, Report 1905-6* Cd., 3102, xxxvi, p. 233.

33. R.J. Kinkead, *Irish Medical Practitioners Guide* (Dublin, 1889) p. 22.

34. *Memorandum* by the Medical Commissioner of the LGB *Royal Commission on the Poor Laws*, etc., *Appendix Vol. X*, op.cit. p. 115.

35. Ibid., p. 223.

36. Surgeon-General Evatt, *A Report on the Poor Law Medical System in Ireland, British Medical Journal, Supplement*, 26 March, 1904, Vol. 1 (pp.47-75) p. 63.

37. Ibid., p. 59.

38. Carnegie United Kingdom Trust, *Report on the physical welfare of mothers and children*. Vol. iv Ireland (Dublin, 1917) pp. 76-7.

39. *Nuisance Removal and Diseases' Prevention Acts, 1848, 1849.*

40. *Sewage Utilization Act, 1865, Sanitary Act, 1866.*

41. *Royal Commission on the Poor Laws, Appendix Vol. 10*, op.cit., Diagram No. 11.

42. Ibid., Diagram No. 14.

43. Ibid., Diagram No. 13.

44. *Report of the Departmental Committee ... to inquire into the Public Health of the City of Dublin*, 1900 Cd. 243 xxxix, 681; Belfast Health Commission, *Report to the LGB* 1908 Cd. 4128 xxxi, 699; *Report upon the Sanitary Circumstances and Administration of Waterford County Borough*, in *Report of the LGB, 1910-11*, 1911, Cd. 5847, xxxii, 1. pp. 407-433; LGB, *Report on the Sanitary Circumstances and Administration of the City of Dublin with special reference to the causes of the high death rate*, 1906.

45. For example, *LGB, Report 1905-6*, 1906 Cd. 3102, xxxvi, 495; *Report 1906-7*, 1907 Cd., 3682, xxviii 1.

46. Sir F.R. Falkiner in Association of Charities, op.cit., p. 64.

47. Harry Eckstein, *The English Health Service: Its Origins, Structure, and Achievements* (London, 1959) p. 38.

48. *Viceregal Commission on Poor Law Reform, Report Vol. III, Evidence and Index*.

49. R.J. Kinkead, op.cit., p. x.

50. For example the *Medical Press and Circular — Irish Poor Law and Lunacy Intelligence*, 5 April, 1905, p.3; 12 April 1905; 3 May 1905.

51. Ibid., 16 June, 1909.

52. Surgeon General Evatt, op.cit.

53. *Medical Press and Circular*, 11 May 1910, p. 484.

54. R.J. Kinkead, op.cit., p. 17.

55. *HC*, 12 February 1907 (169) col. 93.

[56.] *Royal Commission on the Poor Laws*, etc. *Report on Ireland*, op.cit., p. 30.

[57.] R.B. McDowell, *The Irish Administration 1801-1914* (London, 1964) pp. 189-90.

[58.] Sir Henry Robinson, *Memories, Wise and Otherwise* (London, 1924).

[59.] Beatrice to Sidney Webb in *Letters of Sidney and Beatrice Webb Vol. 2, A Partnership 1892-1912*, ed. Norman McKenzie (Cambridge: London, 1978) p. 311.

[60.] Deputy Patrick McGoldrick, *DD*, 19 May 1924 (7) Col. 1601.

[61.] John Redmond claimed that per head of population, Ireland had the most costly civil government of any nation in Europe. *HC*, 12 February 1907 (169) col. 93.

[62.] David W. Miller, *Church, State and Nation in Ireland, 1898-1921* (Dublin, 1973).

[63.] *The Tablet*, 1 July 1911, p. 18.

[64.] Emmet Larkin, 'Socialism and Catholicism in Ireland' in *Church History*, Vol. 33, 1964 (pp. 462-483) p. 481.

[65.] Ibid. and David W. Miller, op.cit., pp. 270-2.

[66.] Helen Burke, op.cit., p. 465.

NOTES TO CHAPTER 2
PROPOSALS FOR REFORM, 1903-1911

[1.] *Viceregal Commission on Poor Law Reform in Ireland, Report, Vol. 1*, op.cit. and *Royal Commission on the Poor Laws and Relief of Distress, Report on Ireland* 1909, op.cit.

[2.] *Royal Commission on the Poor Laws and Relief of Distress, Separate Report* (Minority) 1909, Cd.4499, XXXVII, p. 739 and *Separate Report on Ireland* (Minority) 1909, Cd. 4630 XXXIII 90.

[3.] *Viceregal Commission on Poor Law Reform, Report, Vol.1*, op.cit. facing p.1.

[4.] Ibid.

[5.] Dr T.H. Moorhead, *Viceregal Commission on Poor Law Reform, Report Vol. III, Evidence and Index* 1906, Cd. 3204, L11. 1. p. 14, question 331.

[6.] Ibid., p. 598, questions 17658/9.

[7.] Ibid., p. 22.

[8.] Joseph Lee, op. cit., Dublin, 1973, p. 13.

[9] *Viceregal Commission on Poor Law Reform, Report, Vol. III, Evidence and Index, op. cit.*, p. 194, question 5657.

[10.] Ibid., p. 460, question 13403.

[11.] Ibid., p. 452, question 13122.

[12.] Ibid., especially Dr N.W. Colahan, p. 820, question 24536.

13. Ibid., Dr P.J. Cremen, pp. 916-920.
14. *Viceregal Commission on Poor Law Reform, Report, Vol. 1,* op.cit., p.63.
15. Ibid., p. 34.
16. Ibid., p. 68.
17. Ibid., p. 81.
18. Ibid., p. 24.
19. Ibid., pp. 23-24.
20. *Royal Commission on the Poor Laws,* etc. *Report* 1909, Cd.4499, XXXVII. 1. p. 2.
21. Sir Henry Robinson, op.cit., p. 212.
22. Ibid., p. 218.
23. *Royal Commission on the Poor Laws, Report on Ireland,* op.cit., p. 37.
24. Ibid., p. 87.
25. Ibid., p. 63.
26. Ibid., p. 62.
27. Ibid., pp. 61-64.
28. Ibid., p. 62.
29. Ibid., p. 1.
30. *Royal Commission on the Poor Laws, Separate Report,* op.cit., p. 1006.
31. Ibid. Emphasis theirs.
32. Ibid., p. 1025.
33. Richard Titmuss 'Health' in Morris Ginsberg, ed., *Law and Opinion in England in the Twentieth Century* (London, 1959).
34. About 20,000 of these were in the friendly society section of the Ancient Order of Hibernians. John Redmond *HC,* 14 Nov. 1911 (31) col. 300.
35. *HC,* 4 May 1911 (25) cols. 609.
36. Ibid., col. 616.
37. Ibid., cols. 624-5.

NOTES TO CHAPTER 3
MEDICAL BENEFIT, 1911-1913

1. *HC,* 4 May 1911 (25) cols. 653, 652.
2. Ibid., 1 June 1911 (26) col. 232. The editorial of the *Irish Independent,* 15 May, p. 4 refers to the dissension in the Party on the issue.
3. *Braithwaite Papers,* Paper No. 46, Lloyd George to Braithwaite, 27 March 1911, London School of Economics.
4. W. J. Braithwaite, *Lloyd George's Ambulance Wagon* ed. Sir Henry Bunbury (London 1957) pp. 150-2.
5. *HC,* Bill 198, 1911.
6. An earlier, unpublished, version of the Bill (140-1911) specified that

a sum not exceeding 2s a year would be paid to a medical officer for each deposit contributor resident in his district. *National Insurance Bill file Part 1*. PIN 3: 3, Public Record Office.

7. *National Insurance Bill* file Part 2. PIN 3 : 4, Public Record Office.

8. See for example *Irish Independent* 18 May 1911, p.4 and 12 June 1911, p.4.

9. *Census of Population, 1911* Cd 6663 1912-13 cxviii 1 p. xxvii.

10. *HC*, 24 May 1911 (26) col. 300.

11. Ibid., col. 303.

12. *HC*, 24 May (26) col. 763.

13. Braithwaite, op.cit., p. 161.

14. *HC*, 24 May (26) col. 769.

15. *BMJ Supplement* 1 July 1911, pp. 1-2.

16. Ibid., 3 June 1911, p. 359.

17. Ibid.

18. Ibid., 8 July 1911, p. 52.

19. Ibid. My emphasis.

20. Ibid., 24 June 1911, p. 481. *Irish Independent*, 10 June 1911, p. 6.

21. *Medical Press and Circular*, 5 July 1911, Vol. XCII, New Series, p. 3.

22. *BMJ Supplement*, 22 July 1911, p. 189.

23. *BMJ Supplement*, 8 July 1911, p. 52.

24. *Medical Press and Circular*, 5 July 1911, Vol. XCII, p. 3.

25. *BMJ Supplement*, 8 July 1911, p. 70.

26. *BMJ Supplement*, 22 July 1911, p. 183.

27. Ibid., 24 June 1911, p. 473.

28. *The Tablet*, 1 July 1911, p. 18.

29. *HC*, 25 October 1911 (30) col. 163.

30. David Miller, op.cit., p. 276.

31. James Lardner, *HC*, 14 November 1911 (31) col. 261.

32. Reprinted in *BMJ Supplement*, 22 July 1911, p. 189.

33. Ibid.

34. Braithwaite, op.cit., p. 188.

35. *Medical Press and Circular,* 19 July 1911, Vol. XCII, p. 57

36. For example, as reported in the *BMJ Supplement* 26 August, p. 325, 30 September, p. 367.

37. Braithwaite, op.cit., p. 204.

38. Ibid., pp. 222-3.

39. *HC*, 25 October 1911 (30) col. 149.

40. Ibid., cols. 162-3.

41. Ibid., col. 154.

42. Ibid., 14 November 1911 (31) col. 228.

43. Ibid., col. 224.

44. Ibid., cols. 250-1.

45. Ibid., cols. 260-1.

46. Ibid., col. 261.

47. Ibid., 15 November 1911 (31) col. 442.

48. Ibid., cols. 443-4.

49. Ibid., col. 413.

50. Ibid., col. 415.

51. Ibid., cols. 431-434.

52. Ibid., col. 436.

53. *BMJ Supplement*, 2 December 1911, pp. 547/8.

54. Ibid., p. 547.

55. *HC*, 21 November 1911 (31) col. 1015.

56. *Report of Sir William Plender...into existing conditions in respect of medical attendance and remuneration in certain towns.* Cd. 6305 1912-13 lxxviii 679.

57. Speech reported in the *Freeman's Journal*, 20 December 1911 and quoted in *BMJ Supplement*, 23 March 1912, p. 342.

58. Ibid.

59. *Report of the Committee appointed to consider the extension of Medical Benefit under the National Insurance Act to Ireland.* HC Cd. 6963 1913 xxxvii (1) p.4.

60. M. J. O'Lehane, representing the Irish Trades Union Congress and Irish Drapers' Assistants Association. Ibid. *Appendix 1, Minutes of Evidence*, Cd. 7039 1913 xxxvii. (17) p. 39.

61. Newman Thompson, representing the Union Friendly Society, ibid., p. 42.

62. Richard O'Carroll, representing the Dublin United Trades Council and the Labour League, ibid., p.46.

63. *HC* 10 March 1913 (50) col. 69.

64. *Report of the Committee appointed to consider the Extension of Medical Benefit, etc., Appendix 1, Minutes of Evidence,* op.cit., p. 137.

65. Ibid., p. 47.

66. Ibid., p. 55.

67. Ibid., pp. 12, 48, 96, 137.

68. Ibid., p. 53 especially.

69. Dr O'Sullivan, Waterford, *ibid.*, p. 146.

70. Dr P.G. Lee, ibid., p. 97.

71. Dr Maurice Hayes, ibid., p. 53.

72. Ibid., p. 51.

73. Dr E. Whitley Allsom, ibid., p. 140.

74. *Report of the Committee appointed to consider the extension of medical benefit to .... Ireland,* op.cit.

75. Robinson to Nathan, 28.3.1915, MS Nathan, 449, quoted in Leon O Broin, *The Chief Secretary — Augustine Birrell in Ireland* (London 1969) p.116. Nathan was Under Secretary at Dublin Castle.

76. Richard Titmuss, 'Health' in Ginsberg (ed.) op.cit., p. 300.

NOTES TO CHAPTER 4
MEDICAL SERVICES IN YEARS OF UPHEAVAL, 1913-1919

[1.] For a general text on this important period see F.S.L. Lyons *Ireland Since the Famine* (London, 1971).

[2.] *Report for 1912-13 on the Administration of the National Insurance Act*, Part I (Health Insurance), 1913 Cd 6907 xxxvii (1) p. 451.

[3.] *Report on the Administration of National Health Insurance during the years 1914-17*, 1917-18, Cd. 8890, xvii (31) p. 238.

[4.] *Interim Report of the Departmental Committee on Tuberculosis — 1912-13*, Cd. 6164, xlviii (1) p. 5.

[5] *Final Report of the Departmental Committee on Tuberculosis, Vol. 2*, 1912-13, Cd. 6654, xlvii (47) pp. 173-4.

[6.] *Report of the LGB for Year Ending 31 March 1913*, 1913, Cd. 6978, xxxii (457) p. 56.

[7.] Ibid., p.xxxiv.

[8.] Ibid., p. xxx.

[9.] *Report of the LGB for year ending 31 March 1914*, 1914, Cd. 7561, xxxix (595) p. xxxiii.

[10.] *Report of the LGB for the year ending 31 March 1918*, 1919, Cmd. 65 xxv (1) pp. xlviii — xliv.

[11.] Ibid.

[12.] *Report of the LGB for year ending 31 March 1915*, 1914-16, Cd. 8016, xxv (341) p.xxvi and the *Report of the LGB for the year ending 31 March 1917*, 1917-18, Cd. 8765, xvi (257) p. xxxiv.

[13.] *HC* 25 November 1914 (68) col. 1482.

[14.] Ibid., col. 1260.

[15.] Ibid., April 1916 (81) col. 1720-1.

[16.] *Report of the LGB for year ending 31 March 1918,* op.cit., p.xxx.

[17.] Carnegie United Kingdom Trust, *Report on the Physical Welfare of Mothers and Children*, Vol. IV, Ireland (Dublin, 1917) p. 7.

[18.] Ibid., p. 19.

[19.] Ibid., p. 66.

[20.] Ibid., p. 65.

[21.] HC 8 July 1915 (73) cols. 617-629; 783-799; 13 July 1915 col. 803.

[22.] *Report of the LGB for year ending 31 March 1917* 1917-1918, Cd. 8765, xvi (257) pp. l-li.

[23.] *Report of the LGB for year ending 31 March 1918* op.cit., p. lvi.

[24.] Dr E. Coey Bigger/Carnegie United Kingdom Trust, op.cit.

[25.] Ibid., p. 2.

[26.] Ibid., p. 33.

[27.] *Report of the LGB for year ending 31 March 1919*, 1920, Cmd. 578, xxi (1) p xlvii.

28. *Report of the LGB for year ending 31 March 1920*, 1921, Cmd. 1432 xiv (781) p.xlix.

29. *Report of the LGB for year ending 31 March 1918*, op.cit., p. xxxiv-xxxvi.

30. *Report of the National Health Insurance Commission (Ireland) for the period Nov 1917 to 31 March 1920*, 1921, Cmd. 1147 xv (653) p. 62-3.

31. *Report of the LGB for the year ending 31 March 1919*, op.cit., p. xlix.

32. *HC*, 27 February 1919 (112) col. 1835.

33. Ibid., cols. 1849-52.

34. Ibid, cols. 1852-55.

35. No. 44, 9 Geo. 5.

36. Ibid., Section 10.

37. *Report of the Irish Public Health Council on the Public Health and Medical Services in Ireland*, 1920, Cmd. 761 xvii (1075) p. 3.

38. Ibid., p. 4.

39. Ibid., p. 6.

40. Ibid., p. 8.

41. Ibid., p. 11.

42. Ibid., p. 7.

43. Ibid., p. 16.

44. Ibid., p. 19.

NOTES TO CHAPTER 5
EFFICIENCY, ECONOMY AND THE NEW STATE, 1919-1932

1. This interpretation is based on E. Rumpf and A.C. Hepburn, *Nationalism and Socialism in Twentieth-Century Ireland* (Liverpool, 1977).

2. HC, 26 February 1919 (112) col. 1855.

3. Tom Garvin, *The Evolution of Irish Nationalist Politics* (Dublin, 1981) p. 199.

4. Dorothy Macardle, *The Irish Republic* (London, 1968) p. 838.

5. Ibid., p. 839.

6. J.L. McCracken, *Representative Government in Ireland: A Study of Dail Eireann 1919-48* (London, 1958) p. 31.

7. Garvin, op.cit., p. 199.

8. Quoted in Macardle, op.cit., p. 254.

9. Ibid., p. 255.

10. *Report of the Local Government Department*, 3 May 1921, *Art O'Briain Papers* MS 8460 National Library, Dublin.

11. Restoration of Order (Ireland) Act, 1920.

12. *Report of the Local Government Department*, 3 May 1921, op.cit.

13. *Minutes of Proceedings of the First Parliament of the Republic of Ireland 1919-1921*, Official Record (Dublin, n.d. 1921?) p. 185.

14. *Final Report of the Commission on Local Government*, 1920, in *Minutes of Proceedings of the First Parliament of the Republic of Ireland, 1919-1921, Official Record*, op.cit., p. 218.

15. *Minutes of Proceedings of the First Parliament of the Republic of Ireland, 1919-1921, Official Record*, op.cit., p. 220 et.seq.

16. Ibid.

17. Ibid.

18. Ibid. and p. 260.

19. Quoted in DLGPH, *First Report, 1922-1925*, op.cit., pp. 146.

20. *DD*, 3 June 1931 (38) col. 2267.

21. David Fitzpatrick, *Politics and Irish Life, 1913-1921: Provincial Experience of War and Revolution* (Dublin, 1977) pp. 194-5.

22. *Report of the Local Government Department*, 3 May 1921, op.cit.

23. *DD*, 9 February 1923 (2) col. 1435.

24. *Report of the Local Government Department*, 3 May 1921, op.cit.

25. *Report of the Commission on the Relief of the Sick and Destitute Poor, including the Insane Poor* (Stationery Office, R27/3) p. 11.

26. *HC*, 4 April 1921 (140) col. 17.

27. *DD*, 1 June 1926 (16) col. 93.

28. *DD*, 16 November 1923 (5) cols. 927-8.

29. DLGPH, *First Report 1922-1925*, op.cit., p. 53.

30. *Report of the Commission on the Relief of the Sick and Destitute Poor, including the Insane Poor*, op.cit., p. 14.

31. Ibid., p. 12.

32. Ibid., passim.

33. Ibid., p. 11.

34. Ibid., *Minutes of Evidence* (Stationery Office R27/1-2).

35. *Report of the Commission on the Relief of the Sick and Destitute Poor, etc.* op.cit., p. 19.

36. Ibid.

37. Ibid., p. 31.

38. Ibid., pp. 75-7.

39. Ibid., p. 80.

40. This interpretation is based on that of James Meenan, *The Irish Economy since 1922* (Liverpool, 1970).

41. Terence Brown, *Ireland: A Social and Cultural History 1922-79* (Glasgow, 1981) p. 15.

42. DLGPH, *First Report*, op.cit., p. 27.

43. *DD*, 18 January 1924 (6) col. 383-4.

44. Claire P. Carney, 'Selectivist Social Services: The Origin of Certain Services in the Republic of Ireland with an Evaluation of the Underlying Social

Policy', unpublished Ph.D. thesis, University College Dublin, 1977 p. 245.

45. Under the Local Government Act, 1925.

46. *DD*, 29 May (7) col. 1594-5.

47. These powers were made permanent by the Local Government Act, 1925.

48. *DD*, 3 June 1924 (7) col. 1785.

49. S. Burke, Minister for Local Government and Public Health, *DD*, 19 May 1926 (15) col. 1816.

50. DLGPH, *Third Report 1927-28* p. 100 (Stationery Office, K 24/3) p. 19; Report 1930-31 (Stationery Office K24/6) p. 703, p. 103 and Dr John Shanley 'The State and Medicine' reprint from *The Irish Journal of Medical Science*, May 1929.

51. DLGPH, *Second Report 1925-1927* (Stationery Office, K 24/2).

52. DLGPH, *Third Report 1927-28* op.cit. pp. 37-38.

53. S. Burke, Minister for Local Government and Public Health, *DD*, 4 November 1924 (9) col. 705.

54. Ibid., 19 November 1924 (9) 1240.

55. DLGPH, *Report 1931-1932*, P. 894 (Stationery Office, K 24/7) p. 50.

56. Ibid., p. 63.

57. Ibid., p. 68.

58. Ibid., p. 70.

59. DLGPH, *Fourth Report 1928-1929*, P. 336, (Stationery Office, K 24/4) p. 48.

60. DLGPH, *Second Report 1925-1927*, op.cit., p. 66.

61. Ibid., *First Report 1922-1925*, op.cit., p. 34.

62. *Report of the Commission on the Relief of the Sick and Destitute Poor, etc.,* op.cit., passim.

63. DLGPH, *Fourth Report, 1928-1929,* op.cit., pp. 46-7.

64. Ibid., *Report 1930-1931,* op. cit., p. 61.

65. Ibid., pp. 61-2.

66. Ibid., Third Report 1927-1928, op.cit., p. 41.

67. Ibid., Report 1932-1933, P. 1154, (Stationery Office, K 24/8) p. 53.

68. Ibid., *Fourth Report 1928-1929,* op.cit., p. 57.

69. Ibid., *Report 1929-1930*, P. 495 (Stationery office, K 24/5) p.5.

70. Ibid., *Report 1930-1931*, op.cit., p. 83. In March 1931 £21,310 of the grant of £145,623 allocated in 1912 was still unspent.

71. R.C. Geary,'Mortality from Tuberculosis in Saorstat Eireann', *Journal of the Statistical and Social Enquiry Society of Ireland*, vol. xxii, Oct. 1930, pp. 67-103; T.W.T. Dillon, 'The Statistics of Tuberculosis', *Irish Journal of Medical Science*, Vol. XVI, July 1942, pp. 221-243.

72. DLGPH, *Fourth Report 1928-1929,* op.cit., p. 57.

73. *DD*, 28 May 1924 (7) col. 1424 and 3 June 1924 (7) col. 1732.

74. Ibid., 4 July 1924 (8) col. 468.

[75.] *Committee of Inquiry into Health Insurance and Medical Services, Interim Report,* 1925, (Stationery Office, N 2/1) pp.4-11.

[76.] *Committee on Health Insurance and Medical Services, Final Report, 1927* (Stationery Office, N 2/3).

[77.] Ibid., p. 23.

[78.] Submission of Evidence by the Irish Medical Committee, *Interim Report of the Committee on Health Insurance and Medical Services,* 1925, op.cit., p. 59.

[79.] *Committee on Health Insurance and Medical Services, Final Report,* op.cit., Appendix A — Summary of Views, Expressed by Representatives of the Irish Medical Committee, etc.

[80.] Ibid., p. 24.

[81.] Ibid., p. 32.

[82.] Ibid., p. 31.

[83.] *DD*, 3 May 1933 (47) col. 512.

[84.] *DD*, 20 May 1931 (38) cols. 1489, 1485.

[85.] DLGPH, *The Hospitals Commission, Third General Report 1927,* Stationery Office, p. 45 and *Returns of Local Taxation 1932-33* P. 1310, Stationery Office, p. 14.

[86.] Under the Public Charitable Hospitals (Amendment) Act, 1931.

[87.] Quoted in *DD* 28 April 1933 (47) col. 322.

[88.] See Kevin O'Higgins, *DD*, 9 February 1923 (2) col. 1435.

[89.] Oliver MacDonagh, *Ireland: The Union and its Aftermath* (London, 1977) p. 106.

NOTES TO CHAPTER 6
HOSPITALS FOR THE PEOPLE, 1932-1942

[1.] DLGPH, *Report 1932-33*, pp. 122-23.

[2.] See the Reports of the DLGPH for these years.

[3.] For the economic problems of these years see James Meenan, *The Irish Economy since 1922,* op.cit.

[4.] Richard Corish TD, *DD*, 3 June 1942 (87) col. 903.

[5.] Desmond Roche, *Local Government in Ireland* (Dublin, 1982) p. 105.

[6.] Ibid.

[7.] General R. Mulcahy, DD, 16 June 1942 (87) col. 1039.

[8.] Mr S. MacEntee, *ibid.,* 3 June 1942, col. 883.

[9.] *DD*, 20 November 1946 (103) col. 1144.

[10.] *DD*, 3 June 1931 (38) col. 2273/4.

[11.] Ibid.

[12.] *DD*, 28 April 1933 (47) col. 319-330.

13. Ibid., col. 326.

14. Ibid., col. 323.

15. Ibid., col. 324.

16. Ibid., cols. 323-4.

17. See for example Deputy Fitzgerald-Kenney, Ibid., col. 336.

18. Deputy Fitzgerald-Kenney, Ibid., col. 330.

19. Brian Abel-Smith, *The Hospitals 1800-1948* (London, 1964) pp. 405-423.

20. DLGPH, The Hospitals Commission, *First General Report, February 1936,* P 1976 (Stationery Office, R 56/1) p. 92.

21. DLGPH, The Hospitals Commission, *First General Report,* op.cit. Excludes tuberculosis and mental hospital beds.

22. Ibid., p. 8.

23. Ibid.

24. Ibid., p. 9.

25. Ibid., pp. 11-12.

26. Ibid.

27. Ibid., p. 15.

28. Ibid., p. 17, p. 59.

29. Ibid.

30. Ibid., pp. 57-9.

31. Ibid., p. 59.

32. Ibid.

33. DLGPH *Report 1932-33,* P. 1154 (Stationery Office, K 24/8) p. 132.

34. Ibid., pp. 132-3.

35. Ibid.

36. *DD*, 30 March 1939 (75) col. 567.

37. DLGPH, *Report 1941-42,* P. 6107 (Stationery Office, K. 24/17) p. 92.

38. *DD*, 3 June 1942 (87) col. 895.

39. DLGPH, The Hospitals Commission, *Sixth General Report 1942-44* (Stationery Office, R 56/6) p. 27.

40. S.T. O Ceallaigh, Minister for Local Government and Public Health, *DD*, 31 March 1939 (75) col. 571.

41. DLGPH, The Hospitals Commission, *Fourth General Report 1938* (Stationery Office, R 56/4) p. 7.

42. DLGPH, The Hospitals Commission, *Sixth General Report,* op.cit., p. 5 and *DD*, 8 May 1940 (80) col. 4.

43. DLGPH, The Hospitals Commission, *Fourth General Report 1937,* op.cit., p. 18.

44. Ibid.

45. DLGPH, The Hospitals Commission, *Fifth Report, 1941* (Stationery Office, R 56/6) p. 10.

[46.] DLGPH, The Hospitals Commission, *First Report, February 1936,* op.cit., p. 68.

[47.] See for example the editorial in *JIMA*, Vol. 12, No. 69, March 1943, p. 25.

[48.] Minister for Local Government and Public Health, *DD*, 26 April 1933 (47) col. 103.

[49.] J.H. Whyte, *Church and State in Modern Ireland 1923-1979,* Second Edition (Dublin, 1980) p. 74.

[50.] *DD*, 7 April 1938 (70) col. 1653.

[51.] Ibid., col. 1659.

[52.] Ibid., 18 February 1941 (85) col. 1946.

[53.] Ibid., cols. 1921 and 1930.

[54.] DLGPH, The Hospitals Commission, *Sixth General Report,* op.cit., p.9.

[55.] Ibid.

[56.] *Sale of Food and Drugs (Milk) Act, 1936, Milk and Dairies Act, 1935,* and *Slaughter of Animals Act, 1935.*

[57.] DLGPH, *Report 1931-32,* op.cit., p. 63 and *Report 1942-43* P. 6706, Stationery Office, K 24/18) p. 59. In 1942 the numbers inspected fell to 111,000. Ibid. The total number of children attending national schools in 1940 was 472,145. John Coolahan, *Irish Education: History and Structure* (Dublin, 1981) p. 49.

[58.] DLGPH, *Reports,* passim.

[59.] DLGPH, *Report 1938-39* (Stationery Office, K 24/14) pp. 28-9.

[60.] DLGPH, *Report 1940-41,* P. 5497 (Stationery Office, K 24/16) p. 28.

[61.] Prof. T.W.T. Dillon, 'The Statistics of Tuberculosis', op.cit., p. 229.

[62.] DLGPH, The Hospitals Commission, *Second General Report 1935 and 1936* (Stationery Office, R 56/2) p. 16.

[63.] DLGPH, The Hospitals Commission, *First General Report,* op.cit., p. 43.

[64.] Ibid., pp. 44, 49.

[65.] DLGPH, The Hospitals Commission, *Second General Report,* op.cit., p.18.

[66.] Ibid., p. 21.

[67.] Ibid., pp. 22-3.

[68.] DLGPH, *Report 1939-40,* P. 4731 (Stationery Office, K 24/15) p. 143.

[69.] Prof. T.W.T. Dillon, 'The Statistics of Tuberculosis', op.cit., p. 235.

[70.] *DD*, 16 June 1942 (87) col. 1058.

[71.] Midwives Act, 1931.

[72.] DLGPH, *Report 1933-34,* P. 1840 (Stationery Office, K 24/9) p. 64 and *Report 1939-40,* op.cit., p. 39.

[73.] DLGPH, *Report 1933-34,* op.cit., p. 64.

[74.] DLGPH, The Hospitals Commission, *Fourth General Report,* op.cit., p. 11.

[75.] Ibid.

[76.] DLGPH, *Report 1937-38*, P. 3399 (Stationery Office, K 24/13) p. 57.

[77.] *DD*, 21 April 1936 (61) cols. 1200 and 1202.

[78.] DLGPH *Report 1939-40,* op.cit., p. 40.

[79.] DLGPH, *Report 1941-42,* op.cit., p. 55.

[80.] DLGPH, *Report 1944-45*, P. 7772 (Stationery Office, K 24/20) p. 32.

[81.] *DD*, 7 December 1939 (78) col. 1257.

[82.] Ibid., col. 1206.

[83.] Ibid., 6 December 1939, col. 1000.

[84.] Ibid., col. 1045.

[85.] Ibid., col. 1048.

[86.] *JIMA*, vol. 15, No. 90, December 1944, p. 69.

[87.] The Minister, Sean T. O Ceallaigh defended this policy in the *DD*, 23 April 1936 (61) col. 1614.

[88.] See for example a paper by Dr John Shanley, 'The State and Medicine' reprint from *The Irish Journal of Medical Science*, May 1929. Dr Shanley became an extremely influential figure in medical organisation in the 1930s and 1940s.

[89.] *JIMA*, Vol. 10, No. 56, February 1942, pp. 20-21.

NOTES TO CHAPTER 7
TOWARDS A NATIONAL HEALTH SERVICE, 1942-1945

[1.] K. Nowlan and D. Williams, eds. *Ireland in the War Years and After 1939-51* (Dublin, 1969) and the Reports of the DLGPH for the war years.

[2.] Dr T. O'Higgins, *DD*, 28 October 1943 (91) col. 1406. Dr O'Higgins combined the jobs of CMO for Meath and Dail deputy for many years.

[3.] DLGPH, *Report 1941-42,* op.cit., p. 38.

[4.] Ibid. *Reports 1940-45,* op.cit., passim.

[5.] Ibid., *Report 1937-38,* op.cit., p. 45. *Report 1940-41,* op.cit., p. 41, *Report 1942-43,* op.cit., p. 45.

[6.] Ibid., *Report 1941-42,* op.cit., pp. 177-8, *Report 1942-43,* op.cit., p. 164.

[7.] Dr James Ryan, Minister for Health, *DD*, 24 June 1947, (107) col. 4.

[8.] Information from Dr James Deeny.

[9.] Dr Deeny had the formula for DDT before the chemical was commercially available in Ireland.

[10.] Desmond Roche, 1982, op.cit., p. 58.

[11.] For the depth of feeling about the county managers, see *DD*, vol. 91 passim.

12. *DD*, 16 June 1942 (87) col. 1113.

13. *DD*, 28 October 1943 (91) col. 1349.

14. See for example, *DD*, 3 June 1942 (87) col. 989 and ibid., col. 1068.

15. Sir William Beveridge, *Social Insurance and Allied Services*, November 1942, Cmd. 6404 (London, 1942).

16. See for example, *DD*, 23 October 1943 (91) col. 1383 and after, and the *JIMA*, Vol.12, February 1943, No. 98.

17. Sir William Beveridge, op.cit., p.6.

18. Ibid., p. 162.

19. *A National Health Service*, Cmd. 6502 (London, 1944).

20. Radio Telefis Eireann, *Sean MacEntee, Commemorative Programme*, radio broadcast, 10 January 1984.

21. DLGPH, Memorandum to the Government, *Urgent Problems Relating to Public Health which must be dealt with*, March 1944, Cabinet Files, S 13444A, SPO.

22. Ibid.

23. Ibid., DLGPH, *Bill to amend the Public Health Acts, Need for proposed legislation*, June 1944.

24. Ibid., *Public Health Bill 1944, Scheme of Additional Provisions*, November 1944.

25. See for example Emmet Larkin, 'Socialism and Catholicism in Ireland', in *Church History*, Vol. 33, 1964, pp. 426-483.

26. Anne Fremantle ed., *The Papal Encyclicals in Their Historical Context* (New York, 1963).

27. Ibid.

28. Dermot Keogh, *The Vatican, the Bishops and Irish Politics 1919-39* (Cambridge, 1986), p. 204.

29. Ibid., p. 226.

30. Inaugural speech to the Commission on Vocational Organisation, 5 October 1939, *Document 19, MS 934*, National Library of Ireland.

31. John Whyte, op.cit., p. 74.

32. *Irish Independent*, 8 July 1943.

33. Ibid.

34. Sean P. Farragher, *Dev and his Alma Mater* (Dublin, 1985) p. 191.

35. Joseph Lee, 'Aspects of Corporatist Thought in Ireland: The Commission on Vocational Organisation, 1939-43', p. 339, in Cosgrove and McCartney, eds. *Studies in Irish History* (University College Dublin, 1979).

36. *Report of the Commission on Vocational Organisation*, 1943, (Stationery Office, Dublin, 1944).

37. Ibid., p. 319.

38. This refusal to meet the Assocation came about during negotiations on fees for administering diphtheria vaccine.

39. Ibid., para. 667.

40. Ibid., p. 320.

41. Ibid., p. 104.

42. Commission on Vocational Organisation, *Minutes of Evidence Vol. 13, MS 934*, National Library of Ireland. See also Joseph Lee, in Cosgrave and McCartney, op.cit., p. 340.

43. Notes of an interview between John Whyte and Dr F.C. Ward, 18 June 1966.

44. Dr John Dignan, Bishop of Clonfert, *Social Security: Outlines of a Scheme of National Health Insurance* (Sligo, 1945).

45. Ibid., p. 7.

46. Ibid., p. 36.

47. Ibid., p. 12.

48. Ibid., p. 20.

49. Ibid., p. 25.

50. Ibid., p. 34.

51. Ibid., p. 33.

52. *Irish Independent*, 14 March 1945, referred to in John Whyte, op.cit., pp. 111-2.

53. See John Whyte's comments Ibid., pp. 105-6.

54. Information from Dr Shanley.

55. Dr John Shanley, Presidential address, *JIMA* Vol. 13, July 1943, No. 73, pp. 74-7.

56. Dr John Shanley, 'The Reorganisation of the Medical Services', ibid. Vol. 14, No. 82, April 1944, pp. 40-43.

57. Ibid., p. 41.

58. Ibid., No. 84, June 1944, p. 64. For the dispensary doctors criticism see the letter from Dr J.F. Falvey, ibid., May 1944, No. 83, pp. 55-6.

59. Ibid., June 1944, p. 64.

60. 'A Scheme for a National Medical Service', ibid., Vol. 15, No. 90, December 1944, pp. 66-71.

61. Ibid., p. 70.

62. *Irish Press*, 4 November 1944.

63. *Irish Times*, 6 November 1944.

64. Ibid., 7 November 1944.

65. Vincente Navarro, *Class Struggle, the State and Medicine* (London, 1978) p. 28.

66. My informants, Desmond Roche, John Garvin, and Brendan Kiernan, all confirmed this point.

67. Notes of interview between John Whyte and Dr F.C. Ward, 18 June 1966. Also referred to by John Whyte, op.cit., p. 128.

68. DLGPH, *Report of the Departmental Committee on Health Services* (Stationery Office, Dublin, 1945) Unpublished, 50 copies printed. One on Cabinet file S13444 C, SPO.

69. Ibid., p. 75.
70. Ibid., p. 42.
71. Desmond Roche and John Garvin were my informants.
72. *Report of the Departmental Committee on Health Services,* op.cit., p. 75.
73. Ibid., p. 80.
74. Ibid., pp. 86-7.
75. Ibid., pp. 100-1.
76. Desmond Roche, James Deeny and John Garvin confirmed this point.
77. Information from James Deeny.
78. *Report of the Departmental Committee on Health Services,* op.cit., p. 85.
79. Information from Desmond Roche.
80. Information from James Deeny.
81. Particularly the memorandum from the DLGPH *Health Services*, 26 September 1945, Cabinet Files S13444 C, SPO.
82. DLGPH, 7 December, 1945 and Department of the Taoiseach, Minute 8 December 1945, Cabinet files, S13444 C, SPO.
83. The Royal Irish Academy of Medicine, *Report on Tuberculosis*, 1942 referred to in the White Paper, *Tuberculosis*, January 1946, P. 7368 (Stationery Office, Dublin, 1946).
84. *Irish Independent*, 16 February 1943, quoted in John Whyte, op.cit., p. 79.
85. Information from Dr Shanley.
86. John Whyte, op.cit., p. 79.
87. Information from James Deeny. The commitment was given at a meeting with representatives of Dun Laoghaire Corporation and Prof. Dillon. A participant at the meeting leaked the proceedings to an evening newspaper.
88. DLGPH, *Tuberculosis,* op.cit.
89. *Report of the Departmental Committee on Health Services,* op.cit., p. 100.
90. Terence Brown, op.cit., p. 180.
91. See Dr J. McPolin's extreme views in *JIMA*, Vol. 24, February 1949, no. 140, pp. 30-32.

NOTES TO CHAPTER 8
DRAWING THE BATTLE LINES, 1945-1948

1. DLGPH, *Health Services*, Memorandum to Government, 9 March 1946, Cabinet files, S 13444C, SPO.
2. *Seanad Debates*, 3 April 1946, (31) col. 1245.
3. Public Health Bill, 1945, Explanatory memorandum, November 1945, Cabinet files, S 13444B, SPO.
4. Dr F.C. Ward, Parliamentary Secretary, *DD*, 12 December 1945 (98) cols. 1708-9.

5. J.H. Whyte, op.cit., p. 134.

6. DLGPH, Urgent Problems which must be dealt with, Cabinet files, S 13444, SPO.

7. *JIMA*, Vol. 18, No. 107, May 1946, p. 65.

8. *DD*, 12 December 1945 (98) col. 1701.

9. Ibid., col. 1709.

10. Ibid., col. 1708.

11. Ibid., col. 1731.

12. Ibid., col. 1738.

13. Ibid., 13 December 1945, cols. 1896-99.

14. Letter dated 23 January 1946, Cabinet files, S 13444C, SPO.

15. Referred to in the Taoiseach's letter to Archbishop McQuaid, 6 March 1946, Cabinet files, S 13444C, SPO.

16. Letter from D. O'Suilleabhain, Secretary to the Parliamentary Secretary (Dr Ward) to the Secretary of the Taoiseach, 27 February 1946, Cabinet files, S 13444 C, SPO.

17. Ibid.

18. Ibid. This account confirms the substance of Dr Ward's recollections to John Whyte in an interview in 1966.

19. Letter read to John Whyte by Dr Ward in 1966. Notes of interview made by John Whyte.

20. *DD*, 22 March 1946 (100) col. 352 and ibid. 20 March 1946 col. 166.

21. See contributions by Deputies McGilligan and Costello, Ibid., 3 April 1946 (100) col. 1137 and April 1946, col. 1384.

22. Notes of interview with John Whyte, 1966.

23. See *DD*, 11 April 1946 (100) cols. 1795-1833.

24. Ibid., col. 1789.

25. *JIMA*, Vol. 18, No. 105, March 1946, p. 47.

26. Ibid.

27. *DD*, 5 June 1946 (101) cols. 1320-33.

28. Ibid., 14 December 1945 (98) col. 2093.

29. Letter from Dr Ward to the Chief Whip, Fianna Fail, 10 September 1946, Cabinet files, S 13866A, SP0.

30. Ibid.

31. *Report of the Tribunal appointed by the Taoiseach on the 7th day of June, 1946 pursuant to resolution passed on the 5th day of June 1946, by Dail Eireann and Seanad Eireann*, P 7722 (Stationery Office, Dublin).

32. *DD*, 16 July 1946 (102) cols. 853-4.

33. Speech by Mr MacEntee to the IMA, June 1946, Miscellaneous Memoranda, No. 3, Deeny Papers, RCSI.

34. DLGPH, *Proposals for the Reform of the Health Services*, March 1946, Cabinet files, S 13444C, SPO.

35. Minute signed by J.J. McElligott, Secretary, Department of Finance

to the DLGPH re the draft scheme for the development and reorganisation of the health services, 14 February, 1946. Ibid.

[36.] Ibid.

[37.] DLGPH, *Proposals for the Reform of the Health Services, Supplementary Memorandum*, 23 August 1946, Cabinet files, S 13444D, SPO.

[38.] Ibid.

[39.] Ibid.

[40.] Department of the Taoiseach, Minute of 3 September 1946, ibid.

[41.] Minute of 18 January 1947, ibid.

[42.] Letter dated 16 October 1946, ibid.

[43.] *DD*, 15 November 1946 (103) col. 1025.

[44.] Ibid., col. 1026.

[45.] Information from Dr Oliver Fitzgerald, at the time editor of the *JIMA*, and Dr T.C.J. 'Bob' O'Connell.

[46.] See for example his articles 'Some Aspects of the Sociology of the Medical Profession' in the *JIMA*, Vol. 19, No. 110, August 1946, pp. 118-22 and No. 111 September 1946, pp. 135-44.

[47.] See for example his letter of 13 April 1951 to the Taoiseach, John A. Costello. Cabinet files S 14997 B, SPO.

[48.] Memorandum from Dr James Deeny to the Secretary, DOH, December 1946, Deeny Papers op.cit.

[49.] Memorandum from Dr James Deeny to the Secretary, Department of Health, December 1946, Miscellaneous File No.3, Deeny Papers, op.cit. John Garvin confirmed the Department's attitude to me.

[50.] *JIMA*, Vol. 19, No. 109, July 1946, p. 111.

[51.] Dr J. McPolin, 'Some Aspects of the Sociology of the Medical Profession', op.cit.

[52.] See for example John Whyte, op.cit., pp. 261-5.

[53.] *DD*, 11 February 1947 (104) cols. 749-83, passim.

[54.] *Health Bill, 1947*, Sections 21, 22, 23.

[55.] Ibid., Sections 24, 25, 26.

[56.] *DD*, 1 May 1947 (105) col. 1977.

[57.] Ibid., col. 1979.

[58.] Ibid., 10 June 1947 (106) col. 1508.

[59.] Ibid., 3 July 1947 (107) col. 880.

[60.] Ibid., 27 June 1947 (107) cols. 471-2.

[61.] Ibid., 1 May 1947 (105) col. 1954.

[62.] Ibid., 10 June 1947 (106) col. 1497.

[63.] Ibid., cols. 1498-9.

[64.] Ibid., col. 1499.

[65.] Ibid., col. 1513.

[66.] Ibid.

[67.] Ibid., 3 July 1947 (107) cols. 884-5.

68. *JIMA*, Vol. 21, No.122, August 1947, p. 32.

69. Ibid.

70. Referred to in John Whyte, op.cit., p. 151.

71. Letter from Dr James McPolin to the Taoiseach and to the Minister for Health, 9 July 1947, Cabinet files, S 13444E, SPO.

72. Department of the Taoiseach minute to the DOH, 10 July 1947, ibid.

73. Letter from the Attorney General to the Minister for Health, 28 July 1947, ibid.

74. Minutes of meeting of the Council of State, 13 August 1947, ibid.

75. *JIMA*, Vol. 21, No. 122, August 1947, p. 28, and No. 126, December 1947, pp. 103-4.

76. *Irish Independent*, 22 December 1947, quoted in John Whyte, op.cit., p. 152.

77. Letter of 16 October from Dr O'Neill to Dr McPolin, ibid.

78. *Statement of the Irish Hierarchy on the Health Act, 1947* Cabinet files, S 14997A, SPO.

79. Ibid.

80. John Whyte, op.cit., p. 143.

81. Dept. of Health, *Outline of Proposals for the Improvement of the Health Services*, P 8400 (Stationery Office, 1947).

82. Ibid., p. 22.

83. Ibid., p. 23.

84. Ibid., p. 22.

85. Censorship of Publications Board, quoted in *The Liberal Ethic* (The Irish Times, 1950) p. 57.

86. Information from James Deeny.

87. Ibid.

88. Ibid.

89. The term was coined by Sir Horace Plunkett; quoted in *The Liberal Ethic*, op.cit., p. 32.

90. Letter from the Taoiseach to Dr James Staunton, 16 February 1948, Cabinet files, S 14997 A, SPO, Dublin.

91. *JIMA*, Vol. 20, No. 119, May 1947, p. 259.

92. Ibid., p. 260.

93. Ibid., Vol. 21, No. 122, August 1947, p. 19.

94. Ibid., No. 126, December 1947, p. 103.

95. Ibid., Vol. 22, No. 127, January 1948, p. 2.

NOTES TO CHAPTER 9
THE SPORT OF POLITICS, 1948-1951

1. Noel Browne, *Against the Tide* (Dublin, 1986).
2. *JIMA*, Vol. 22, No. 128, February 1948, pp. 26-7 for Browne's criticism of Deeny's paper. Several informants mentioned the incident of the stormy meeting.
3. *DD*, 6 July 1948 (111) col. 2301.
4. Ibid. 8 July 1948, col. 2580-1.
5. Department of Finance *Memorandum on Health Expenditure*, 31 December 1948, Cabinet files, S13444G, SPO.
6. *DD*, 8 July 1948 (111) cols. 2543, 2557 and 11 July 1950 (122) col. 1292.
7. *First Report of the DOH 1945-49*, Pr. 42 (Stationery Office, 1950).
8. James Deeny, *Tuberculosis in Ireland*, Report of the National Tuberculosis Survey (1950-53), (Dublin, 1954) p. 231.
9. Ibid.
10. Ibid., p. 232.
11. *DD*, 8 July 1948 (111) col. 2566, and *Memoranda 1957*, No.18, Deeny Papers, RCSI.
12. *First Report of the DOH*, op.cit., p. 45.
13. *Tuberculosis in Ireland*, op.cit., p. 233.
14. Ibid., p. 21.
15. Ibid.
16. Ibid., p. 240.
17. Ibid., p. 235.
18. Ibid., p. 240.
19. *DD*, 6 July 1948 (111) col. 2273.
20. Ibid., col. 2274, and *First Report of the DOH,* op.cit. p. 22.
21. Central Statistics Office, *Statistical Abstract of Ireland, 1952*, Pr. 1212, Stationery Office, p. 173. The figure refers to the financial year 1948-9.
22. *DD*, 6 July 1948 (111) col. 2274 and 1 July 1949 (116) col. 1823.
23. DOH, Memorandum, 9 June 1948, *Amendment of Health Act, 1947*, Appendix A, Cabinet files, S13444G, SPO.
24. Ibid.
25. Minutes from Dr James Deeny to Mr Murray, Ass. Secretary, DOH, 12 April 1949, Miscellaneous File No. 6, Deeny Papers, op.cit.
26. Note of 25 June, 1948, Cabinet files, S13444G, SPO.
27. Information from Dr Noel Browne. Confirmed in Browne, op.cit., p. 153.
28. J.H. Whyte, op.cit., p. 203.
29. *DD*, 10 June 1953 (139) cols. 1021-2.
30. DOH, *Discussions between the Minister for Health and the Irish Medical*

Association regarding Mother and Child Health Service, Sequence of Events, March 1951, Cabinet files, S14447A, SPO and *DD*, 5 April 1951 (125) col. 668.

31. On 27 March 1951 the Taoiseach's Department could find no record of the submission to the government of proposals for a mother and child service. *Cabinet files, S13444G,* SPO. See also *DD*, 12 April 1951 (125) col. 738. Dr Ryan later claimed that Mr Costello only received a copy of the scheme on 7 November 1950. *DD* 10 June 1953 (139) col. 1024.

32. A copy of the scheme is appended to J.H. Whyte, *Church and State in Modern Ireland, 1923-1970* (1st Edition) (Dublin, 1971) Appendix A.

33. *JIMA*, Vol. 26, No. 146, August 1949, p. 17.

34. Ibid., Vol. 24, No. 144, June 1949, p. 99.

35. Ibid., vol. 26, No. 154, April 1950, p.66 and *DD*, 23 April 1953 (138) col. 701.

36. Ibid., Vol. 25, No. 149, November 1949, p. 67.

37. Ibid., No. 148, October 1949, p. 50.

38. *DD*, 11 July 1950 (122) col. 1221.

39. Ibid.

40. Noel Browne op.cit., pp. 87-8.

41. Information from Dr Deeny. Relations subsequently became so bad between the Minister and the profession that one doctor prominent in the IMA at the time commented to me that they would have 'brought in Lucifer himself to defeat Browne'.

42. *JIMA*, Vol. 23, No. 136, October 1948, p. 63.

43. Ibid., Vol. 29, No. 174, December 1951, p. 130.

44. Ibid.

45. Minutes of a meeting between representatives of the IMA and the Minister for Health, held in the Custom House on 24 October 1950, Cabinet files, S14997A, SPO.

46. Ibid.

47. *JIMA*, see for example, Vol. 24, No. 143, May 1949, pp. 81-2.

48. Ibid., Vol. 26, No. 156, June 1950, p.93 and No.155, May 1950, p. 76.

49. Ibid., Vol. 28, No. 163, January 1951, pp. 17-18.

50. See for example the President's speech in ibid. Vol. 27, No. 158 August 1950, pp. 17-19.

51. *Discussions between the Minister for Health and the IMA regarding Mother and Child Service, Sequence of Events,* March 1951, op.cit.

52. *JIMA*, Vol. 27, No. 161, November 1950, pp. 73-4.

53. Ibid., No. 162, December 1950, p. 111.

54. Ibid. The percentages have been corrected from the original.

55. Ibid.

56. Referred to in a letter from Dr Delaney, Medical Secretary of the IMA to the Taoiseach, 12 December 1950, Cabinet files, S14997A, SPO.

57. *Irish Times*, 4 April 1951.

58. DD, 11 July 1950 (122) col. 1298 and Minutes of a meeting between the representatives of the IMA..., 24 October 1950, op.cit.

59. DD, 11 July 1950 (122) col. 1298.

60. J.H. Whyte, op.cit. (1980) p. 207.

61. Informants close to the Minister at the time have confirmed to me that the Minister was the author.

62. *The Mother and Child Scheme — Is it needed?*, Cabinet files, S14997A, SPO.

63. Ibid.

64. Information from a doctor formerly prominent in the IMA.

65. *Irish Independent*, 12 February, 1951.

66. Information from a doctor formerly prominent in the IMA.

67. *Irish Press*, 15 February 1951.

68. Dr O'Higgins continued to be a senior officer of the IMA despite his ministerial office and J.A. Costello's daughter was married to a brother of the editors of the IMA Journal.

69. DD, 12 April 1951 (125) col. 749.

70. See Mr MacBride's 'apologia' on the Cabinet files, 7 April 1951, S14997B, SPO.

71. Noel Browne op.cit., p. 144.

72. Ibid., p. 146.

73. Ibid., p. 145.

74. Ibid., p. 153.

75. Letter from the Bishop of Ferns, Dr James Staunton, Secretary to the Hierarchy, to the Taoiseach, 10 October 1950, Cabinet files, S14997A, SPO.

76. Ibid.

77. Ibid.

78. Ibid.

79. Ibid.

80. Ibid.

81. *Memorandum of observations of the Minister for Health*, 24 March 1951, Cabinet files, S14497A, SPO.

82. For Dr Browne's account see DD, 12 April 1951 (125) col. 669 and Noel Browne, op.cit., p. 161. Mr Costello gave the bishops' account in DD 12 April 1951 (125) cols. 739-40. Noel Browne discusses the conflicting accounts in *Against the Tide*, op.cit., pp. 161-2.

83. DD, 12 April 1951 (125) col. 742.

84. Ibid., col. 747.

85. Ibid.

86. Letter from the Taoiseach to the Minister for Health, 21 March 1951, Cabinet files, S14497A, SPO.

87. Minutes of meeting between the IMA and the Taoiseach, Mr Costello

and the Tanaiste Mr Norton on 29 November 1950 in Leinster House, Cabinet files, S14997A, SPO.

88. *DD*, 12 April 1951 (125) col. 748. On that occasion he gave the date of the meeting with the IMA as 27 November.

89. Ibid., col. 749.

90. Letter from the Minister for Health to the Taoiseach, 16 December 1950, Cabinet files, S14997A, SPO.

91. Ibid.

92. *Discussions between Minister for Health and IMA regarding Mother and Child Service, Sequence of Events,* op.cit.

93. Memorandum from IMA to Secretary DOH, 3 February 1951, Cabinet files, S14497A, SPO.

94. Ibid.

95. Letter from the Secretary, DOH to the Secretary, IMA, 19 February 1951, Cabinet files, S14497A, SPO.

96. *Discussion between Minister for Health and the IMA regarding Mother and Child Service, Sequence of Events,* op.cit.

97. Letter from the Secretary, DOH to the Secretary, IMA, 5 March 1951 and letter from the Minister for Health to the Taoiseach, 5 March 1951, Cabinet files, S14497A, SPO.

98. *Mother and Child — What the New Service means to every Family,* Cabinet files, S14497A, SPO.

99. *DD*, 12 April 1951 (125) col. 753.

100. *Irish Independent,* 17 March 1951.

101. Script of radio announcement by Dr Noel Browne, Minister for Health on the Mother and Child Services, broadcast from Radio Eireann on 8 March 1951, Cabinet files, S14497A, SPO.

102. Information from Dr Browne.

103. *DD*, 12 April 1951 (125) col. 757.

104. Letter from the Secretary of the DOH to IMA, 13 March 1951, Cabinet files, S14497A, SPO.

105. Letter from Mr P. McGilligan, Minister for Finance to Dr N. Browne, Minister for Health, in J.H. Whyte, op.cit. (1980) p. 427.

106. *DD*, 12 April 1951 (125) col. 757.

107. Ibid., col. 758.

108. Letter of 15 March 1951 from John A. Costello to Dr Noel Browne, Cabinet files, S14497A, SPO.

109. Ibid.

110. Letter from Dr Noel Browne to the Taoiseach, 19 March 1951, Cabinet files, S14497A, SPO.

111. Copy on Cabinet files, S14997D, SPO.

112. Letter from the Secretary DOH to the Secretary of the IMA, 21 March 1951, Cabinet files, S14497A, SPO.

[113.] Letter from the Taoiseach to the Minister for Health, 21 March 1951, Cabinet files, S14497A, SPO.

[114.] Note of a telephone conversation with the Minister for Health made by the Taoiseach, 22 March 1951, Cabinet files, S14497A, SPO, and *DD*, 12 April 1951 (125) cols. 765-767.

[115.] Ibid.

[116.] Memorandum of Observations of the Minister for Health, 24 March 1951, Cabinet files, S14497A, SPO.

[117.] Information from Dr Browne. Confirmed in Noel Browne, op.cit., pp. 163-4.

[118.] Letter from Dr McQuaid to the Taoiseach, April 1951, Cabinet files, S14497A, SPO.

[119.] Ibid.

[120.] See for example newspaper advertisements in the national press on 21 March 1951; the statement by the President of the IMA to the Taoiseach, undated, but presented on 29 November 1950, Cabinet files, S14497A, SPO, and the presidential address by Dr P.T. O'Farrell to the annual general meeting of the Association, *JIMA*, Vol. 27, No. 158, August 1950, p. 17.

[121.] M. MacInerny, 'Noel Browne; A Political Portrait', *Irish Times*, 10 October 1967, quoted in J.H. Whyte, op.cit. (1980) p. 225.

[122.] *DD*, 12 April 1951 (125) col. 780. Noel Browne, op.cit. has a graphic account of the decisive Cabinet meeting, pp. 176-7.

[123.] Letter from Sean MacBride to Dr Noel Browne, 10 April 1951, Cabinet files, S14497B, SPO.

[124.] *JIMA*, Vol. 28, No. 168, June 1951, pp. 91-2.

NOTES TO CHAPTER 10
COMPROMISE, 1951-1957

[1.] *JIMA*, Vol. 28, No. 168 June 1951, p.91.

[2.] Letter from the Taoiseach to Dr McQuaid, 9 April 1951, Cabinet files, 14497A, SPO.

[3.] See for example *DD*, 10 July 1951 (126) cols. 1231-2.

[4.] *JIMA*,Vol. 29, No. 170. August 1951, p. 22 and *DD*, 10 July 1951 (126) col. 1227.

[5.] Ibid., col. 1228.

[6.] Ibid., col. 1219 and *Proposals for Improved and Extended Health Services*, Foreword. Pr. 1333 (Stationery Office, July 1952).

[7.] The phrase was coined by General MacEoin, Minister for Justice, referring to anticipated objections to legalising adoption.

[8.] *DD*, 30 July 1953 (141) col. 1149.

9. *JIMA*, Vol. 29, No. 170, August 1951, p. 23.
10. *DD*, 11 July 1951 (126) cols. 1340-1.
11. *DD*, 17 July 1951 (126) col. 1636.
12. Ibid.
13. Ibid., 26 February 1953 (136) cols. 1900-2.
14. See for example the article by Professor Abrahamson in *Irish Independent*, 6 April 1953.
15. *JIMA*, Vol. 30, No. 178, April 1952, p. 84.
16. Ibid., Vol. 29, No. 174, December 1951, pp. 129-36.
17. Ibid., p. 132.
18. Letter dated 29 July 1952, Ibid., Vol. 31, No. 183, Sept. 1952, p. 274.
19. *DD*, 26 February 1953 (136) col. 1909.
20. DOH, *Health Service*, 24 June 1952, Cabinet files S13444H., SPO. and Central Statistics Office, *Statistical Abstract of Ireland 1958*, Pr 4564, p.204.
21. Ibid. *Memo for the Government-Health Services*, 11 July 1952.
22. *JIMA*, Vol. 30, No. 180, June 1952, p. 178.
23. Ibid., Vol. 31, No. 186, December 1952, p.368.
24. *Proposals for Improved and Extended Health Services*, July 1952, Pr. 1333 (Stationery Office, 1952).
25. DOH, *Health Service*, 24 June 1952, op.cit.
26. *Proposals for Improved and Extended Health Services,* op.cit., p.12.
27. DOH, *Health Service,* 24 June 1952, op.cit.
28. James Meenan, *op. cit.*, p. 286. The *Report of the Advisory Body on the Establishment of a Voluntary Health Insurance Scheme* estimated in 1956 that there were 460,000 persons in the upper income group or 16% of the population, implying that 84% were eligible for hospital and specialist services. Pr. 3571 (Stationery Office, 1956).
29. DOH, *Health Service*, 24 June 1952, op.cit.
30. Ibid.
31. DOH *Memorandum for ... Government regarding certain objections raised to proposals for improvement of the Health Services*, 10 November 1952, Cabinet files, S13444I, SPO.
32. Ibid.
33. DOH *Improved and Extended Health Services: Discussions with representatives of the Irish Medical Association*, 3 October 1952, Cabinet Files, S13444I, SPO.
34. Ibid., Vol. 31, No. 186, pp. 364, 367.
35. Ibid., Vol. 31, No. 186, December 1952, p. 367 and Vol. 32, No. 190, April 1953, p. 127.
36. Ibid., p. 370 and Vol. 32, No. 190, p. 120.
37. DOH, *Improved and Extended Health Services: Discussions with representatives of the Irish Medical Association ...*, 3 Oct 1952, op.cit.

NOTES TO CHAPTERS

38. Ibid. *Memo. for ... the Government regarding certain objections raised to proposals for improvement of the Health Services, op. cit.*

39. *JIMA*, Vol. 31, No. 185, Nov. 1952, p. 332 and *DD*, 23 April 1953 (138) col. 703.

40. Letter from P. O Cinneide, Secretary, DOH, to the Secretary, IMA, 21 October, *JIMA*, Vol. 31, No. 185, November 1952, p. 333.

41. Ibid., Vol. 31, No. 186, December 1952, p. 369.

42. Ibid., Vol. 32, No. 185, November 1952, and No. 186, December 1952.

43. Much of the correspondence is reprinted in *JIMA*, Vols. 31 and 32, Nos. 185-187, Nov. 1952-Jan. 1953.

44. Notes of interview between Dr J.H. Whyte and Dr McQuaid in 1969.

45. DOH, *Improved and Extended Health Services: Discussion between the Minister for Health and the Archbishop of Dublin on the 16 Sept. 1952*, Cabinet files, S 13444 J, SPO.

46. Ibid.

47. Ibid.

48. The lack of sympathy between Dr McQuaid and Dr Ryan is clear from the interviews they gave to J.H. Whyte in 1969 and 1966 respectively. Mr Lemass expressed his difficulty in understanding the bishops' objections when he met the episcopal committee on 10 December 1952.

49. See for example his request of 11 Nov. 1952, Cabinet files, S 13444 I, SPO.

50. DOH, *Improved and Extended Health Services: Discussions between the Minister for Health and the Archbishop of Dublin ... on the 6th October 1952*, Cabinet files, S 13444 J, SPO.

51. Ibid.

52. Letter from Archbishop McQuaid to the Tanaiste, 6 Nov. 1952, Cabinet files, S 13444 J, SPO.

53. DOH, *Improved and Extended Health Services: Discussions between the Tanaiste, the Minister for Health and the Archbishop of Dublin ..., on the 10 Dec. 1952*, Cabinet files, S 13444 J, SPO.

54. Ibid.,

55. *Health Bill, 1952* as published, Feb. 1952.

56. Ibid. Section 4.

57. Dr J. Ryan, Minister for Health, *DD*, 26 February 1953 (136) col. 1958.

58. Untitled memorandum, dated 7.5.1953, Cabinet files S 13444 J, SPO.

59. Ibid.

60. J.H. Whyte, op.cit., p. 284.

61. *DD*, 26 February 1953 (136) cols. 1903-4.

62. Ibid. The Minister was referring to the medical dynasties which controlled appointments in many voluntary hospitals.

318

63. Ibid., col. 1904.

64. Ibid. cols. 1905, 1907.

65. Reported in *JIMA*, Vol. 32, No. 188, Feb. 1953, p. 68.

66. Information from T.C.J. O'Connell, confirmed by the Minister in *DD*, 11 June 1953 (139) cols. 1115-6.

67. The Minister's reluctance to compromise is clear from the editorial of the *JIMA*, Vol. 32, No. 190, April 1953, pp. 119-21.

68. Ibid.

69. *Irish Independent*, 9 April 1953, quoted in *DD*, 15 April 1953 (138) col. 127.

70. Quoted in *DD*, 16 April 1953 (138) col. 301.

71. *JIMA*, Vol. 32, No. 190, April 1953, p. 120.

72. Ibid.

73. *DD*, 26 March 1953 (137) cols. 1315, 1317.

74. J.H. Whyte, op.cit. p. 281.

75. *JIMA*, Vol. 32, No. 190, April 1953, p. 127.

76. *Irish Independent*, 6-13 April 1953.

77. J.H. Whyte, op.cit., p. 284.

78. Ibid.

79. Ibid., p. 285.

80. Ibid., Appendix C.

81. *DD*, 26 February 1953 (136) col. 1897.

82. Copy of *Public Statement by the Hierarchy on the Health Bill, 1952*, 14 April 1953, in J.H. Whyte, op.cit., Appendix C.

83. *JIMA*, Vol. 32, No. 192, June 1953, p. 190.

84. Lord Longford and T.P. O'Neill, *Eamon de Valera* (London, 1970) p. 442.

85. Notes of an interview between Dr Ryan and J.H. Whyte in 1966. Dr Ryan also commented to Dr Whyte that the bishops often seemed very ill-informed.

86. DOH, Untitled memorandum, 17 April 1953, Cabinet files, S 13444 J, SPO.

87. Lord Longford and T.P. O'Neill, op.cit., p. 447.

88. Mr de Valera was aware of the role played by the profession in Dr Browne's downfall. Ibid., p. 436.

89. It is clear from the attitude of the Fine Gael speakers on the money resolution of the Health Bill, 1952 on Thursday 16 April 1953 that they knew that the Hierarchy was about to come out against the Bill.

90. Dr McQuaid was out of the country from 4 April to 6 June 1953. Notes of an interview with J.H. Whyte, August 1969.

91. Dept. of the Taoiseach, minute by the Secretary to the Government of the details of Mr de Valera's visit to Drogheda, 18 April 1953, op.cit. and J.H. Whyte op.cit., p. 289.

92. Ibid.

93. Ibid.

94. Dept.of the Taoiseach, Note by the Secretary to the Government of the Outcome of the Conference of 22 April 1953, Cabinet files, S 13444 K, SPO.

95. For a discussion of the conflicting claims of both camps, see J.H. Whyte, op.cit. pp. 294-8. More recently, Ronan Fanning has stressed the extent of concessions made to the Hierarchy, *Irish Times*, 13-14 February 1985.

96. *DD*, 9 June 1953 (139) col. 780; 17 June 1953 (139) cols. 1511, 1609.

97. Ibid., 18 June 1953 (139) cols. 1693-6 and 25 June 1953 (139) cols. 2056-71.

98. Ibid., 11 June 1953 (139) col. 1226 and 29 July 1953 (141) cols. 1054-5.

99. Ibid., 16 July 1953 (140) cols. 1422 and 29 July 1953 (141) col. 1119.

100. Ibid., 18 June 1953 (139) col. 1651-2.

101. In his interview with J.H. Whyte, Dr Ryan accepted that he had rejected about seventy per cent of what the bishops demanded.

102. *DD*, 11 June 1953 (139) col. 1215.

103. Letter of 9 May 1953 from Archbishop Kinnane to the Taoiseach, Cabinet files, S 13444 J SPO.

104. Ronan Fanning, op.cit.

105. *JIMA*, Vol. 32, No. 192, June 1953, p. 192.

106. Information from Mr T.C.J. O'Connell. He was accompanied by Professor Cunningham, Professor of Obstetrics and Gynaecology at University College, Dublin.

107. Letter of 27 June 1953 from the Taoiseach to Archbishop Kinnane, Cabinet files, S 13444 K SPO.

108. Ibid. Letter of 29 June 1953 from the Secretary to the Government to the Secretary, DOH and *DD* 30 July 1953 (141) cols. 1111-2.

109. *JIMA*, Vol. 33, No. 194, August 1953, p. 49.

110. Ibid., p. 50.

111. Ibid., p. 53.

112. Information from Mr T.C. J. O'Connell.

113. Ibid., p. 53.

114. Petition to the President, 28 October 1953, Cabinet files, S 13444 K, SPO.

115. Information from T.F. O'Higgins.

116. Ibid.

117. Information from Mr T.C. J. O'Connell and T.F. O'Higgins.

118. *DD*, 7 July 1954 (146) col. 1340-1.

119. Ibid., col. 1320.

120. *Report of the DOH 1954-55*, Pr. 3319 (Stationery Office; 1956) pp. 21, 27.

121. *Report of the Advisory Body on the Establishment of a Voluntary Health*

Insurance Scheme, Pr. 3571. (Stationery Office; 1956) p. 5.

122. Ibid., pp. 24-5.

123. *Voluntary Health Insurance Act, 1957.*

124. Information from Mr T.C. J. O'Connell who was a member of the board of the VHI at the time.

125. Whyte, op.cit. and Fanning, op.cit. and *Independent Ireland* (Dublin, 1983).

126. The Hospitals Trust, *Ireland's Hospitals* (n.d. 1956?) pp. 26-7.

NOTES TO CHAPTER 11
TAKING HEALTH OUT OF POLITICS, 1957-1970

1. F. S. L. Lyons, op. cit., p. 573.

2. *Programme for Economic Expansion*, Pr. 4796 (Stationery Office, 1958).

3. Whyte, op.cit., pp. 333-5.

4. Neither the First, nor the *Second Programme for Economic Expansion 1963-4* (Pr. 7239) referred explicitly to social policy.

5. *Irish Times*, 30 March 1965.

6. Information from Dr James Deeny.

7. Central Statistics Office, *Statistical Abstract of Ireland 1957*, Pr 4107, Stationery Office, p. 199.

8. Ibid., *1958*, Pr. 4564, p. 204.

9. *Report of the Department of Health, 1957-8*, Pr. 4914 (Stationery Office; 1959).

10. *DD*, 26 June 1957; (163) col. 131.

11. *Report of the Study Group on the General Medical Service*, 12 February 1962, Deeny papers, op.cit.

12. Ibid., p. 24.

13. Letter from the Secretary of the DOH to the IMA, 15 June 1959, reproduced in the *JIMA*, Vol. xlv, No. 265, July 1959.

14. Ibid., No. 268, Oct. 1959.

15. *JIMA*, Vol. xlv, No. 268, Oct. 1959, p. 116. Letter from P. O Muireadhaigh, Assistant Secretary, DOH.

16. Ibid., No. 270, Dec. 1959, p. 183.

17. My medical informants agree that Mr Doolin cannot be given the benefit of the doubt on this occasion.

18. The Labour Party, *Policy Document on Health*, 1959.

19. See Deputy O'Higgins' motion, *DD* 23 November 1961 (192) cols. 720-46.

20. Ibid., col. 746.

21. Ibid.

22. Ibid., col. 1492.
23. Select Committee on the Health Services, *Memorandum from the DOH describing the Irish Health Services*, pp.8-9.
24. Ibid., p. 9.
25. Ibid., *Digest of Submissions and Oral Evidence tendered to the Committee on the General Medical Service*, March 1963.
26. Ibid., *Memorandum from the DOH on submissions made on the General Institutional and Specialist Services*, October 1962, p. 14.
27. Ibid., p. 16. *A Hospital Plan for England and Wales*, Cmnd. 1602 (HMSO; 1962).
28. Ibid. passim.
29. Ibid., *Memo ... on the General Medical Services,* op.cit., p. 18.
30. Ibid., *Memo. ... on the General Institutional and Specialist Services,* op.cit., p. 18.
31. Ibid., *Memo. ... describing the Irish Health Services,* op.cit., p. 63.
32. Central Statistics Office, *Statistical Abstract of Ireland 1957,* op.cit., p. 199; *1958,* op.cit., p. 204; *1964,* Pr. 7781, p. 235. The figures are the net expenditure by local authorities and grants in aid to the Hospital Trust Fund.
33. Ibid. *1962* p. 266 and *1966*, Pr. 8950, p. 271.
34. Department of Local Government, *Returns of Local Taxation, 1954-5* Pr. 3769 (Stationery Office) p. 19 and *1965-66* Pr. 9666, Stationery Office, p. 16.
35. Select Committee on the Health Services, *Memo ... describing the Irish Health Services,* op.cit., p. 66.
36. Ibid., pp. 66-7.
37. Oireachtas, *Interim Report of the Select Committee on the Health Services,* T 186, February 1962 and *Second Interim Report of the Select Committee on the Health Services,* T 189, January 1963.
38. Fine Gael, *Winning Through To A Just Society*, 1965.
39. The Labour Party, *Election Manifesto*, 1965.
40. *The Health Services and their Further Development*, Pr. 8653 (Stationery Office; January 1966).
41. Ibid., p. 16.
42. Ibid.
43. Ibid., pp. 31-2.
44. Ibid., p. 32.
45. Ibid., p. 43.
46. Ibid.
47. Ibid., p. 59.
48. Ibid., p. 62.
49. Ibid., p. 65.
50. Ibid., p. 67.
51. *DD*, 1 March 1966 (221) col. 610.
52. Ibid.

[53.] *DD*, 23 February 1967 (226) cols. 1772-4.

[54.] *Irish Times*, 18 April 1967, quoted in J.H. Whyte, op.cit., p. 300.

[55.] Ibid.

[56.] Ibid.

[57.] Ibid., 1 March 1966 (221) col. 677.

[58.] The Health Bill, 1969 as introduced provided for a minimum of 50 per cent of elected public representatives. *DD*, 6 May 1969 (240) col. 512.

[59.] Central Statistics Office, *Statistical Abstract of Ireland 1970-71*, Prl 1974, pp. 238, 281.

[60.] Consumer Price Index used as deflator. Ibid., *1969*, Prl. 1101, p. 325.

[61.] Ibid., *1970-71*, op.cit., p. 238.

[62.] Ibid., *1972-73*, Prl. 4053, p. 314-5 and Select Committee on the Health Services, *Memorandum from the DOH describing the Irish Health Services*, op.cit, p. 27.

[63.] See census returns for occupation in *Statistical Abstract of Ireland 1959*, op.cit, p. 51; *1966*, Pr. 8950, p. 45; *1969* op.cit., p. 51 and *1974-1975* Prl 6072 p. 52. My estimate is a conservative one.

[64.] W.E.J. McCarthy, J.F. O'Brien, V.G. Dowd, *Wage Inflation and Wage Leadership* (Dublin, 1975).

[65.] Central Statistics Office, *Statistical Abstract of Ireland 1970-71,* op.cit., p. 240.

[66.] Department of Local Government, *Returns of Local Taxation*, 1969-70, Prl. 2345, Stationery Office, p. 16 and *Reports of the Department of Local Government 1962-3* and *1969-70* (Stationery Office).

[67.] *JIMA*, Vol. XL, No. 360, June 1967, pp. 221-2.

[68.] Consultative Council on the General Hospital Services, *Outline of the Future Hospital System*, Prl. 154 (Stationery Office, 1968).

[69.] Ibid., p. 31.

[70.] Ibid., p. 27.

[71.] Sir Anthony Esmonde, *DD*, 17 April 1969 (239) col. 1755.

[72.] Deputies Reynolds and Bruton, Ibid., 1 May 1969, cols. 343, 361.

[73.] Information from a former official of the DOH.

[74.] *Senate Debates*, 12 May 1966, (61) col. 354.

[75.] Ibid., col. 355.

[76.] For example, Deputies Hogan, Esmonde, Gibbons, and O'Connell.

[77.] *Senate Debates*, 25 May 1966 (61) cols. 467-8 and *DD*, 31 March 1966 (222) col. 462.

[78.] *Senate Debates*, 25 May 1966, (61) col. 468.

[79.] *DD*, 16 April 1969 (239) Col. 1653.

[80.] Ibid.

[81.] Ibid., col. 1634.

[82.] Ibid.

[83.] Ibid., col. 1638.

84. *Health Bill, No. 4, 1969.*
85. *DD*, 16 April 1969 (239) col. 1643.
86. Ibid., cols. 1648-9.
87. Ibid., col. 1650.
88. Ibid., 6 May 1969 (240) col. 511.
89. Ibid., 16 April 1969 (239) col. 1653.
90. Ibid., cols. 1692-1701.
91. Ibid., Health Bill, 1969, Committee Stage, Vols. 241-243, passim.
92. Ibid., 27 November 1969 (242) col. 2066.
93. Ibid., cols. 2270-1.
94. *Health Contributions Act, 1971.*
95. *DD*, 30 June 1971 (255) col. 177.
96. Brendan Hensey, *The Health Services of Ireland*, 2nd edition (Dublin, 1972) p. 86 and DOH, *Statistical Information on the Health Services*, 1980 (Stationery Office, 1980) p. 72.
97. Brendan Hensey, (1972) op.cit., p. 28.
98. See for example Deputy Moore *DD* 2 March 1966 (221) col. 789.
99. John Curry, *Irish Social Services* (Dublin, 1980) p. 145.

NOTES TO EPILOGUE
PAYING RESPECTS TO THE PAST

1. Hugh Heclo, op.cit., p. 1.
2. Hirobumi Ito, 'Health Insurance and Medical Services in Sweden and Denmark 1850-1950' in Arnold J. Heidenheimer and Nils Elvander, eds., *The Shaping of the Swedish Health System* (London, 1980).
3. Ibid. and Arnold J. Heidenheimer, Hugh Heclo and Carolyn Treich Adams, *Comparative Public Policy — The Politics of Social Choice in Europe and America*, 2nd ed. (London, 1983).
4. For an analysis of current high levels of expenditure on health services see A. Dale Tussing, *Irish Medical Care Resources: An Economic Analysis* (Dublin, 1985).
5. In 1976 Ireland had the highest number of cases treated per acute hospital bed of any EEC country. (Dept. of Health, *Statistical Information on the Health Services, 1978*). Since the country is not underendowed with hospital beds this represents a high admission rate. Given the young age profile of the population, this is surprising. The picture is confirmed by the National Economic and Social Council which found a much higher hospital admission rate for middle aged persons in Ireland than in Britain. (NESC, *Health Services: The Implications of Demographic Change*, Dublin 1984).
6. VHI, *27th Annual Report and Accounts* (Dublin, 1984) p. 17.

7. A referendum in 1983 amended the Constitution to prohibit abortion under any circumstances. Clerical and medical support in favour of the referendum was an important factor in the campaign. The Health (Family Planning) Act, 1979 made the purchase and sale of contraceptives legal for the first time but contraceptives, including non-medical contraceptives, could only be purchased at chemists with a doctor's prescription. The Minister consulted with the Hierarchy before publishing the Bill (*Dail Debates* 14 February 1985, cols. 2592-3). The Health (Family Planning) (Amendment) Act, 1985 which permits the purchase of non-medical contraceptives without a medical prescription, caused great controversy and was only passed by a narrow margin. Sterilisation for family planning purposes is available in a few public hospitals.

8. R. M. Titmuss, *Commitment to Welfare* (London, 1968) p. 92.

Sources & Bibliography

A. **Interviews**

B. **Collected Papers – Unpublished**
1. Personal Papers
2. Other Unpublished Papers

C. **Official Publications**
1. British (Including publications relevant to Ireland prior to 1921)
2. Irish

D. **Journals and Newspapers**

E. **Books and Articles**

F. **Theses**

A. Interviews

Interviews conducted for this study and earlier related research:

Dr Noel Browne, Minister for Health 1948-51.

Dr James Deeny, Chief Medical Officer, Departments of Local Government and Public Health/Health 1944-66.

The late Dr John Garvin, senior official, Departments of Local Government and Public Health/Health up to 1947.

Dr Oliver Fitzgerald, Editor, Medical Association of Eire Journal, 1944-52.

Dr Brendan Hensey, former Secretary, Department of Health.

The late Brendan Herlihy, former Assistant Secretary, Department of Health.

Mr Brendan Kiernan, former Legal Adviser, Departments of Local Government and Public Health/Health.

Dr Thomas Murphy, former Medical Officer, Department of Health.

The late Mr T.C. J. O'Connell, former prominent member of the Irish Medical Association.

Mr Michael Mulvihill, former Private Secretary to Dr Noel Browne, Minister of Health.

Mr Thomas F. O'Higgins, Minister for Health 1954-57.

Dr John Shanley, former President, Irish Medical Association.

Mr Desmond Roche, Secretary, Departmental Committee on the Health Services, 1945.

I am grateful to my father, T.J. Barrington, for information about the period when he was an official of the Department of Local Government and Public Health and Private Secretary to Mr Sean MacEntee, Summer 1945 to late 1946.

Mr Thomas F. O'Higgins kindly supplied me with a written account of the difficulties he faced in implementing the Health Act, 1953.

I am especially grateful to Professor J.H. Whyte for giving me copies of notes he made of interviews with the following during research for his work, *Church and State in Modern Ireland 1923-1979*:

Mr J. Darby, senior official, Department of Health;

the late Mr James Dillon, Minister for Agriculture, 1948-51, 1954-57;

the late Dr John Charles McQuaid, Archbishop of Dublin, 1940-72

the late Dr E.G.T. MacWeeney, Senior Medical Officer, Departments of Local Government and Public Health/Health;

the late Dr James Ryan, Minister for Health and Social Welfare 1947-8, 1951-4, Minister for Finance, 1957-65;

the late Dr F.C. Ward, Parliamentary Secretary to the Minister for Local Government and Public Health, 1932-46.

B. Collected papers – unpublished

1. Personal papers

Braithwaite, W.J. The London School of Economics and Political Science.

Deeny, Dr J., Library of the Royal College of Surgeons in Ireland.

Gavan Duffy, Charles MS 15,440 [Formal papers on the proceedings of Dail Eireann, 1919-1923], National Library of Ireland.

Johnson, Thomas MS 17, 124 [Draft of Democratic Programme as submitted at their Request to the Sinn Fein Leaders, January 1919] National Library of Ireland.

O'Briain, Art MS 8460, National Library of Ireland [Report of Local Government Department, 3 May 1921].

Redmond, John MSS film 1059-85, Bodleian Library, Oxford.

2. Other unpublished papers

Dail Eireann – Select Committee on the Health Services
   Memorandum from the Department of Health on Submissions made on the General Institutional and Specialist Services, Sept. 1962
   Memorandum from the Department of Health on Submissions made on the Domiciliary, Maternity and Infant Care Service, Child Welfare Service and School Health Examination and Treatment Service, Sept. 1962.
   Memorandum from the Department of Health on Submissions made on the General Medical Services, Oct., 1962.
   Memorandum from the Department of Health describing the Irish Health Services, Dec., 1962.
   Digest of Submissions and Oral Evidence tendered to the Committee in regard to the General Institutional and Specialist Services.
Departmental Committee on The Health Services, Report, 1945. (50 copies printed by Stationery Office). Copy on Cabinet file S13444C, State Paper Office.
Ministry of Pensions and National Insurance, *National Insurance Bill 1911*:
   Part I — to Second Reading PIN 3:3
   Part II — Committee Stage (Commons) PIN 3:4
   Part III — Report to Third Reading (Commons) PIN 3:5
   Public Record Office, London.
Cabinet Papers, State Paper Office, Dublin
   Allegations against Dr F.C. Ward, Parliamentary Secretary to the Minister for Local Government and Public Health, Tribunal of Inquiry, 1946, S 13866.
   Dublin Fever Hospital Board Dissolution 1945, S 13692.
   Department of Health Staff, S 14152.
   Health Act 1947, Views of the Roman Catholic Hierarchy, S 14227.
   Hospitals Sweepstakes, Reports of Committee of Reference, S 3237/9.

Public Charitable Hospitals Act, 1933, S 3237/13.
The Mother and Child Health Scheme, S 14997.
Reorganisation of the Health Services, S 13444.

C. Official publications

1. British (including publications relevant to Ireland prior to 1921).

Act for the more effectual Relief of the Destitute Poor in Ireland, 56 1 and 2 Victoria 1838 *Statutes at Large,* Vol. 14.

Beveridge, Sir William, *Social Insurance and Allied Services*, Cmd. 6404, London, 1942.

Bill to provide for altering and reforming the Administration of the Poor Law System in Ireland 1910 (4) iv. 491, 1912-13 (9) IV.577.

Bill to provide for Insurance against Loss of Health and for the Prevention and Cure of Sickness and for Insurance against Unemployment: etc. 1911 (198) iv. 1.

Census of Population, 1911:
  General Report, 1917-18 Cd. 8491, xxxv 483.
  General Report (Ireland), 1912-13 Cd. 6663, cxviii 1.

Committee appointed to consider the Extension of Medical Benefit under the National Insurance Act to Ireland, Report, 1913, Cd. 6963 xxxvii, p.1. Appendices, same volume, p. 213.

Viceregal Commission on Poor Law Reform in Ireland, Report 1906 Cd 3202 li 349,
  Vol. 2 Appendices to Report 1906 Cd. 3203 li 441,
  Vol. 3, Evidence and Index 1906 Cd. 3204 lii 1.

Committee on Irish Finance Report, 1912-13 Cd. 6153, xxxlv.

Departmental Committee on Tuberculosis, *Interim Report*, 1912-13 Cd. 6164, xlviii 1.
  Final Report, Vol. 1, 1912-13 Cd. 6641, xlviii 29.
  Appendix to Final Report, Vol. 11, 1912-13 Cd. 6654, xlviii 47.

Irish Public Health Council, *Report on the Public Health and Medical Services in Ireland*, 1920 Cmd. 761 XVII 1075.

Local Government Board — Ireland, *Annual Reports*, 1904-05 to 1919-20, British Parliamentary Papers, 1905 — 1921.

Standing Committee on the Medical Treatment of Children Bill, Report, 1919 (73) VI 729.

Minister for Health, *A National Health Service*, Cmd. 6502, London, 1944.

National Health Insurance Commission, *Report for 1912-13 on the Administration of the National Insurance Act, Part I (Health Insurance)* 1913 Cd 6807 xxxvi 1. [Part V, National Health Insurance Commission (Ireland) p. 419].

National Health Insurance Commission, *Report for 1913-14 on the Administration of National Health Insurance*, 1914 Cd 7496 lxxii 3. [Part V. Ireland, p. 377].

SOURCES & BIBLIOGRAPHY

National Health Insurance Commission, *Report on the Administration of National Health Insurance during the years 1914-17*, 1917-18 Cd. 8890 xvii 31. [Ireland, p. 163].
National Health Insurance Commission (Ireland), *Report for the Period Nov. 1917 to 31 March 1920*, 1921 Cmd. 1147 XV 653.
Poor Law Commissioners, *Ireland: Report on Medical Charities*, 1841 (324) xi 1.
Parliamentary Debates, Vols. 120 (March 1903) to 167 (May 1923).
Report of Sir William Plender to the Chancellor of the Exchequer on the Result of his Investigation into Existing Conditions in respect of Medical Attendance and Remuneration in Certain Towns, 1912-13 Cd. 6305 lxxviii 679.
Royal Commission on the Poor Laws and the Relief of Distress, Report, 1909 Cd. 4499 xxxvii 1.
Report on Ireland, 1909 Cd. 4630 xxxviii 1.
Appendix Vol.10 Evidence (with Appendices) relating to Ireland 1910 Cd. 5070 L. 195.
Standard Time Rates of Wages in the U.K., at 1st January 1912, 1912-13 Cd. 6054, xcii 573.
Standing Committee A on the Ministry of Health Bill *Report*, 1919 (61) v. 517.

2. Irish

Advisory Body on the Establishment of a Voluntary Health Insurance Scheme, Report Pr. 3571, Stationery Office, 1956.
Commission on the Relief of the Sick and Destitute Poor, including the Insane Poor. Report, R 27/3, Stationery Office, 1927. — *Minutes of Evidence*, R 27/1-2, Stationery Office, 1925.
Commission on Vocational Organisation, Report, R 76/1, Stationery Office, 1944.
Committee of Inquiry into Health Insurance and Medical Services.
Interim Report, N 2/1, Stationery Office, 1925.
Appendices to Interim Report, N 2/2, Stationery Office, 1925.
Final Report, N 2/3, Stationery Office, 1927.
Central Statistics Office, *Statistical Abstract of Ireland*, 1949 — 1972-73, Stationery Office.
Consultative Council on the General Hospital Services, *Outline of the Future Hospital System*, Prl. 154, Stationery Office, 1968.
Dail Eireann, *Minutes of Proceedings of the First Parliament of the Republic of Ireland 1919-1921 Official Record*, Dublin, n.d. 1921 (?).
Dail Eireann, *Debates*, Vol. 1, 1922 to Vol. 255, 1971.
Department of Finance, *Estimates*, Various years, Stationery Office.
Department of Health, *Health Progress 1947-53*, Pr 2086, Stationery Office, 1953.
Department of Health, *Health Services and their Further Development*, Pr 8653, Stationery Office, 1966.
Department of Health, *Outline of Proposals for the Improvement of the Health Services*, P 8400, Stationery office, 1947.

Department of Health, *Proposals for Improved and Extended Health Services*, Pr 1333, Stationery Office, 1952.

Department of Health, *Reports*, 1945-49 to 1957-8, Stationery Office.

Department of Health, *Statistical Information Relevant to the Health Services*, 1976 to 1983, Stationery Office.

Department of Local Government, *Reports* 1955-56 — 1967-71, Stationery Office.

Department of Local Government and Public Health, *Reports*, 1922-25 to 1944-45, K Series, Stationery Office.

Department of Local Government and Public Health, The Hospitals Commission, *Reports* 1 to 7, 1936 to 1947, Stationery Office.

Department of Local Government and Public Health/Department of Local Government *Returns of Local Taxation*, 1932-33 — 1970, Stationery Office.

Department of Local Government and Public Health, *Tuberculosis*, P. 7368, Stationery Office, 1946.

Department of Local Government and Public Health, *Report of the Conference between the Department of Local Government and Public Health and Representatives of Local Public Health and Public Assistance Authorities*, K29, Stationery Office, 1930.

Health Act, 1947.

Health Act, 1953.

Health Act, 1970.

Health Bill, 1969, Explanatory Memorandum, 3/69, Stationery Office, 1969.

Health Contributions Act, 1971.

Local Government Act, 1925.

Local Government (Temporary Provisions) Act, 1923.

McKinsey and Co. Ltd., *Towards Better Health Care*, Vols. 1-3, Department of Health, 1971.

Ministers and Secretaries Act, 1924.

New Ireland Forum, *The Economic Consequences of the Division of Ireland since 1920*, Stationery Office, 1983.

Public Assistance Act, 1939.

Public Hospitals Act, 1933.

Public Services Organisation Review Group, *Report*, 1969.

Seanad Eireann, *Debates*, particular volumes consulted where necessary.

Select Committee on the Health Services, *Interim Report*, T 186, Feb., 1962. *Second Interim Report*, T 189, Jan., 1963.

D. Journals and newspapers

Irish Free State Medical Association Journal (1937-41) *Medical Association of Eire Journal* (1961-52) *Irish Medical Association Journal* (1952-74). Vols. IX, July — December 1941 to LXIII, 1970.

Irish Independent. May 1911 to August 1912. Other issues consulted as necessary.
Journal of the British Medical Association. May 1911 to June 1912.
The Medical Press and Circular. Vols. LXXIX, February 1905 to Vol. CXLIII.
The Medical Press and Circular, Weekly Supplement, *Irish Poor Law and Lunacy Intelligence.* Most issues between 1905 and 1909 read.

E. Books and articles

Abel-Smith, Brian *The Hospitals 1800-1948,* London, 1964.
———— *Value for Money in the Health Services,* London, 1976.
Andrews, C.S. *Dublin Made Me: An Autobiography,* Cork, 1979.
Association of Charities, *Dublin Charities,* Dublin, 1902.
Ayers, G.M. *England's First State Hospitals,* London, 1971.
Barrington, T.J. *From Big Government to Local Government,* Dublin, 1975.
———— *The Irish Administrative System,* Dublin, 1980.
Berkhofer, Robert F., *A Behavioral Approach to Historical Analysis,* New York, London, 1969.
Birrell, Augustine *Things Past Redress,* London, 1937.
British Medical Association, An Investigation of Contract Medical Practice in the United Kingdom, *British Medical Journal Supplement,* 22 July 1905, pp. 1-96.
Braithwaite, W.J. *Lloyd George's Ambulance Wagon. The memoirs of W.J. Braithwaite,* London, 1957.
Brown, Terence *Ireland — A Social and Cultural History, 1922-79,* London, 1981.
Browne, Noel *Against the Tide,* Dublin, 1986.
Burdett, H.C. *Pay Hospitals and Paying Wards Throughout the World,* London, 1880.
Burke, Peter *Sociology and History,* London, 1980.
Carr, Arthur S., Comyns, Garnett, W.H. Stuart, and Taylor, J.H. *National Insurance* 2nd edn., London, 1914.
Coey Bigger, E. *Report on the Physical Welfare of Mothers and Children,* Carnegie United Kingdom Trust, Dublin, 1917.
Chubb, B. *The Government and Politics of Ireland,* Stanford and London, 1970.
Collis, W.R.F. *The State of Medicine in Ireland,* Dublin, no date but probably 1943/4.
Coogan, T.P. *Ireland Since the Rising,* London, 1966.
Coolahan, John *Irish Education: Its History and Structure,* Dublin, 1981.
Curry, John *The Irish Social Services,* Dublin, 1980.
Daly, Mary E. *Social and Economic History of Ireland since 1800,* Dublin, 1981.
Dangerfield, George *The Strange Death of Liberal England,* London, 1966.
Davis, Richard *Arthur Griffith and Non-Violent Sinn Fein,* Tralee, 1974.
Deeny, James "The Recent Epidemiology of Typhoid in Ireland" in *Journal of the Medical Association of Eire,* Vol. 19, No. 111, Sept. 1946.

——————— "The Spread of Tuberculosis in an Irish Town — a Study of Slow-Motion Contagion" in *Journal of the Medical Association of Eire*, Vol. 21, No.126, Oct. 1947.

——————— "The Professional Civil Servant" in *Administration*, Vol. 1, No. 3, Autumn 1953, pp. 57-63.

——————— and Murdock, Eric T. "Infant Mortality in the City of Belfast" in *Journal of the Statistical and Social Inquiry Society of Ireland*, Vol. XVII, 1943-44, pp. 221-240.

Dicey, A.V. *Lectures on the relation between Law and Public Opinion in England in the Nineteenth Century*, 2nd Edn., London, 1952.

Dignan, Bishop J. *Social Security: Outlines of a Scheme of National Health Insurance*, Sligo, 1945.

Dillon, T.W.T "The Statistics of Tuberculosis" in the *Dublin Journal of Medical Science*, 6th series, No. 199, July 1942.

Eckstein, Harry *The English Health Service: its Origins, Structure, and Achievements*, London, 1959.

Evatt, G. Surgeon-General "A Report on the Poor Law Medical System in Ireland with special reference to the Dispensary MedicalService",in *British Medical Journal Supplement*, 26 March 1904, Vol. 1, pp. 47-75.

Fanning, R. *The Irish Department of Finance 1922-1958*, Dublin, 1978.

——————— *Independent Ireland*, Dublin, 1983.

——————— "Real Story Behind 'Mother and Child'", in the *Sunday Independent*, December 11, 1983.

——————— "Fianna Fail and the Bishops", in *The Irish Times,* 13-14 February 1985.

Farley, D. *Social Insurance and Social Assurance in Ireland*, Dublin, 1964.

Farrell, B. *The Founding of Dail Eireann: Parliament and Nation Building*, Dublin, 1971.

Ferguson, Thomas *Scottish Social Welfare 1864-1914*, Edinburgh, London, 1958.

Fine Gael *Winning Through to a Just Society*, Dublin, 1965.

Finnane, Mark *Insanity and the Insane in Post-Famine Ireland*, London, 1981.

Fitzpatrick, D. *Politics and Irish Life*, Dublin, 1977.

Fleetwood, John F. *History of Medicine in Ireland*, 2nd edn., Dublin, 1983.

Ford, P. *Social Theory and Social Practice*, Shannon, 1968.

——————— and Ford, G. *Select List of British Parliamentary Papers Vol. 1 1833-1899*, Rev. ed., Shannon, 1969.

——————— and Ford G. *A select list of reports of inquiries of the Irish Dail and Senate, 1922-72*, Dublin, 1974.

Fremantle, Anne *The Papal Encyclicals in their Historical Context*, New York, 1963.

Garvin, Tom *The Evolution of Irish Nationalist Politics*, Dublin, 1981.

Geary, R.C. "The Mortality from Tuberculosis in Saorstat Eireann, A Statistical Study" in *Journal of the Statistical and Social Inquiry Society of Ireland*, Vol. XVII, October 1930, pp. 67-103.

SOURCES & BIBLIOGRAPHY

Gilbert, Bentley B. *The Evolution of National Insurance in Great Britain — The Origins of the Welfare State*, London, 1966.
———— *British Social Policy 1914-1939*, London, 1970.
Greaves, C.G. *The Life and Times of James Connolly*, London, 1972.
Gwynn, D.R. *The Life of John Redmond*, London, 1932.
Hardy, Nelson, H. *The State of the Medical Profession in Great Britain and Ireland in 1900*, Dublin: London, 1900.
Halevy, E. *History of the English People 1905-1914 — The Rule of Democracy Book 1*, New York and London, 1952.
Heclo, Hugh *Modern Social Politics in Britain and Sweden — From Relief to Income Maintenance*, New Haven: London, 1974.
———— "Policy Analysis" in *British Journal of Political Science*, No. 2, 1972, pp. 83-108.
Heidenheimer, Arnold J. "The Politics of Public Education, Health and Welfare in the USA and Western Europe: How Growth and Reform Potential have differed" in *British Journal of Political Science*, No.3, 1973, pp. 315-340.
———— and Elvander, Nils *The Shaping of the Swedish Health System*, London, 1980.
————, Heclo, Hugh and Adams, Carolyn Treich *Comparative Public Policy — The Politics of Social Choice in Europe and America*, 2nd edn, London, 1983.
Hensey, Brendan *The Health Services of Ireland*, 1st edn., Dublin, 1959: 2nd edn., Dublin, 1972; 3rd edn., Dublin, 1979.
Inglis, Brian *A History of Medicine*, London, 1965.
Irish Catholic Hierarchy "Statement on the National Insurance Bill", in *The Tablet*, July 1, 1911, p. 18.
Irish Medical Association *Summary of the objections of the Association to the Minister's proposed Mother and Child Scheme*, no date but probably early 1951.
Kaim-Caudle, P.R. *Social Policy in the Irish Republic*, London, 1967.
Kelly, John "Noel Browne: A myth of martyrdom?" in the *Sunday Press*, December 7, 1986.
Kinkead, Prof. R.J. *Irish Medical Practitioners Guide*, Dublin, 1889.
Keogh, Dermot *The Vatican, the Bishops and Irish Politics 1919-39*, Cambridge, 1986.
The Labour Party *Policy Document on Health*, Dublin, 1959
The Labour Party *Outline Policy: Health, Social Welfare*, Dublin, January 1969.
Larkin, Emmet *James Larkin 1876-1947 Irish Labour Leader*, London, 1965.
Larkin, Emmet "Socialism and Catholicism in Ireland" in *Church History*, XXXXIII December 1964, pp. 462-83.
Lee, J.J. *The Modernisation of Irish Society 1814-1918*, Dublin, 1973.
———— (ed.) *Ireland 1945-70*, Dublin, 1979.
———— "Aspects of Corporatist Thought in Ireland: The Commission on

Vocational Organisation 1939-43'' in Cosgrove and McCartney, eds., *Studies in Irish History*, Dublin, 1979, pp. 324-46.

Levenson, S. *James Connolly*, London, 1973.

Levy, Hermann *National Health Insurance: A Critical Study*, Cambridge, 1944.

Lewis, J. *The Politics of Motherhood*, London, 1980.

Litton, Frank (ed.) *Unequal Achievement: The Irish Experience 1957-1982*, Dublin 1982.

Longford, Earl of and O'Neill, Thomas P. *Eamon de Valera*, London, 1970.

Lyons, F.S.L. *The Irish Parliamentary Party 1890-1910*, London, 1951.

———— *John Dillon*, London, 1968.

———— *Ireland Since the Famine*, London, 1970.

MacArdle, D. *The Irish Republic*, 4 edn. London, 1968.

McCarthy, W.E.J., O'Brien, J.F. and Dowd, V.G. *Wage Inflation and Wage Leadership*, Dublin, 1975.

McCracken, J.L. *Representative Government in Ireland: A Study of Dail Eireann 1919 — 48*, London, 1958.

MacDonagh, O. *Ireland: The Union and Its Aftermath*, 2nd edn., London, 1977.

———— ''The nineteenth century revolution in government'', in *The Historical Journal*, Vol. 1, No.1, 1958, pp. 52-67.

McInerney, Michael ''Noel Browne: Church and State'', in *University Review*, V, 2, Summer 1968, pp. 171-215.

———— ''Dr Noel Browne: A Political Portrait'', in *The Irish Times*, 9 October 1967.

MacManus, F. ed. *The Years of the Great Test 1926-39*, Cork, 1967.

McDowell, R.B. *The Irish Administration*, London, 1964.

McKenzie, Norman ed. *The Letters of Sidney and Beatrice Webb Vol. II Partnership*, Cambridge: London, 1978.

McPolin, J. ''Some Aspects of the Sociology of the Medical Profession'' in *Journal of the Medical Association of Eire*, Vol. 19, No. 110 August 1946, and No. 111 Sept., 1946.

Maltby A. and J. *Ireland in the Nineteenth Century: A Breviate of Official Publications*, Oxford, 1979.

Maltby, A. and McKenna, B. *Irish Official Publications: a Guide to Republic of Ireland Papers with a breviate of Reports 1922-72*, Oxford, 1980.

Maxwell, Robert J. *Health and Wealth — An International Study of Health Care Spending*, Lexington, 1981.

Meenan, F.O.C. ''St Vincent's Hospital: Origins and Early Development'' in *Irish Medical Journal*, November 1985, Vol. 78, No. 11, pp. 329-332.

Meenan, J. *The Irish Economy Since 1922*, Liverpool, 1970.

Miller, David W. *Church, State and Nation in Ireland 1898-1921*, Dublin, 1973.

Mommsen, W. ed. *The Emergence of the Welfare State in Britain and Germany*, London, 1981.

Morgan, Kenneth, O. *David Lloyd George 1863-1945*, Cardiff, 1981.

Moos, S. "A Pioneer of Social Advance — William Henry Beveridge",in *Durham University Journal*, Vol. LVI, December 1963, pp. 2-13.

Moss, W. *Political Parties in the Irish Free State*, New York, 1933.

National Economic and Social Council *Some Major Issues in Health Policy*, Dublin, 1977.

———— *Health Services: The Implications of Demographic Change*, Dublin 1984.

National Tuberculosis Survey/Deeny, James *Tuberculosis in Ireland*, Dublin, 1954.

Navarro, Vincente *Class Struggle, The State and Medicine: an historical and contemporary analysis of the medical sector in Great Britain*, London, 1978.

Newman, C.E. *The Evolution of Medical Education in the Nineteenth Century*, London, 1957.

Nowlan, K. and Williams, D. (eds.) *Ireland in the War Years and After 1939-51*, Dublin, 1969.

O'Brien, Eoin *Conscience and Conflict, A Biography of Sir Dominic Corrigan*, Dublin, 1983.

O Broin, Leon *The Chief Secretary — Augustine Birrell in Ireland*, London, 1969.

O'Carroll, J.P. and Murphy, J.A. *De Valera and His Times*, Cork, 1983.

Organisation for Economic Cooperation and Development *Social Expenditure 1960-1990, Problems of Growth and Control*, Paris, 1985.

Parris, H. "The Nineteenth Century Revolution in Government. A Reappraisal Reappraised", in *The Historical Journal*, Vol. III, No. 1, 1960, pp. 17-37.

Phelan, Denis *A Statistical Inquiry into the Present State of the Medical Charities of Ireland*, Dublin, 1835.

Popper, K.R. *Objective Knowledge — an Evolutionary Approach*, Oxford, 1972.

———— *Conjectures and Refutations*, London, 1969.

Poynter, F.N.L. *Medicine and Science in the 1860s*, London, 1968.

Robins, J.A. "The Irish Hospital, an Outline of its Origins and Development", *Administration*, Vol. VIII, No. 2, 1960, pp. 145-165.

———— *Fools and Mad*, Dublin, 1986.

Robinson, Sir Henry *Memories: Wise and Otherwise*, London, 1924.

———— *Further Memories of Irish Life*, London, 1925.

Roche, Desmond *Local Government in Ireland*, Dublin, 1982.

———— "Tuberculosis: The Attack Develops" in *Administration*, Vol. 1, No. 3, 1953, pp. 83-89.

Rumpf, E. and Hepburn, A. *Nationalism and Socialism in Twentieth Century Ireland*, Liverpool, 1977.

Ryan, Desmond *James Connolly*, Dublin, 1924.

Shanley, John P. "The State and Medicine" reprint from *The Irish Journal of Medical Science*, May 1929.

———— "The Reorganisation of the Medical Services" in *Journal of the Medical Association of Eire*, Vol. 14, No. 82, April 1944 pp. 40-43.

———— "The History of the Irish Medical Association", in *Journal of the Irish Medical Association*, Vol. 62, No. 385, July 1969, pp. 237-244.

336

Smith, F.B. *The People's Health 1830-1910*, London, 1979.

Taylor, A.J.P. *Lloyd George, Rise and Fall*, Cambridge, 1961.

Thane, Pat *Foundations of the Welfare State*, London, 1982.

————— ed. *The Origins of British Social Policy*, London, 1978.

The Hospitals Trust *Ospideil na hEireann — Ireland's Hospitals*, Dublin, no date, 1956?

The Irish Times *The Liberal Ethic*, Dublin, 1950.

Titmuss, R.M. "Health" in Morris Ginsberg, ed. *Law and Opinion in England in the 20th Century*, London, 1959, pp. 299-318.

————— *Commitment to Welfare*, London, 1968.

————— *The Gift Relationship*, George Allen Unwin, London, 1970.

————— *Social Policy — An Introduction*, London, 1974.

Tudor Hart, J. "Bevan and the Doctors" in *The Lancet* Vol. iii for 1973, pp. 1196-1197.

Tussing, A. Dale *Irish Medical Care Resources: An Economic Analysis*, Dublin, 1985.

Voluntary Health Insurance Board *Twenty Seventh Annual Report and Accounts*, Dublin, 1984.

Whyte, J. *Church and State in Modern Ireland* 1st edn., Dublin, 1971, 2nd edn. Dublin, 1980.

White, T. De Vere *Kevin O'Higgins*, London, 1948.

Widdess, J.D.H. *The Royal College of Surgeons in Ireland and its Medical School*, 2nd edn., Edinburgh: London, 1967.

————— *A History of the Royal College of Physicians in Ireland*, Edinburgh: London, 1963.

Wohl, Anthony S. *Endangered Lives — Public Health in Victorian Britain*, London, 1983.

World Bank *Atlas*, 1979.

F. Theses

Barrington, Ruth "The Shaping of Policy on the Irish Health Services 1961-1970", Master of Arts minor thesis, University College Dublin, 1973.

Burke, Helen "The Poor Law in Ireland in the Nineteenth Century with particular Reference to the Social Services provided by the South Dublin Union", unpublished Ph.D. thesis, University College Dublin, 1976.

Carney, Claire P. "Selectivist Social Services: The Origin and Development of Certain Services in the Republic of Ireland with an Evaluation of the Underlying Social Policy", unpublished Ph.D. Thesis. University College Dublin, 1977.

Williams, P.M. "The Development of Old Age Pensions Policy in Great Britain 1878-1925", unpublished Ph.D. thesis, 1970, University of London.

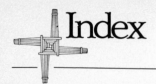

Index

voluntary hospitals, sweepstakes
Hospitals Commission 117, 135,
267
report 120-4, 130
proposals on tuberculosis 162
Hospitals Trust Fund 117, 122,
123, 125, 225
and tuberculosis sanatoria 163 *see
also* sweepstakes
housing 13, 20
Hughes, James 172
Hurson, J. 107, 139

IMA (Irish Medical Association)
16-18, 153, 255, 283
and health insurance, 1911 44-57
and Catholic Church 148-9, 166,
234
and Shanley plan 152-4
official scheme 154-5, 157
on Public Health Bill, 1945
170, 174
on mother and child scheme 202,
204-14
on voluntary health insurance
224-5
on 1952 White Paper 229-30,
232-4
see also medical profession
infant mortality 75, 78, 131, 132,
137, 145-6, 191
infectious diseases 4, 12, 22, 73,
74, 132, 138
powers to control 133, 142-3,
167, 168-74, 185, 186, 187
under control 248-9, 250
Irish administration 1, 14, 18-19,
22
see also Local Government Board
Irish Independent 42, 50
Irish Insurance Commission 52, 59,
68-9, 80
Irish Medical Association *see* IMA
Irish National Foresters 35, 60

Irish Party 1, 18, 19-20, 22, 67,
71, 73, 77
and the Catholic Church 21
on health insurance, 1911 39-57
and British government 39-40,
48-9
Irish Press, The 155
Irish Public Health Council 81-6,
87, 90, 101, 107, 110
Irish Red Cross 161-2
Irish Republican Army 67
Irish Times, The 155

Jubilee nurses 11-12, 228-9

Keady, P.J. 156, 159
Kelly, Dr Denis (Bishop of Ross)
30

Labour Party (Irish) 95, 97, 106,
273, 275
on Health Act, 1953 245
impetus for change 257-8, 260
Lardner, James 20, 59, 60
League of Nations 130
Larkin, Emmet 21
Lavery, Cecil 201
Lemass, Sean 230
Liberal Party 19, 20, 34-7, 38, 39,
89
lice infestation 139-40, 169, 171-2
Limerick 14, 179-81, 184-5, 191
Lloyd George, David
and health insurance, 1911
35-8 *passim*, 40, 41, 43, 46-56
passim, 81
and health services 65
Local Appointments Commission
101, 199, 274
local authorities 5, 11, 12, 13-14,
19, 31, 100-2, 114
see also county councils; boards
of guardians; boards of health
and public assistance